RECONNECT TO THE ROOTS OF INNATE WELLNESS
& SACRED FEMININE WISDOM

YOUR BODY

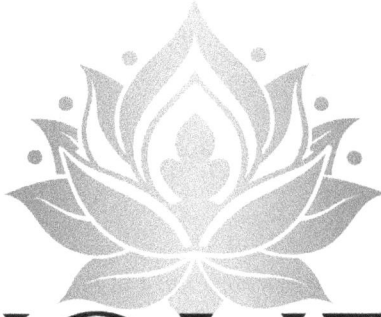

YOUR POWER

DR MICHELLE BOYCE, DC

FLOWER *of* LIFE PRESS

PRAISE

'Your Body, Your Power *by Dr Michelle Boyce, DC, is an absolute gem for anyone looking to cultivate a holistic approach to well-being. Michelle combines cutting-edge research with time-honored wellness practices, making it practical and accessible for both beginners and seasoned health enthusiasts. Each chapter is filled with actionable steps and easy-to-follow advice that anyone can incorporate into their daily routine—from nutrition and movement to mental health and stress management. What sets this book apart is Michelle's emphasis on integrating physical, emotional, and spiritual health in an achievable, empowering, and deeply resonant way. It's a true roadmap for any woman looking to prioritize her health in a balanced, sustainable way.'*

—Hallie Lifson, Priestess, Therapist, Teacher of Erotic Arts and Spiritual Practice

'Dr Michelle has done something extraordinary in this book by naming something we all know exists, that something you can fall into if you don't consciously opt out of, the "Modern Disease of the Modern Woman." Not only has Michelle given it a name, but she has also laid down a roadmap for choosing something altogether different, healing, and transformative! Personally, this book couldn't have come at a better time for me; I am incredibly grateful! Thank you, Michelle!'

—Dr Kelly Melnikova-Rhodes MChiro (Chiropractor)

'Reading Your Body, Your Power *feels like having a good conversation with your older sister. It feels relatable, encouraging, and confronting at the same time. The book teaches you many new things and offers new insights about your body from a female perspective. It invites you to take better care of yourself and love yourself more.'*

—Sara van Lieshout, Women's Empowerment Coach

'Your Body, Your Power *by Dr Michelle Boyce, DC, is the "body manual" women often wish we'd been born with! Michelle has given us a practical and comprehensive guide to our body's interwoven physical, emotional, and even sexual responses that form the basis of our life experiences. Centered on the too-often overlooked unique ways a woman's body works, this book fills in the frustrating gaps in care that women face when addressing health and well-being. But, this is no boring or dry textbook; instead, it's like having the wise big sister you never knew you needed to explain all the changes women face as we move through the various stages of life. Chock-full of relatable examples and case studies, practical exercises, and digestible information, this is a book I know I'll return to again and again.'*

—Rima Bonario, Th.D., Author, Teacher, Coach, Speaker

'This is a book that every woman should have on her bookshelf! In Your Body, Your Power, *Michelle blends her wonderfully practical approach to women's health, developed over decades of experience as a health practitioner, with her deep spiritual knowledge of sacred holistic healing. She empowers us as modern women to reclaim sovereignty over our bodies and rediscover the lost wisdom that has always been accessible and resides within our uniquely beautiful feminine vessels. By examining the sociological and cultural factors that may have led women to suffer from the "Modern Disease of the Modern Woman," Michelle lovingly offers practices for rebalancing our bodies and re-establishing the connection between brain and body through movement, emotional fluidity, nervous system balancing, and a uniquely feminine spiritual perspective. This is a life-changing book, and I am so grateful to Dr Boyce for bringing this much-needed wisdom to life!'*

—Kirsty Jandrell, Priestess

FLOWER *of* LIFE PRESS

Your Body, Your Power: Reconnect to the Roots of Innate Wellness & Sacred Feminine Wisdom
By Dr Michelle Boyce, DC

Published by Flower of Life Press
www.floweroflifepress.com

Flower of Life Press books may be ordered through booksellers or by contacting:
support@floweroflifepress.com

Cover and Interior design: Astara Jane Ashley

Library of Congress Control Number: Available upon request.

ISBN: 979-8-9909775-7-0

---

*Visit **www.drmichelleboycedc.com/resources** for additional book resources and practises.

DEDICATION

'When sleeping women wake, mountains move.'
~Chinese Proverb

To all the women who came before me and who will come after me, may you remember your body's power and innate wisdom as a portal to who you truly are.

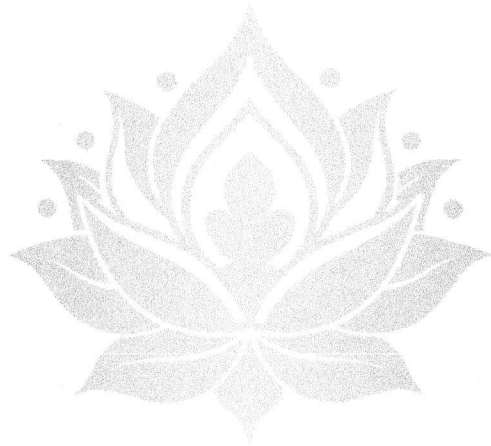

TABLE OF CONTENTS

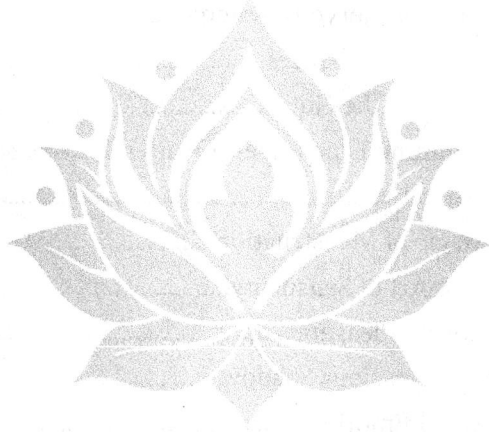

INTRODUCTION

Enlightenment is just a change in perception.

From a very young age, I knew I wanted to help people. I did it intuitively, listening to my friends and trying to heal my dolls and Barbies with potions and prayers. But my path into the world of holistic health wasn't straight. I took a few detours along the way, first deciding to train as a medical doctor. This was short-lived when I quickly realised that I didn't want to just treat the symptoms—I wanted to get to the root cause of people's pain and sickness. I had learnt first-hand that there wasn't a pill for every ailment, and when there was, it usually came with side effects.

This book is a culmination of over fifteen years of practise in my clinic, helping women and their families heal and thrive. I help women with chronic pain and stress when all else has failed. In fact, I'm usually the last stop for those who have tried all the medical routes, only to be left feeling unheard, unhelped, and more confused than ever.

The 'Modern Disease of the Modern Woman' (MDMW) is a term I came up with in my practise after helping thousands of women go from exhausted and wired to thriving and alive. I believe that most women intuitively know that they are struggling with something more than just physical pain.

When I started working as a Chiropractor, I began to see a pattern. Many of my patients presented with a cluster of health problems that seemed to be unrelated to their pain. When reading their energy bodies, I would see patterns of psychological, emotional, and spiritual tension and stress that were contributing to their pain. These women were feeling tired AND wired, using substances like caffeine to amp up and wine to calm down. They experienced poor memory, brain fog, sleep problems, digestive issues, and exhaustion most of the time.

Many said there was so much to do, yet so little time. They felt frazzled and over-emotional with chronic PMS and weight problems that they couldn't fix—regardless of the diet plan or supplements they tried. They felt stressed and anxious and lacked joy. To them, self-care was just one more task on the to-do list that wasn't getting done.

Even though my patients felt like they were striving to be all things to all people, they still felt like failures. They never felt good enough and then felt guilty for feeling resentful or frustrated. They rarely said no and lacked boundaries, juggling many commitments while trying to smile and look picture-perfect for the outside world. Perfection and control were their default way of managing everything, including themselves. Does any of this sound familiar? This is the **Modern Disease of the Modern Woman.**

Pain may be the reason many women step into my office, yet lurking underneath that pain is a massive mountain of stress, tension, and disconnection that they are either unconscious of or have kept buried because they have no time to deal with it.

Stress is not new—it's always been part of our lives. The problem women face today is the unrelenting and often unrealistic demands that modern life places on them. Today's advanced technology is amazing, yet the endless beeping and notifications keep us working and busy mentally—and sometimes physically—day and night.

When I was growing up, there were no cell phones, which meant my mum could travel in her car or on the bus, read a book, listen to music, and wind down from the day. Today, we are busy answering emails, replying, and ping-ponging messages, rarely free even when we think we are. We are constantly plugged in like little Duracell bunnies, only recharging briefly when we're lucky enough to fall asleep.

Compared to even 100 years ago, science has made some of the most significant breakthroughs in treating disease, yet we have the highest rates of heart disease, cancer, and autoimmune diseases than ever before. Depression and anxiety are at an all-time high, and let's not forget metabolic syndrome and type 2 diabetes. Where did it all go wrong?

Today, women's opportunities for liberation are immense; we've conquered so much, yet we are still stuck and caged in a prison-like system because we are continually trying to prove our worth. This prison is like a wheel, giving us a rush as we run around *doing, doing, doing,* all the while feeling the need to control everything and never resting or slowing down. It's a feeling of desperation that keeps us constantly amped up and 'on'— because otherwise, our whole world and life will fall apart. We are always looking to the external world for our worth and value. And after aeons of oppression and suppression, why wouldn't we?

Today's modern woman is subject to enormous physical, emotional, and hormonal demands. Each woman is the sum total of all her parts—physical, chemical, emotional, psychological, and spiritual—and when we are not well, it affects our loved ones, our long-term health, and our happiness. The impact of this modern disease on the modern woman and her family is high.

Most of my clients just want to feel normal again and at home in their bodies, but with the influence of social media, the body has become an enemy. In reality, most of us do not look or feel how the adored Instagram or social media influencers tell us we should. We see mums bouncing back into size ten jeans after giving birth, sipping smoothies, and looking radiant while claiming they have an amazing relationship and job, telling us we can have it all… Our actual results are disappointing, and we are left feeling like a failure. That deep shame and guilt cause us to reach for the fridge to binge, numb out by shopping or watching TV, or drinking too much wine.

My patients have been my greatest teachers, inspiring me to invent new and profound ways to help women heal. I have also experienced this modern disease myself. I began to share my principles of healing with my patients, and once they became aware of what was making them sick and how they could change it, I began to see massive shifts in their results.

My personal healing journey and initiation into my priestess lineage helped me develop new ways to see the female body and heal its pain. I went back in time to when the female body was worshipped and adored for its healing power, intuition, and sacredness, all of which had become redundant and long forgotten in so many of the women I was treating.

Our bodies have been owned, used, and abused collectively—and it's still happening today. If you've picked up this book, perhaps you feel it, too. The amount of body shame, judgement, and disconnect is truly alarming. Many women hate their bodies—or loathe at least one part of it. Somehow, we believe our whole life will be better if we can change it.

Why are we thinking and behaving in ways that are chronically affecting our health?

There is not one answer that fits all, yet some common factors exist. The answer lies in our biochemistry, beliefs, repressed emotions, and core wounds—most of which we're unaware of! So many of us are racing around believing that feeling pain or being tired, bloated, or sick is the norm, and we can't even remember what 'good' feels like.

Once you begin to step off the hamster wheel and understand how you got here in the first place, you, too, will start to understand your behaviour, beliefs, and emotions—and where you've been keeping them locked away. Even though you haven't been thinking of them, these repressed qualities are working subconsciously through and in your life, driving your choices and behaviours. The backbone for true long-term health is learning to bring all parts of your mind, body, and spirit back into balance. In my experience, most women don't know what they want. But let me tell you this: *It's okay, and it's not your fault.* We've been brainwashed to believe that following a patriarchal blueprint is the ONLY way and that wanting anything else is selfish and over-demanding—and no one likes or loves a woman like that, right?

When we slow down and get back into our bodies, we begin to understand where all that juicy stuff we were looking for has been hiding. We have been taught to look outside ourselves when everything we need is within us. We need to reconnect with the power that lives within each of us. It's already there. We don't need to buy it or be jealous of anyone else; we have our own superpower just waiting for us to embody. We simply need to turn it on.

In this book, I'm going to walk you through how and why you feel the way you do and, most importantly, what you can do about it. My intention is that you will start to make the shifts that help you move from a busy, wired, and tired state to a calmer, more balanced one so that you can feel like you again. You have this power—it's waiting inside of you.

Throughout this book, you may notice I use words such as Goddess, God, Source, Universe, or Soul to represent your inherent spiritual nature and ability to access a greater power. Feel free to substitute a word that works for you in these instances. Healing is all about YOUR experience and relationship to your body and LIFE, and I invite you to explore which word resonates for you and works within your belief system.

I use the word 'She' to refer to your body. Your body has its own life force that is separate from your mind. She knows how to heal, create, sense, and intuit better than you can think. This is a journey back to her innate healing wisdom and aliveness.

This book is not a quick fix. It's about venturing slowly into places where you haven't been fully present. If applied and understood on a cellular level, the tools and information in this book will change your life and health. Your new life will cost you your old one; you can't stay the same and expect your life to change. Many of us are scared to pay the price of that change because we fear the unknown. Remember that you always have a choice about the changes you make. So let's get started!

Ask yourself:

- What is the cost of not taking action to change my life?
- What is it costing me to play safe while lying and denying to myself and to others about how I *really* feel?

PART ONE
LET'S GO ON A JOURNEY

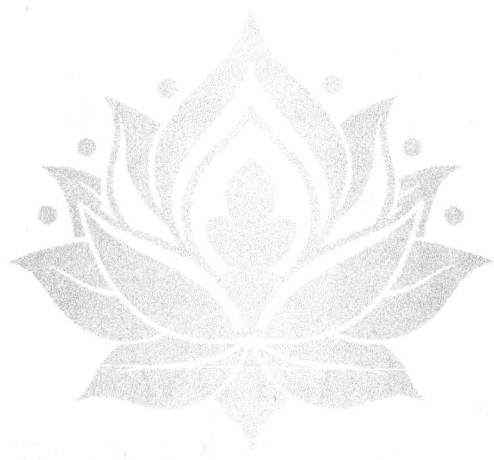

CHAPTER 1

THE MODERN DISEASE OF THE MODERN WOMAN

We need to stop looking at what is in front of us to discover what is inside of us.

Most of us aren't aware of the patterns that control our lives. We need to begin to recognise that the way we are experiencing life right now, whether negative or positive, is built upon a foundation of beliefs, thoughts, emotions, and programming that's been on repeat since we were little girls.

We often navigate life without much awareness, accepting everyday occurrences as normal. However, these seemingly ordinary experiences actually serve as subtle indicators that we are accumulating and retaining tension.

Our bodies are brilliant at adapting, but when the stress and tension are present for longer periods, we start to experience pain, and it's our body's way of saying, 'Hello, I'm struggling here… can you give me some help?' Most of the time, we haven't got time—it's inconvenient, there's so much to do and think about, we are already running late, and it will have to wait. So, we take pain medication to block the pain and get on with our busy lives.

However, as the pain and numbness intensify, symptoms become increasingly bothersome. Perhaps it manifests as a rigid neck, persistent headaches, or a dull ache in the lower back. The impact on our daily lives becomes evident, and we become fixated on the escalating symptoms within our bodies. When the pain worsens, our focus shifts externally, seeking solutions and changes to alleviate the symptoms that enable us to continue our hectic lives. Frustration sets in when various treatments prove ineffective, leading us to experiment with different approaches, such as stretching, needling, and massage, only to find that the relief is temporary. Concerns escalate, and thoughts of underlying illnesses like cancer surface, prompting visits to doctors who prescribe medications or cortisol injections, offering temporary respite for a few weeks to a month. However, the pain inevitably resurfaces, and the cycle of chronic pain takes hold, leaving us in a state of uncertainty about what steps to take next.

When we have pain, we reduce our movement, which leads to less function, which creates more pain, and so the cycle goes… Add in some mild depression, tiredness, anger, and frustration, and you have a recipe for long-term illness.

The cycle needs to be broken. With chiropractic care and my 'Sheology' system, we can directly impact the nervous system, reduce pain, and, more importantly, rewire the connection between the body and the brain for better coherence.

Sheology

Sheology is a system that I created which represents our female biology. It offers a women-centred approach to health and well-being. It is my prescription go-to medicine for the Modern Disease of the Modern Woman. Our unique female biology, nervous system, physiology, and biochemistry differ from a man's. I have seen time and time again that when women align with the wisdom codes in their DNA, transformation, healing, and miracles happen. We often follow a cookie-cutter, medicalised masculine approach, but it is failing us. Many women I meet think something is wrong with them, but *nothing* is wrong with them. The map they are following is simply not designed to take them in the right direction. The feminine way is non-linear. There are different landmarks on the way, and learning to recognise and know this about yourself will change everything. There are eight pillars in Sheology:

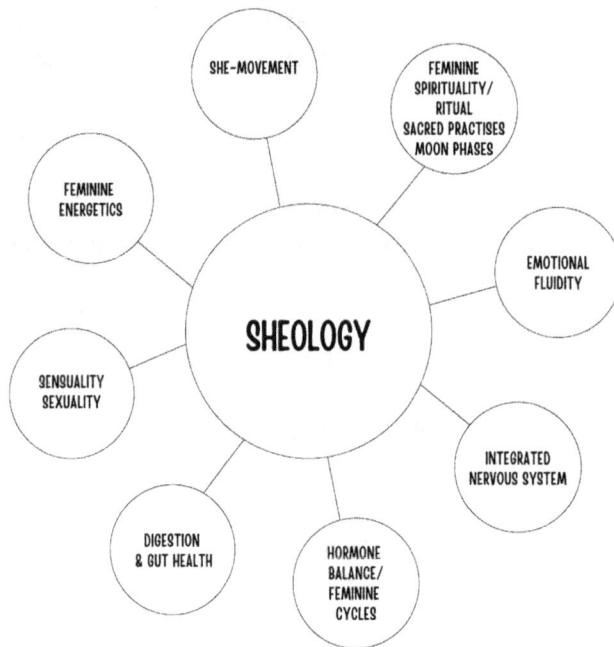

The aim of Sheology is to reclaim, rebalance, and reconnect the physical, mental, and emotional body, restoring wholeness to the centrepoint of the sacred self. Health means freedom from physical, mental, and emotional imbalances. The body, mind, and emotions share an intimate relationship, and many conditions women struggle with today are due to mental stress, burnout, repressed anger, grief, depression, blame, guilt, anxiety, disconnection, suppression of sexual desire, and other psychosomatic disturbances. The practise of Sheology can help transform you into a strong, healthy human, restoring balance and harmony to the body, mind, and soul—leading to self-realisation.

Many women are suffering physically, mentally, and emotionally, and I want you to feel the aliveness, reconnection, and bliss that I am privileged to witness every day in my clients. Sheology is the path back to *you,* and I can't wait to share how your body works. I am so grateful to be on this journey together and that you have chosen this book as a guiding light back to your body.

True healing comes when we remember, re-embody, and realign with the wisdom of the feminine body. By reclaiming our roots, cycles, and Sheology practises, we move beyond the band-aid medical solutions that fail to heal today's chronic health conditions that increasingly impact our bodies and lives. It's time for us to empower ourselves with the knowledge, tools, and practises that address the root causes of pain, chronic illness, and separation from self. This includes what we eat, knowing which foods help us heal or make us sick, how we move, self-regulate, think, and express our emotions, and how tuned in we are to our sacred connection. These factors affect conditions like stress, hormonal disruption, chronic pain, and health problems. *Your Body, Your Power* offers a holistic approach to healing the feminine body using food, movement, feminine cycles, sacred practises, and 'She-Movement.'

Rewiring doesn't happen overnight. This book is designed to fit into your life and not add more stress to your never-ending to-do lists. Responsibility for your health is a key requirement for success and real change. My deepest desire is that you:

- Remember the wisdom within, the cycles of birth, death, and rebirth, and the changes reflected in nature and deeply embodied in your Sheology.
- Feel and follow the ebb and flow of the earth, which mirrors your feminine body, from your monthly cycle and births to your journey into wise womanhood.
- Know that you are energy and more than just the physical body you can touch and see.
- Remember 'HER-story,' the magic and sacredness of the vessel you inhabit in this lifetime.
- Embody your physicality, roots, beliefs, and personal power.
- Feel and embody your sensuality, sexuality and repressed emotions that are your birthright.
- Integrate all the depths and fullness of your mind, body, emotions, and soul.
- Reclaim your inner Shakti who wants to guide, walk, and dance with you through this beautiful life.
- Re-align and reset your body, mind, and sacred self with the support of the knowledge and practises within these pages.

The feminine lives through your body, not in your mind.

She-Movement

Learning to self-regulate your nervous system directly influences how you feel and how you heal, and this is what we do in 'She-Movement.' She-Movement is based on my years of research, professional training, personal experience, and work with clients. It's a unique and integrated practise of sensuality, Shakti awakening, movement, neuroscience, psychology, and physiology that addresses a woman holistically. It teaches women to self-regulate their nervous system, improving overall health and specifically supporting them physically, emotionally, chemically, and psychologically. I've found that while these techniques help support any woman at any stage of life, they are particularly potent in the perimenopausal and menopausal years.

In the process of healing, it's essential to address the entirety of the body, not just a specific area. For example, when a patient presents with neck pain, my approach extends beyond focusing solely on the neck. I examine her overall posture, nervous system, and spine. My rationale is grounded in the understanding that the apparent pain often compensates for an underlying issue that extends beyond the immediate discomfort. This perspective goes beyond the physical aspect, delving into the spiritual and emotional dimensions of one's being, recognising that the root cause of the pain may reside in a deeper realm within the body.

Imagine you experience an improvement in your well-being, a common outcome in about 90% of cases. What prevents a recurrence? If there's no alteration in your unconscious beliefs, patterns, and actions, and if you neglect to address the persistent rush, stress, and disruptions to your nervous system, the issues may resurface or even manifest differently in your body.

True healing transcends quick fixes and reactive measures; it involves delving into the core of the symptoms, reaching not just your physical self but connecting with your soul. It's an internal process that requires exploring where you may have deviated from your true essence.

Prevention is better than cure.

Healing is a journey. It's the path to knowing yourself, cultivating intimacy with yourself, learning how to surrender, honour your intuition, and connect to your soul.

First, let's assess what you are currently experiencing:

Physical signs your body is telling you to regulate your nervous system:

- Holding your breath and breathing high and shallow
- Gripping your fingers or toes, fists clenched
- Legs crossed, perched on the edge of the chair
- Crossing arms and legs
- Tightening of jaw, hips, and fists
- Shutting down—no eye contact
- Tired but wired
- Sitting more than 4 hours a day at a computer
- Problems falling asleep

- Waking up around 2 a.m.
- Sugar cravings
- Can't lose weight
- Suffering from PMS
- Loss of interest in sex
- Painful sex or numbness
- Can't relax
- Change in bowel movements
- Feeling anxious
- Stiffness and pain in the shoulders, neck, and back
- Waking up exhausted, with a feeling of dread
- Normal activities are taking more effort than they used to

Non-physical signs:

- Changing the subject
- Numbing out
- Concentration problems, zoning out
- Avoidance (scrolling, shopping)
- Procrastination, small tasks feel overwhelming
- Projection and blaming others
- Judging others
- Easily snappy and irritated at others
- Body shame and judgement
- Distractions and addictions
- Frustration, anger
- Negative self-talk
- Going over scenarios in your head, second-guessing what you said
- Thinking people are against you
- Worried about what people think of you
- Need to control, overthink, worry, organise, plan, and rearrange constantly
- Can't turn your brain off; there is a constant buzz of anxiety
- Startle easily
- Highly sensitive to noise
- Feel like you are drowning

How many applied to you? If it's more than five, you are likely struggling with the Modern Disease of the Modern Woman.

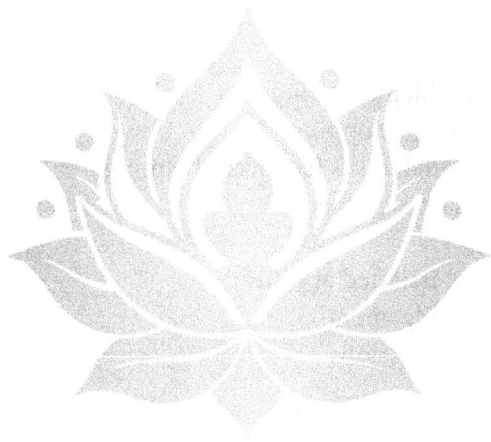

CHAPTER 2
YOUR BODY

Changing the way we perceive and experience the body is challenging,
but it's no more difficult than staying within a body or belief system
that does not nourish the whole woman.

Deep inside us is a powerful treasure that holds the magic to transform, create, ignite, and heal. We all hold this alchemy that, once found, can transform and transmute pain and disease out of our bodies. It is the magic that opens the curtains, parts the veils, and shines a light on our soul, slowly and gently awakening it from its deep slumber.

As the sun pierces through the clouds, your essence, sexuality, and sensuality break open your golden cage. You spread your wings and fly free. You are the phoenix rising, the butterfly emerging from the cocoon, the snake shedding her skin. You are life itself—you are she, and she is you. Life looks you deep in the eyes and says, 'Welcome home. I've been waiting patiently for you to awaken. Are you ready now to be the woman you were born to be?'

Deep inner knowing, gnosis, and expansion occur as the veils part, and linear time becomes cyclical as you remember who YOU are. Slowly, you are handed an ethereal key to Pandora's Box, the key to life itself.

Pandora's Box is a Greek myth symbolising women bringing evil into the world. It was a box never to be opened, locked away within each of us, generation after generation. In modern society, it is associated as the source of all trouble and wrath, a curse that will come upon anyone who dares to open it.

Even though Pandora's Box is hidden within you, tucked away and out of sight and mind, it's still there. It holds the remembrance and codes of crystalline feminine power that have been shut away due to lifetimes of fear, persecution, and lies.

Deep down, you may have known it was there but ignored the nudges, pulls, and pushes to remember. Life is easier if it remains unfound. Life is simpler if it remains closed. You feel safer wearing the masks.

This power contained within is your *Shakti*—your life force. It's your femininity, sensuality, and sexuality. You experience it in your breath, laughter, orgasms, in your hips as you dance, in sunsets, and in the sound of a newborn baby's cry. It is the joy and ecstasy of being alive, feeling the sun on your face and the wind in your hair.

It's the part of you that's missing, dulled down, bound and kept quiet, not able to feel and express the true magnetism of who you are. It's your soul; it's 'She'—it's *you*.

Shakti is the living energy of the Goddess, the power within the feminine. Shakti (the Yin, or divine feminine energy) is the wife of Shiva (the Yang, or divine masculine energy.) Together, they create the perfect balance of life.

Today, many of us are stuck in the Shiva, masculine energy, and we have become out of alignment because we lack the balance of the feminine.

Shiva without Shakti is like ideas, work, and drive without wisdom, passion, and flow. Shakti without Shiva is disorganised and lacks direction.

We need both structure and flow to thrive. A river needs its banks so it can flow from one place to another without flooding. Without this structure, it becomes a stagnant lake. Shakti is the energy of sexuality that manifests and creates all life. We access our Shakti life force when we are expressive, fluid, passionate, and joyful. But so many of us have created blockages to this life force within.

Cultural norms and upbringing have shaped unrealistic expectations about our appearance, behaviour, and identity, nearly suffocating our true selves. Free expression has been manipulated and controlled around our bodies, sensuality, and sexuality. Whether we are conscious of it or not, we are bound to the rules of the patriarchy.

Your body is the way back to this wisdom. It's the gateway to your soul and to the truth of who you really are. We've been taught that the answers are somewhere to be found outside of ourselves—in things, people, and religion—but it's been inside us all along.

I am here to guide you back to the power that already exists within. It's about creating independence and resilience rather than dependence and reliance. When you receive what once was lost and learn how to use that magic and power, you remember who you truly are, and everything changes and transforms.

However, the fear is real! Some women ask me, 'What if I open Pandora's Box and activate my power, but I can't control it? What if something bad happens to me?' We've been taught to fear the untamed part of ourselves, favouring predictability, control, and restraint. When we don't choose ourselves, we remain caged, stuck in survival mode as a people-pleaser, fitting nicely and neatly into an imposter lifestyle. We end up feeling bitter, resentful, full of judgement and self-righteousness, shaming others who dare to be and have all that we secretly want and desire—but are too afraid to claim for ourselves.

Projection becomes your protection.

Being wild, free, and unapologetic is dangerous and unpredictable. It's the unknown that scares you, so numbing becomes your existence. Are you too afraid to open your box because of what others might think? It's time to open Pandora's Box and come home to yourself.

Meditation

On this journey, I'm asking you to let your body lead and awaken to the sensations within that are intuitive and your birthright. It's time to cut away the dead, outdated beliefs, the stagnant emotions of blame, guilt, shame, and lack. It's time to thrive, not just survive. Your body is the portal into your soul, and your Shakti energy should not be constrained, controlled, or kept safe in a golden cage. The guilt, shame, and dislike you have about your body have been passed down! It's time to let it burn and love your body for all it is and does for you in every moment. When complete, journal what comes up for you.

Close your eyes, find a comfortable seated position with your spine straight, and take some deep breaths. Now, bring your awareness to your womb area. You can place your hand here if this helps. Imagine you're sitting inside of your womb. Sit there and be with all that is. When you're ready, imagine yourself getting up inside your womb and looking around. Open the windows and let in the fresh air, the energy of spring cleaning... getting rid of the dust that has settled. The new light lets you see the dust and shadows more clearly. Look around. What needs to be thrown away? What can stay, and what needs a repaint or some much-needed TLC?

Take Back Your Body

It's time to take back your body so you can love, honour, and respect her for who she is. All your magic, power, and intuition lie deep within her, and we need to start treating her like the goddess she is. Listen and let her lead you to the wisdom and power within. It's time to journey to the depths of the wild, fierce, abundant, and sacred places she longs to show you.

The body is how we experience life, pleasure, and even God! It's not out there like some off-planet being—it's within you, patiently waiting for you to come home. Acknowledging her existence means dropping the roles, parting the veils, and seeing yourself and life through her eyes. There is no more hiding, no more excuses, no buts, maybes, or later or when I have time. She's here with loving, fierce compassion; she sees behind the masks, excuses, and patterns and gently shakes you awake. When we don't listen, the gentle shaking becomes a fierce roar, an illness, or pain. She makes us take notice because you only start to truly live when you wake up to the power within. You begin to see with new eyes and feel with an open heart all that you are. You know in every cell of your being that you are *both* human and divine.

It's remarkable how we've been conditioned to fear and resent our bodies. Messages from social media, television, and magazines, both culturally and through our bloodlines, dictate that our bodies must conform to a specific appearance and behaviour to be loved, accepted, and successful. This narrative begins in childhood, passed down from mothers and grandmothers, woven into our lineage, embedding itself in our blood, breath, and bones. Consequently, we find ourselves engrossed in the pursuit of an unattainable standard. This preoccupation distracts us from what truly matters, becoming a means through which the patriarchal system manipulates and controls us; we don't have time to get around to what's *really* important—our purpose for being here. The constant pursuit of trying to look a certain way and the relentless over-achieving keeps us disconnected from our inner strength, and we fail to recognise the magic we already are. These manufactured illusions that we aspire to are a big part of the Modern Disease of the Modern Woman; they create a deep discontent with our bodies. In this state, we are essentially brainwashed and asleep.

Our worth and love are invaluable; no price is high enough to pay for them. When we embrace every aspect of ourselves, we stand tall in wonder at the perfectly divine vessel we inhabit. It's crucial to take a stand for ourselves and women collectively, dismantling limiting beliefs and breaking through blocked emotions. Opening our hearts, bodies, and voices is essential to reclaiming our power and defeating the patriarchal forces that have held us captive for too long.

The pain in our bodies serves as a wake-up call, urging us to start truly living instead of merely existing within the confines of a rule book that binds us. This pain represents a significant void we attempt to fill with distractions. Our body is our temple, not meant to conform to external standards but to nurture, nourish, and sustain our soul in this lifetime. Amid diets, self-punishment, restrictions, and abusive habits, we often lose sight of this fundamental truth.

Remember: She (your body) is a sacred vessel. Women usually believe these are their only choices:

1. Have a strict diet regime and calorie count, and become obsessed with everything we eat and drink, or...
2. Think 'screw it', and just go all out, eating whatever we want because we are so fed up with controlling ourselves and thinking our body has given up on us.

Both leave us hungry for more because neither is truly fulfilling or sustaining. Many of us swing from one end of the pendulum to the other, leaving us exhausted and lost, always fighting and chasing our tail. Do you know this feeling? You feel terrible, are tired and grumpy, and can't access your power. You have given away your energy physically and spiritually, chasing and maintaining a collective illusion.

There are many important reasons why we should care for and feed our bodies. Foods that nourish us have nothing to do with what we look like or how much we weigh. Our beautiful, precious organs—our heart and breasts, our lungs that breathe, our brain, our kidneys—do I need to say more? We must feel love and compassion for all our parts and stop taking them for granted.

Stop weighing your worth!

Many women are slaves to the number on the scale, and it can negatively influence our mood, our health, and the way we speak to ourselves and those we love. Instead of letting the number you see on the scale measure your self-worth, ask yourself, 'How else can I measure how good I feel?' Feeling good is a key part of the puzzle of caring for ourselves. When we are kind, compassionate, and strive for balance, we make better choices and become more flexible, whereas restrictive diets of binging, numbing, and calorie counting keep us locked up and caged within. It's all a mirror; how free or restrictive we are is reflected back at us in every area of our lives. A tight, stiff body represents a tight, stiff, unfulfilled mind and life.

I want you to start focusing on your health, not your size. One size certainly doesn't fit all and depends on your culture, age, and DNA. Remember that skinny girls aren't always healthy, just like curvy women aren't always fat. Skinny fat is on the increase, with women completely unaware of underlying health problems because they've been so focused on the number on the scale or their jeans size. The fat around your internal organs is a greater indicator of many chronic diseases.

There has been body diversity since the beginning of time, and we need to accept and celebrate our bodies as the sacred vessels they are and be grateful for all they give, remembering them as the divine container of magic and innate intelligence. This is your soul's home while you are here on this planet. We must start treating it with the respect and love it craves and deserves. When we start taking care of ourselves on a micro level, we begin affecting the macro level, and that's how we heal ourselves and this planet. We can stand up and shine our light, taking back our bodies and health.

Body shame carries a negative vibration and affects our health. It influences how we feel and act—and if we get sick. It's time to change the narrative and focus on what we feel rather than what we look like. The time has come for us to be the author of our own lives—not just the reader.

The Golden Rule: Balance

I teach most of my patients to live by the 80/20 rule. Eliminating all sources of joy from our lives can be as harmful and stress-inducing as using food to suppress our emotions. It's about recognising when you are full and asking yourself what you're truly hungry for. Sometimes, it will be genuine hunger, but we all know that when we are staring into the fridge, we are just looking for something to fill the loneliness or numb how we feel. Ask yourself, 'What is the trigger? What emotion am I feeling now?' Be patient and kind, and perhaps journal, take yourself for a walk, or phone a friend, but start noticing your patterns. Breaking a pattern takes work—sometimes you will win, and sometimes you will fail. Be kind and forgiving, and next time, try again, remembering you never fail; you only learn.

Moving away from what we look like and the need for outside validation frees up energy, and that's when miracles start to happen. Miracles occur when we focus on what we want rather than what we don't want. When you start loving your body, showing up every day, and treating her with kindness, love, and respect, your body begins to feel it and, eventually, starts to believe it. At first, the positive, loving conversation you're having with your body won't feel real, and you may feel stupid or frustrated, but slowly, you begin to see the changes. When we plant seeds, it takes time for the seed to sprout. It needs sun and water. Your body is the same. When you plant these new positive, loving seeds, your words, feelings, and thoughts help them to grow. The seeds grow when you show gratitude and focus on everything your body does for you. I love to touch my womb and thank her for my beautiful children, my legs for carrying me everywhere, my hands for their healing, my tongue for taste, and my breasts for the milk that fed my children. I'm grateful I can smell the roses, have arms to hug my babies, and speech to tell them I love them. We all have something to be grateful for.

Many of us may find ourselves despising certain aspects of our bodies, often expressing our frustration through harsh words, blaming our insecurities on stretch marks, C-section scars, cellulite, bloating, or the size of our bottoms. It's important to acknowledge and accept these feelings within yourself and to be present with where you are in this moment while recognising that such changes in perception won't happen instantly.

Exercise

Write down what in your body you're grateful for and why. Stand in front of the mirror daily and say it aloud—feel it as you speak it.

Meditation

Close your eyes and take three long, deep breaths, breathing in through your nose and out through your nose.

Feel your sit bones heavy on the floor or chair; relax your shoulders.

Feel into your body. Where have you been holding resentment towards your body or wishing it was different in some way?

Place your hands on or around that part of your body, or use a hand mirror to view it.

Breathe into it. See it, feel it, feel everything, see everything with your mind's eye.

Let any pain, anger, or resentment rise to the surface. Don't judge or fight it. Let it be.

Now, I want you to hold and connect with this part of you as if you were holding a newborn baby or animal.

Feel the wonder and miracle of what this part of you is and how it was created.

Hold it with care, protection, and love; rub this part of you—give her your attention and affection. Hold her in love.

Now, say out loud or silently, 'I may not love you right now, I may be ashamed of you, I'm sorry, and I'm willing to see you differently and change my feelings towards you.

I'm open to accepting that my distrust and shame around you is learnt and not real.

I choose to write a new story for us.

I love you; I am you. I choose to love all of me.

Thank you for all that you do for me.

This is Earth School—and your body is your teacher. Repeat this process a few times a week until you feel the new imprints within.

Sacred Nourishment

Make eating a sacred practise. Many of us are on the run, grabbing lunch on the go or eating bent over our computers. This isn't kind or loving to our digestive system.

Take your time, perhaps light a candle and eat off your good plates—stop saving them for other people and special occasions. You are important; every time you nourish your body, see it as a special occasion. Take time to chew your food and taste it. Inhaling our food on the run and multitasking leads to gas and a bloated stomach a few hours later.

- Don't drink while you eat—this affects your stomach acid and digestive tract, which means you can't break down or absorb all the vital nutrients your body needs.
- Be in the moment—no electronics or phone calls.
- Be with your body.
- Remember, eating is a sacred energy exchange with life. Everything we put in our bodies has energy, and we absorb that energy, so be mindful of what you're eating. When you cook, do it with love and the intention to nurture and sustain rather than rush and just fill. Putting something in your mouth is intimate. The only other time you might place something in your body is when you are intimate with yourself or your partner.

You Must Be Healthy to Lose Weight

When your body does not feel safe, it will not lose weight. I usually dislike talking about losing weight, as so many women spend their lives and precious energy trying to be thinner and achieve weight loss goals to feel happy. But I'm doing so here to bring light to this topic.

It's time to stop the 'yo yo' diets and restrictions because unless we're looking at our stress hormones, nothing is going to work. When we are living with chronic stress, we will always hold onto access fat and feel bloated. This is because of the chemical and neurologic cascade of events that take place in the body when we are under stress. Our body wants to store fat when stressed because it wants to survive. There is little time to rest and digest when the mind and body are under attack; we bloat and have painful gas, headaches, and weight gain.

The liver becomes overloaded and can't clear toxins and excess oestrogen, so the body stores even more fat. With more toxins circulating around the body, it tries to protect us by storing them in adipose tissue, the backs of our arms, upper back, and thighs. We see this as cellulite, but it's more than that—the body is trapping the fat, free radicals, and toxins away from our vital organs; it is actually protecting us.

Most of us are not meant to be supermodels, and there will never be one size that fits all. But being honest with yourself about your health is so important. You know if you overeat sugar, binge, drink too much wine, or overeat chocolate. You know what it feels like to live in your body. Switching the brain and refocusing the weight issue to a health issue will give you back our power. I always ask, 'How can we get you from surviving to thriving?' Forget about losing weight. When you focus on health and vitality, your body finds a balance that's right for you.

When the Inside Works, the Outside Shines

What if you were to look at the parts of your body that make you sad and frustrated as beautiful messengers from the body asking you to wake up and make different choices? You may need to realise how magical you are, eat, drink, move, think, take a breath, believe, or perceive in a different way than you are currently.

What if the daily headache you get mid-afternoon does not indicate that you need to take a painkiller but a nudge to move, change your posture because you've been sitting at your computer for hours, or drink some water? Do you think the bloated stomach or acid reflux you get every time you eat your sandwich or drink that third cup of coffee is your body telling you it's happy you consumed it? No, it's trying to tell you the opposite—it's uncomfortable, it's struggling, and all the pain and symptoms are not normal even though you've convinced yourself they are.

When our cravings get control over us, we don't listen to reason and don't want to hear the advice our body is desperately trying to give us. We ignore these messages for far too long, which is when worse health conditions emerge. We focus on what the body looks like on the outside, and we beat ourselves up because we're not happy with how we look or feel. But the problem is not on the outside—it's on the inside, and we can influence and help it immensely when we start to listen and make different choices.

There will always be days and weeks when making healthy choices feels hard. Acknowledge and honour it. Don't beat yourself up and judge yourself because those judgements keep you stuck in the negative cycle you find yourself stuck in. Start to become curious, asking yourself, 'I wonder what led me to do or want that? How has my day been? How am I feeling?' When we show up with curiosity rather than judgement, we allow our hearts to open, and we can listen to the real answers.

The foundation for healing disease and pain and reconnecting to our vitality starts with what we put in our mouths. The food we choose and the fluids we drink can either give or take from our precious energy.

When Diets Become Band-Aids

So many of us have fixated on losing weight at some point in our lives and have tried diets and strict exercise regimes only to find that we either become obsessed and over-restrictive with food or fail. We end up putting it all back on again, hating ourselves and our bodies even more than before. Our sense of failure creates more negative self-talk and unhappiness.

Diets don't work. However, addressing why we can't lose weight and the emotional components does. We all know what we must do to lose weight—there are enough books, diets, and information out there telling us what and how much to eat, yet we can't stick to it, and we fail.

We are really failing ourselves because no diet or size is going to make you happy— you need to get comfortable and develop a loving relationship with your body first. Deep down, a core wound wants to hold onto the weight for protection; it's hiding you to keep you safe so you feel protected and don't have to feel pain. You've lost trust in your body and perhaps find yourself in an abusive relationship with yourself. No wonder she has disconnected from you; who wouldn't if spoken to in the manner you address her? You're weary of the rules and restrictions, feeling a strong desire to break free from this cycle, even though societal expectations may suggest otherwise. The rebel within you, the voice of reason, acknowledges this isn't right. Yet, you continue convincing yourself that you'll conform and start afresh on Monday, adhering to the notion of being a 'good girl.'

Diets are restrictive and controlling and are not always—if ever—focused on health. You may say you want to lose weight to be healthy, but you need to be healthy to lose weight. Health starts in the body, in your mind and heart. When you change how you feel about her, are loving and kind, and make better choices, she will come back to life.

She, your body, is brilliant. She knows what to do. She always has since the beginning of time, before magazines, scientists, and doctors existed. She thrives when you love her and feed her with bright, seasonal, plant-based foods. When you give her the vitamins, minerals, healthy fats, protein, and the love she requires, your body works for you rather than against you. A diet full of toxins that lacks vitamins and nutrition will affect your whole system—how you think, feel, and behave. It creates a breeding ground for disease, chronic illness, and pain. When our digestion is not working, neither is our brain. *All the chemicals and hormones needed for our energy and mental health are made in the gut;* just think about that for a moment. It doesn't matter how many positive affirmations you say or how often your body isn't able to produce the life-enhancing chemicals it needs for you to be happy.

When it comes to food, nature knows best. When it comes to medicine, nature knows best, and when it comes to your health, she also knows best.

Humans are prone to making mistakes, as evident in the standard Western diet or the 1990s food pyramid. Attempting to fix a genetic blueprint crafted by God and the universe will inevitably fall short. We often seek convenience with easy, quick, ready-made meal options, but genuine health demands care, time, dedication, and love.

Your body craves taking the time to plan and prepare meals with love, understanding your body's needs, and selecting fresh, vibrant, and nutritious ingredients. It yearns for you to treat it as the sacred vessel it is, forging a partnership that allows it to function optimally and become the body you desire and deserve.

Nothing, and I mean absolutely nothing, can compare to the holistic benefits that real food provides—physically, mentally, and emotionally.

Science has firmly established the protective benefits of a plant-based diet. It provides us with all the vitamins and minerals our body needs to thrive. Eating real food is essential for healing and reconnecting with our bodies. By eating real food, you reduce the harmful substances that live in processed Frankenstein foods. These foods disrupt your natural bodily rhythms, biochemistry, endocrine system, and hormones.

Real Food…

- Allows your body to access and absorb nutrients efficiently and simply.
- Supports optimum PH levels, which reduces disease.
- Decreases your exposure to chemical loaders found in food.
- Enhances and supports liver detoxification, the key organ for eliminating excess oestrogen (think PMS).
- Balances hormones.
- Supports and maintains all the natural systems in the body.
- Gives you energy, a clear head, balanced healthy emotions, and keeps you connected to your true feelings and intuition (toxic food can make you feel badly).

You can't sustain yourself when processed food makes up the majority of what you eat. Your body will start to switch to survival mode. We get sick, develop pain, and have low energy—all precursors to chronic illness. I want you to thrive, and your body wants to thrive. It's time to switch your internal program and shift from surviving to thriving. You were born to shine. What you put into your body gets projected out there into the world. Personally, I'd rather be bright, vibrant, and shiny rather than dull, sick, and tired.

It's challenging to be kind, compassionate, and patient with yourself and others when filling yourself up with stimulants and food that mess with your body's intrinsic chemistry. The reality is that when we choose health, we are choosing to show up for those we love.

Our Health Choices Influence Our DNA and Genes

This topic is near and dear to my heart. Some of us want to give up because we believe that our destiny regarding our health and potential for developing certain diseases is already laid out for us. I used to think the same. I believed that my DNA was a ticking time bomb waiting to erupt and give me all the health problems my family had.

But the good news is DNA is not your destiny; you have so much control over which genes get expressed, and you have that control over your food, lifestyle choices, and emotional health. Your body may be at a genetically high risk for certain diseases, but it doesn't have to be a signed and sealed deal. Often, I see women using this as an excuse, 'Why bother? I'm destined to get fat or develop heart problems; it's in the family.'

My personal experience and all the research say this is not true; it's dinosaur thinking, and it can be used as an excuse to hide behind when we aren't showing up for ourselves and our health the way we know we should be.

My father is overweight and has metabolic syndrome. He has been taking high blood pressure medication for thirty years, is type 2 diabetic since his late forties, and suffers from a cascade of health problems. His mother, my nan, and her mother all had the same issues. My mum was also diagnosed with high blood pressure at age thirty-two and has been on a cocktail of medication since then. She is also type 2 diabetic but changed her health choices and didn't have to medicate. Yet, she always needs to keep on top of it.

My younger sibling shares the same genetic make-up as me, is also overweight, and suffers from high blood pressure and type 2 diabetes. So why not me? Why bother with my health if my DNA says this is my destiny?

What they all have in common is that they make the same lifestyle choices and food choices. Lack of movement, stress, lifestyle choices, and toxic overload have led them down this path. Due to my health scare and understanding of health, I chose differently and made different food and lifestyle choices and have no metabolic disease. I still have a life and love a glass of wine, chocolate, and pizza, but I do it in balance and listen and respect my body so she can look after me. It's a relationship. It's also epigenetics, which is currently the new way scientists look at what causes one person to develop an illness rather than another. It literally means 'above the genes.' You can, for example, have a set of twins separated at birth who both share the same DNA but are exposed to different environmental, emotional, and health choices. Studies have shown that the lifestyle choices we make affect which and how our genes get expressed. This is because epigenetics helps determine the production of the proteins in our cells. The healthier our lifestyle, stress levels, and diet, the less likely we are to switch on genes that lead to disease, illness, and weight gain.

It's empowering and liberating to know that you have the power to profoundly influence your health. Knowing that you can reduce your risk of developing chronic illness or degenerative disease while having a healthy body and mind you love simply by creating balance, making better lifestyle choices, and choosing a high plant-based diet is a miracle.

Counting the Cost

When things aren't going right with your health and body, you must be honest and ask yourself, 'How am I treating her? Am I treating her with love, respect, and honour? Or am I neglecting, abusing, and ignoring her?'

Your body is a mirror; your health gets reflected through how your body feels and ultimately, how connected you are to your soul.

The word 'but' often marks the beginning of a woman's hesitancy, indicating that she might not be fully committed to healing. In matters of our health, there should be no room for 'buts.' Instead, it's about a resounding 'YES, help me; I want to feel fully alive, healthy, and connected to the truth of who I am.' If we confront the 'but' honestly, we recognise it as an excuse—an attempt to justify why we believe we can't embark on this journey. Truthfully, I have a whole box of those excuses myself. Beneath it all, there's fear. We're afraid we can't do it or that we'll fail.

Rather than lamenting about being ignored, unheard, misunderstood, and dissatisfied with your life, consider turning the focus inward. Ask your body how she feels, inquire if she's content with how you've been treating her, and explore what changes she desires. This makes for a wonderful journal exercise—invest time to connect and listen deeply to the underlying truths. Embracing the truth has the power to liberate you, transforming your body, health, and life.

I acknowledge the abundance of information available, and here I am, encouraging you to make changes. Yet, let's pause for a moment. Imagine we're in a beautiful forest with birds singing on a fresh spring morning. As you gaze into my eyes, feel the love and compassion I have for you. I see you—the struggles, the pain… and I love every part of you. You and I are intertwined; we are one. Your battles are my battles; we are all internally struggling.

Regrettably, misinformation is rampant, leaving women feeling confused and frustrated—a collective trauma that affects us all, regardless of how we cope with it. This confusion has us stuck and frozen, unable to make decisions because we've lost sight of what's right for us. This, in turn, fosters more body shame, self-disconnection, abuse, depression, and pain.

I want you to understand that with all your pain, scars, and hurt, you are already whole and complete. You are enough just as you are. The choice is yours to love your body in this very moment and tap into her ancient wisdom. To move forward with anything in life, there must be an acceptance and appreciation of where we are right now, not when we get healthy or achieve our goals, but in all our messiness. She patiently waits for you to feel her, longing to be loved, nurtured, and fed on a soul level. Consider what feels right for you. What does she need and long for?

How does **She** *want to move?*

Just as one body shape doesn't universally apply to everyone, neither does a singular approach to exercise. In different phases of my menstrual cycle, there are times when I crave HIIT training and weightlifting, while other times, my body yearns for activities like dancing, walking, and gentle yoga. This preference can also vary with the changing seasons for all of us. Imposing rigorous exercise routines is another way we try to control and inadvertently detach from our bodies. For some, it constitutes a form of self-abuse.

Developing a loving relationship with your body involves tuning in to how she feels each day, week, and year. Just as obsessively tracking calories, counting steps, measuring distances, running, and lifting weights can become another way of measuring our worth, reinforcing the notion that we must achieve something to be loved and accepted. This stems from a part of us that may feel unworthy or not good enough. I like to align myself with the cycles of the moon and my menstrual cycle, along with listening to how I feel.

For example, in the winter, I slow my exercise down and do everything lightly. My body naturally wants to slow down and hibernate, and I've noticed when I ignore this, I get sick more often. Spring is the time when I start to do more. I naturally have more energy and feel more alive, which is reflected in my movement choices. Summer is the time when I exercise more and challenge my limits. I'm full of energy, and my body thrives on more energetic workouts. When Autumn begins, I'm rebalancing, slowing down, and usually rolling my yoga mat out more and doing Pilates.

When we listen to our bodies and consider our menstrual cycle or the moon's cycle, we use the cycles and nature's rhythms to help us connect to our bodies. Remembering that we are cyclic feminine beings helps us honour the cycles within and around us. We are not linear beings; we can't live in summer or full moon energy the whole year, or we will burn out. Knowing we have more energy to use for exercise when the moon is full or when we are ovulating enables us to make better health choices. We can embrace this time and move our bodies in a way that reflects and honours our hormones.

During the dark moon or when I menstruate, I rest, listen, and journal. It's not a time to push and prove that I can still do it all, even on my period. The old tampon adverts and sanitary towel commercials have brainwashed us into believing that our periods aren't meant to stop us from doing anything. We're told we can still function at 100% capacity and work to our maximum. I wonder who made this up? Because it wasn't Mother Nature! My guess is that it's a way to make us feel guilty about having periods and shame when we feel tired or when our energy is low. It's another form of patriarchal control where we feel less when we can't do what we think a man can do. This is because we have been taught that our worth is based on what we do and achieve, making periods inconvenient for many of us. Most women are suffering from PMS and other hormonal problems, and they don't know why.

The truth is that when we don't honour our cycles and take our rest, our body takes it anyway, which will cause far more problems than just taking an early night or missing your 5km hike or run.

Our body is meant to rest and slow down during this time. It doesn't mean your whole world has to come to a grinding halt, though! You must honour your cycle, energy, and body—listen to how you feel. Missing that one spin class is not going to turn your world upside down, and if it does, then there are bigger problems that need addressing.

The pressure from the media to be stick-thin and bikini-ready after a baby is also another way we are bombarded by abuse. It's unrealistic and unhealthy, and who does it really serve? Certainly not your health or your baby's health!

How many of us are stuck killing it running, spinning, and trying to burn calories, wearing away our joints and self-esteem? Self-control and denial can do us more harm than good! The thinking is distorted. For example, if twenty minutes of jogging equals one chocolate digestive, and you burn those calories, you can eliminate the guilt of eating it!

It's time for some new perspective! How about this? If you want the chocolate digestive, choose to eat it and do not beat yourself up or feel guilty about it. The answer is learning to come to grips with what you're *really* hungry for. Sometimes, it is the chocolate cake; if so, eat it! But don't give yourself a guilt trip over it—that's more toxic than eating the damn thing! There is no good or bad, right or wrong. There is, however, consciousness to everything you do, and behaving unconsciously and making choices from this place is where things start to go wrong.

The 'I've earned it' attitude is another way we control and restrict ourselves. If I can just burn that extra 100 calories, then I've succeeded. But this never gives the true feeling you're looking for. In fact, it likely leaves you chasing your tail and stuck on the merry-go-round of yo-yo dieting and self-hatred.

Why Exercise?

I love exercise! I love how it makes me feel—the energy and vitality it gives me—and it's one of the best drugs for balancing our insulin and hormone levels if done correctly. The reason we need to move goes far beyond the reason to simply burn calories or fit into our jeans again.

Exercise lowers your risk of developing type 2 diabetes. This metabolic disease is rapidly rising culturally and has devastating chronic health consequences that most of us aren't even aware of. After we exercise, our blood sugar levels decrease. Exercise helps take circulating blood sugar glucose from the bloodstream and puts it into working muscles and organs. A great way to achieve this is to take a walk after eating.

Our muscles take up 70-80% of glucose from our food. Therefore, the higher your muscle mass, the more you can clear excess glucose from the bloodstream. Therefore, the more muscle we can maintain as we age, the more insulin receptors we have, which lowers our risk of type 2 diabetes. As we age, women lose muscle mass every year, so it's so important for us to use and build muscle.

Engaging in exercise stimulates our skeletal muscles to produce insulin. This is beneficial as it reduces the workload on the pancreas, leading to lower insulin production and decreased insulin levels. Simply put, less insulin is required in the bloodstream to regulate glucose, minimising its conversion into fat and contributing to diabetes prevention.

Furthermore, exercise contributes to maintaining a healthy waist-to-hip ratio, another crucial factor in reducing the risk of developing this disease.

Visceral fat, also known as abdominal fat, is one of the major contributors to insulin resistance and type 2 diabetes. These fat cells store energy, toxins, and hormones, interfering with insulin use.

Secondly, we breathe deeply when we exercise, activating our diaphragm, the bell of muscles sitting under our ribs. These muscles can become lazy as stress and computer work means we breathe high using only the muscles in our upper chest and neck, which leads to neck and arm pain. When we start to breathe more deeply into our lower ribs and abdomen, we use our diaphragm in the way it was designed to be used.

Your diaphragm was intended for breathing, not as a cushion to lounge on while working over your laptop. When we begin to breathe correctly, we begin to lower our cortisol levels, which means your body thinks it's safe and you burn fat. When we are always stressed and do exercise that pushes us further into stress, like running or spinning, we burn glucose instead of fat. This is because the body is stuck in fight or flight. This makes it hard to lose weight and is the reason so many women think it's impossible to lose weight.

Specific exercises that stimulate the parasympathetic nervous system and convey to our brain that we are in a safe environment enable us to tap into our fat reserves and burn fat. When we are running from that tiger, we only use glucose stored in our muscles as fuel, as it's quick and readily available—certainly not the time to slow down and start using your fat storage as fuel!

How you move directly affects your cortisol levels and chronic stress hormones. Cortisol is the culprit that is laying down the visceral fat around your belly and internal organs, which makes you a target for metabolic disease. Your body is trying to protect you; it feels and perceives your stress and puts the fat there so you can get out of danger. Real or perceived because, let's face it, we are not being chased by tigers anymore but rather pressing deadlines, emails, and to-do lists.

By reducing cortisol levels, we decrease the abdominal fat that gets lovingly stored around your belly, indirectly reducing your hunger and food intake. It's all in our bio-chemistry… I told you the body was magic!

Ways to recognise you are stuck in cortisol mode:

- You're wired and tired.
- No matter how much you exercise or diet, you can't shift the excess fat.
- You crave sugar.
- You feel you would die if I took away your coffee.
- You feel a quicker heart rate after caffeine.
- You are anxious, on edge, and are easily startled.
- You wake up at night and can't get back to sleep.
- You overthink and worry about everything.
- Your breathing is high up in your chest and fast.
- You feel disconnected from your body.
- You experience a 4 p.m. sugar crash.
- You use alcohol to calm down and relax.
- Everything feels urgent.
- You say there aren't enough hours in the day.
- You say *yes* when you want and need to say *no*.
- You have become too serious and have lost the ability to laugh.

The Solution

Through our movement choices, we can influence our cortisol levels. Choose yoga, walking, Pilates, resistance training, or qi gong. These enable us to breathe from our diaphragm, lower our sugar levels, and use fat as fuel. Most women get scared and can't or don't want to believe this. They fear putting on more weight and get stuck in their heads, doubting how this can possibly work. But it's biochemistry, and it does work. Try it, and start following your cycle and feeling into what your body needs. Swap some high-intensity training for nurturing walks, yoga, and anything requiring breathing deeply and connecting. You will lower your cortisol, burn stubborn and unhealthy fat, balance your hormones, reduce your PMS and chronic pain, and likely find some joy. It's so worth it. You are worth it.

Case Study: Mandy

Mandy sought my help, fatigued and burdened with persistent shoulder and lower back pain. A vibrant Brazilian woman residing in the Netherlands for the past 15 years, she initially presented a foreboding demeanour—a mix of anger, irritation, and complacency. Mandy seemed like a volcano on the brink of eruption, suppressing her feelings.

Dealing with patients like Mandy requires caution in communication, as they tend to be defensive and resistant to advice. With a busy life—juggling two children and full-time work—Mandy sought a quick solution to alleviate pain and maintain her powerhouse status. However, the pain she endured had deep-seated roots that developed over the years through bodily compensations and stress patterns.

Mandy initially resisted the need to change her thought processes and movement patterns. Instead, she preferred addressing symptoms while ignoring the underlying issues. As we worked together, she experienced some relief, and our relationship deepened. The real Mandy emerged, and she began to open up.

Mandy was determined to be perceived as serious and unemotional, adhering to a black-and-white, rational approach. Suppressing her emotions stemmed from a desire to be seen as more Dutch and less South American, driven by ancestral judgement. An abandoned childhood fuelled a rejection wound, leading her to adopt a defensive stance, attacking to self-protect.

This internal struggle took a toll on Mandy. Her body remained tense, ready for confrontation, and she struggled to relax. Denying her true self, emotions, and cultural roots, she contorted herself to fit an incompatible shape and culture. The pain she felt was a manifestation of the stress and constraint she imposed on her body.

Mandy transformed by optimising her nervous system through chiropractic adjustments and encouraging reconnection with her body through 'She-Movement' practises. She rediscovered the joy of movement, walked freely, indulged in foods she loved, and allowed her emotions to flow. The pillow release technique, a method I taught her, became a powerful outlet for the repressed pain, unexpressed emotions, and words she held back for years. Mandy learnt that positive or negative emotions need to be in motion, not repressed, to prevent them from draining one's life force.

Honouring your genetics and ancestral bloodline is also key to healing the body. Women for centuries have learnt how their body needs to move, feel, and express itself. For centuries, rituals and cultural lineages have been used to help women remember who they are and how to live a full, abundant life from within. Many of us have forgotten and feel shame about these rituals; some have no remembrance. We are starved and cut off from the umbilical cord of our ancestors, but knowing where we came from and who we are is vital to our health and well-being. How did they move/what rituals did they perform? What did they eat and believe? What wisdom codes do they have to share with you? In my sacred sexuality course, we go deep into the ancestral walls and remember and rebuild these lost linages. We get the blood pumping physically and metaphysically into our roots, hearts, and the womb from which we all came.

Inside each of us is a confident, secure, powerful, magical woman, and my mission is to help you reconnect and reclaim her power.

We are SO hard on ourselves. Striving to meet expectations, do what's right, and be everything for everyone else, we often come up short when it comes to our own needs. Saying 'no' creates guilt, and saying 'yes' when we should say 'no' leaves us conflicted. Given how stretched thin we are, the concept of boundaries is elusive. We find ourselves feeling hollow and barely holding on. The shame we hold in our bodies and lack of self-worth breaks my heart.

Our internal thoughts and inner dialogues are programmed to be negative and full of self-judgement, creating a persistent sense of inadequacy. We are so tired; we try so hard and just don't understand why we feel the way we do. In my practise, when women enter, their posture and energy reveal a lot about their self-perception. The body becomes a truthful mirror reflecting the soul, with no room for deception. It raises the question: Why do many of us seem lifeless and lack vitality behind our eyes, which are often considered windows to the soul?

This happens because we've lost sight of our true selves, disowned the feminine aspects devalued in our culture, and adopted a protective mask to navigate the demands of life. Over time, this survival strategy creates a disconnection that wears down our bodies, much like the sea shapes the pebbles on the beach. The repercussions manifest in our health, relationships, parenting, and work—every aspect of our lives serves as a mirror.

Wearing a smile as a façade gives the impression of having it all together; we keep others at a distance while inside, we suffer. This pretence costs us our health and energy. Internally, it can feel like a slow decline, witnessing our dreams, desires, and passions fade away. It's not surprising that we cling to the hope that a change in diet or weight loss could be the solution to all our problems. Our fixation on external solutions becomes a way of avoiding confronting our inner feelings.

You have so much beauty, power, and potential inside you, waiting for you to re-discover your magic. It's time to start living the life you were born to live.

Inner Smile Practise

(This practise comes from Mantak Chia's Taoist spiritual practises.)

Begin by bringing a wide smile to your face. Make it the biggest, most beautiful smile you can. If you don't feel like smiling, fake it until you do. The energy of smiling will begin to change your frequency, raising your vibration and energy. You will feel nourished and healed as the practise balances your energy field.

Start to smile at different parts of your body. Imagine the external body and your internal organs and cells, such as your heart, liver, and spleen. Thank them for all that they do. Feel the gratitude spreading throughout your entire body, filling you with a sense of peace. If there is a part of your body you are struggling with because you are sick, tired, or in pain, send more love and smiles to this area and see it glowing with health and vitality.

If you struggle with stress, insecurity, anger, or negativity, your emotional body will benefit from this practise, especially if you have a negative relationship with a specific part of your appearance. Smiling into what you dislike will change your relationship with that body part over time because you are building new neural pathways and changing the emotional body and, therefore, how you think and feel. You are filling up with love.

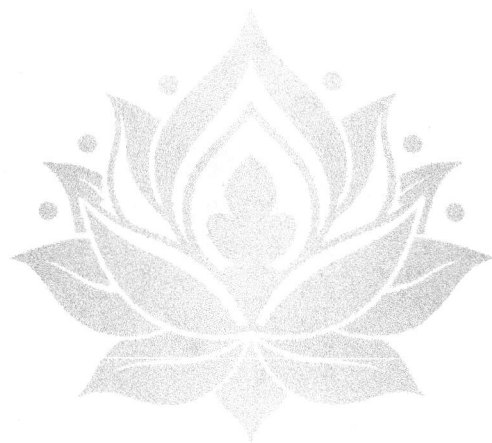

CHAPTER 3
WHAT IS PAIN?

'These pains you feel are messengers. Listen to them.'
—Rumi

Based on my experience, pain includes the following aspects: Physical, Emotional, Spiritual, and Mental. I've found that all these aspects are intertwined, which can make treating and healing pain a complex process—regardless of whether it's raging back pain, chronic headaches, a frozen shoulder, or pain radiating down your leg. In this chapter, I share stories and science so you can understand from a foundational standpoint. So take it slowly, and don't worry if it feels overwhelming—I've broken it down into bite-sized pieces so you can more easily digest it.

Pain is the language of your body. It is one of the channels the body uses to tell us that we are out of balance. Chronic pain, whether it's physical or emotional, is trying to show us that we can't stay the same. We need to change, grow, open, and live a more balanced life. If we can understand this language, we can always learn and grow from what our body tells us. Learning to hear your body's voice and trust it can save your life in many ways.

In a crisis, fear takes over and becomes louder than our intuition. We become stuck in the mind, cut off from what is happening in our body, analysing and rationalising rather than being present with the feeling. The Universe, God, Goddess, Love (insert your word for higher power) is always speaking to you through your body—always within and present. When we take the time to tune in and trust our bodies and our feelings, we can save ourselves a lot of time, energy, and pain.

Tuning into Our Feelings and the Impact of Ignoring Our Emotions

Many of my patients tend to store rage and resentment in their spine. This presents as a stiff and often painful lower back. Usually, the most gentle, placid, and loving women suffer the most from this problem. This woman walks around trying to do everything perfectly—being nice, good, people-pleasing, and doing her best while pleasing everyone but herself. She may experience bursts of anger, aggression, and often uncontrollable floods of tears, usually during her monthly cycle. These symptoms reach a pinnacle during her perimenopausal and menopausal years when she's often unable to control it or hold everything back anymore.

After releasing anger and frustration, she acts like everything is 'fine,' as if nothing has happened. So she puts everything she feels behind her—literally in her back—depositing it there where it builds up and festers until it blows a leak, and suddenly, she explodes and gets sick. Does this sound familiar?

PMS is usually a time when women feel out of control. Perhaps we boldly speak the truth about how we are feeling as it begins to surface and make itself known during this time. However, when we actively connect to our feelings and emotions with a regular She-Practise, we can let off steam and anger in a way that is not harmful to ourselves or others.

Not speaking or feeling one's truth builds up emotion and pain that manifests in the body. Not all lower back pain has a physical origin. Stuck energy, or stagnant shakti, gets lodged in our kidneys. This stuck kidney energy manifests as lower back pain. The build-up of emotions stored in the kidneys can become too much and then be referred to the lower back.

Case Study: Mary

Mary came to me suffering from chronic lower back pain and pain in her coccyx. She was in so much pain she couldn't sit down and was really struggling. Her whole lower back was sensitive to any touch, and even the slightest contact would make her shout out in pain and cry. Mary had been like this for years, suffering silently until her body just wouldn't let her sit on it anymore. In her words, she was an emotional wreck and couldn't even talk about how she was feeling because she was so emotional. Her mother had passed away from cancer a few years back. She was caring for her father—and she resented it. Mary had been mentally abused by her father and held deep anger and unresolved, unexpressed emotions towards him. The continual denial, guilt, and self-loathing she had for herself and how she felt about her father was blocked up within her kidneys and was eating her up inside. She had been trying to get pregnant for years, which was another source of her anxiety. She thought if she could be a good enough daughter, she would be rewarded and be a mum. Mary was feeling helpless and felt punished in some way for being a bad daughter, and she believed this was why she couldn't get pregnant.

The body is always listening and feeling, so what Mary was projecting onto herself became her reality and prevented her from moving on in life. Helping Mary work through the physical and emotional blockages changed her life. The physical pain was a symptom of something so much deeper than just 'pain in her lower back' and likely the reason other treatments she had tried over the years hadn't worked.

By releasing her emotions, feeling her feelings, and doing deep releases and sacred work, Mary could finally let go of her grief and resentment. She was able to create boundaries with her father and accept the situation for what it was. She healed the relationship from her perspective and let go of the emotions she was carrying. The best part about this story is that after three months of doing this work, she fell pregnant naturally.

The flowing energy of our kidneys is so important when trying to conceive, affecting our energy, hormones, and cellular functions. So, in Mary's case, there was no room or space to create a new life before she did the inner work.

⁓✻⁓

Pain Speaks to Us

We are taught to fear pain from a young age, yet pain can be one of our greatest teachers and friends. There is, however, a difference between good pain and bad pain. They have one thing in common: they are trying to get your attention to let you know something is wrong. Pain teaches us how we need to be careful and pay attention; however, most people fear pain and switch to a coping strategy or learnt behaviours around pain, which makes them go numb, become stuck, be a victim, play stupid, or feel powerless.

Knowing that your body has an intelligent way of getting your attention is empowering. Usually, chronic pain is what happens when we've been ignoring the warning signs for weeks or months—or even years. The body always gives us subtle clues about how it feels, but most of us are too busy to feel and hear them. Your body, after trying to accommodate and twist itself into every available position, begins to talk louder until it's shouting, and this is how we end up with chronic pain. Only now, we have a ton of compensation within our bodies, making the fire and pain feel hotter and hotter. This happens when we've been living in our heads, outside our bodies, and we've missed all the subtle clues our bodies gave us along the way.

Think about a time when you asked your kids to do something, and you said it nicely, but they didn't respond. We start to feel tight and agitated and begin to talk louder and louder. Eventually, you find yourself screaming to be heard, losing your composure, and resembling the person you vowed never to become. Strikingly, this parallels the way your body responds, too.

Disconnection from the Body

When women say to me, 'I don't know how this happened; I woke up like this,' or the classic, 'I just bent over to pick something up, and my back went,' I usually hide a compassionate smile because it never 'just happens.'

There were likely signs of stiffness, reduced mobility, and a few aches and pains. Still, you were either too busy or blocked it with a pain killer, lovingly ignorant to how your posture had changed or how you've been sitting in dysfunctional patterns bent over and twisted like a pretzel. The body always seeks balance and tries to accommodate us, but most women are completely disconnected from their bodies and voices.

Case Study: Lucy

Lucy was unable to have children. She had done everything she could to get pregnant, but nothing had worked out. She had chronic lower back pain and felt nothing physical below the waist except pain and numbness. Her social conditioning meant that she felt worthless as a woman because she couldn't have a child. Her body's response had been to wall off her heart, pelvis, and womb around that numbness and loss. When we worked through the emotional numbness, she was so grateful to be free of pain, but most importantly, she became more alive and more herself. By confronting the numbness and walking into and through her pain, she was able to free herself.

~❦~

People deal with pain in several ways:

- Ignore the pain and push through, pretending it's not real or something they will get to later when they have time.
- Mask the pain with painkillers so they can keep on doing everything they perceive they need to do. I call this wanting the 'quick fix.'
- Use pain medications like sweets and form a dependency.
- Self-diagnose or use Google to tell them what's wrong.
- Fear the pain and become a victim.
- Want someone outside themselves to fix it or heal them quickly and conveniently—don't want to take responsibility.
- Think they have some serious problem and spend their lives getting X-rays and MRIs, visiting the best surgeons and doctors, hoping to find the right answer.
- Identify *as* the pain—who are you if you don't have pain?
- Only focus on one part of their body and don't see the whole of themselves. Just treating symptoms.
- Are unaware of their own inner healer and power of the mind, body, and spirit.
- Use pain as a badge of honour to get sympathy or an excuse not to live fully.

None of the above will relieve your pain or get to the root cause of the problem and prevent it from returning.

Pain isn't the problem.

This gets most people's minds spinning, 'the pain is not usually the problem.' Women look at me blankly when I tell them this; they think I don't understand or realise how much pain they are in and how it's affecting their life, but I do, and still, I say, 'The pain is not the problem.'

The pain is a symptom, which sometimes means that pain in your lower back usually comes because of dysfunction, restriction, and compensation from somewhere else in the body, which has been building up over a long period of time. What you are feeling is the symptom, meaning if I just treat the pain, the problem will not go away.

Dysfunctions within the body and spine build up over time until they become chronic. The pain you experience is just the tip of the iceberg or a needle in a haystack. The fact is, you're not aware of what's lurking beneath, and this is why so many women get stuck in the pain cycle, causing more stress, wind up, and even more pain.

Whenever I get a client with chronic pain, I always feel excitement because I know she's about to uncover so many pieces of herself. We will not be masking the symptoms anymore. She will get to the root of the problem and herself.

The Nervous System

Your nervous system is housed within your spine and brain, and its route to your organs and body is via your spine. Most of us are only aware of a trapped nerve when we experience pain and google what a referred pain may be. Your nervous system is under constant strain and demand and will be compromised if your posture, stress, and lifestyle choices are not optimal. This also leads to digestive problems, heart problems, anxiety, difficulty breathing, high blood pressure, and so much more. Yet we don't equate this with our spine; we only get interested in our spines when we have pain and go to a good chiropractor.

Your spinal cord and nervous system need so much more love and attention from you than you know. Chiropractic, my first love, is such a profound and innately intelligent way of turning your nervous system on and removing subluxations so the brain can communicate with your spine and body, preventing disease and pain. Just like you look after your teeth and go to the dentist, you should look after your spine and nervous system, even more so in our modern-day world. Regular chiropractic adjustments will create profound changes in your physical health, well-being, and energy and help to prevent disease within your body. However, not all chiropractors are alike, so I suggest you find one that is vitalistic and educates you about your nervous system. If you want to get to the root cause of your problem, search for a chiropractor who works from a holistic perspective.

Pain Manifests Physically in the Body

All pain in the body, whether emotional, spiritual, or mental, shows up as physical. A broken heart can show up as high blood pressure or clogged arteries, heart disease, or breathing problems. How we experience physical pain is unique to each of us. Grief, for example, can show up as numbness and pain in the body. Sexual trauma can show up as a disconnection from your womb and pain and numbness during or after sex. Sometimes, it can even show up as an eating disorder.

Case Study: Tami

Tami was 45 when she had her third miscarriage. She had a healthy boy but longed for another baby. She had decided later on in life she wanted to be a mum, and she had an urgency to get pregnant as her biological clock was almost empty. When she became pregnant with this baby, she felt it was different. She had all the pregnancy signs and symptoms. She was tired and felt sick, and she was certain she was carrying the little girl her heart longed for. The day before the first echo, she had a dream that her baby girl had died. She woke up and could hardly breathe. She noticed that the whole left side of her body was numb and stuck in a strange position. Her chest and ribs ached, and she felt as though she had been in a fight where she had lost. She felt battered and bruised. Confused, sad, and in pain, she went to her ultrasound, which confirmed what the dream had told her.

The pain began to get worse over the next few weeks, and she wasn't able to work or even hug her children. She felt numb inside, and the pain was the only feeling that let her know she was still alive. She blamed herself and was desperate to hold on to the foetus within. After three weeks, she slowly began to lose the baby naturally as her body miscarried the child, and her emotions began to move. She cried, sobbed, and broke her heart, and slowly, the pain in her body began to change. At first, it changed its intensity, and then it moved around her body. She realised that the pain was her protection, protecting her from her broken heart, because when she finally let go of her baby girl and her dream, she let go of the walls of past regrets, blame, and control that she held in her heart. She had never wanted children before and had only decided to start a family in her late thirties; the grief that she held was for the lost time and regret. Her process was accepting, forgiving, and learning to let go of what she thought made her life perfect. She started to focus on the love she had for her boy, and her pain and numbness began to dissipate. She grieved her loss and held a ceremony where she felt her feelings, didn't push them away, and was able to give her grief a place. Together, we blessed her womb and detoxed the energy, clearing out her root chakra so she could create trust and a relationship within her womb again.

❧

Tami's story is a beautiful example of how grief and trauma show up in the body and how our body tries to protect us. Instead of numbing out and pushing the feelings away, Tami faces and embraces the pain, and by doing so, she has prevented a more serious issue from occurring down the line. So many women lose trust and end up resenting their bodies. The pain and grief get stored within the body, the walls around the heart close up, and our body's posture becomes a pain magnet.

Learning to walk through the door of pain and know the freedom on the other side is empowering and life-changing, and it involves a whole-body approach.

Just fixing Tami's pain wouldn't have been enough for her to heal or integrate fully. Maybe her physical pain would be less, but the emotional, mental, and spiritual pain would have stayed and eventually showed up somewhere else in the body. A mix of numbness and pain is common and not always a neural problem. It's a paradoxical state accessed only when we address our emotions and physical pain together. Emotional numbness, for example, can prevent us from dealing with deeper issues like grief. In Tami's case, it was her grief about not being able to have her second child. She'd lost one of her greatest desires, and a huge part of her cultural conditioning told her that her body was too old and she was past it. My point is there is never just one layer but many.

Pain and Suffering—Messages from Your Soul

There is a deep visceral pain that comes with the constant disapproval and rejection of ourselves, a sense of having lost something unnamed and unknown.

What if we feel down, in pain, and suffer because we've lost touch with our Soul? In an increasingly chaotic world, both inside and out, our spiritual health suffers. We often find ourselves questioning why life is so hard without realising that we might be experiencing a disconnect from our Souls. I call this a 'spiritual crisis,' which is often mistaken as a psychological crisis. We have lost access to our soul language, unable to understand her messages or even recognise her voice. We use psychological, medical and physiological terminology to describe how we feel or get a diagnosis or label reflecting this. We troll the internet to investigate our feelings further when all the answers lie within us. Deep down, we know something is off, and we feel lost to ourselves.

This disconnect can lead to a personal crisis as we struggle with life's challenges that can't be solved by positive thinking alone. More times than not, we're facing a deep spiritual crisis, disconnected from ourselves and the earth, feeling lost and without guidance.

Feeling stuck, fearful, and confused is a sign we're not in tune with our inner voice. We might know deep down what's wrong but ignore it, leading to a cycle of self-betrayal that harms our well-being. This can manifest as tiredness, anger, frustration, and eventually, physical sickness and mental health issues like depression or chronic pain.

In our society, we often prioritise the mind over everything else, but our soul is the driving force of our lives and the reason we are here. Decisions made solely with the mind can leave us feeling unfulfilled, as we miss out on the broader, beautiful aspects of life. Fear of change keeps us stuck in routines, separate from the soul-aligned experiences we unconsciously crave.

Often, we think about illness, pain and suffering as coming towards us, happening to us, but what if your current situation is coming from your soul, happening *for* you rather than against you? You are the co-creator of your current reality, and the meaning you give to your pain or suffering determines whether you experience more pain and suffering. When we perceive pain as breadcrumbs and messages from the soul, the pain stops becoming pain and instead becomes a great opportunity for change and growth.

'The wound is the part through which the light enters.'
—Rumi

If you're struggling, it might be time to connect to your soul and delve into the deeper aspects of who you are—returning to your true self and discovering your vibrant life force.

Healing Soul Pain

This is the deepest kind of pain, buried underneath all the other niggles, pains, aches, and emotions. It's the emptiness you've been trying to fill for your entire life. Perhaps you've tried filling it with relationships, work, things, food, places, experiences, and even with your kids. It's that missing part of you that got buried and put away. Occasionally, you get to taste it, feeling it as the seasons change, in the stillness that lives in an early morning walk, or as you gaze up at the stars and moon late at night. It's in sunsets and laughter, the feeling you can't quite describe, yet you long for it in every cell of your body.

This longing never goes away, but to live in this modern-day world, we end up silencing her. We numb out her cries because they are too painful and annoying, and we know that when we go there, it will require us to change and take action. We are afraid our perfect castles may come crumbling down around us, and then what? Who would we be without everything we have tried so hard to build?

The first step in healing from spiritual pain is recognising that whatever addictive behaviour you are using to feel better isn't going to work. Start feeling what the pain is really about. When did you stop feeling connected to your soul? What is it that needs to change for you to reconnect?

Ask yourself, 'Is my pain tied up with my desperate inner hunger to connect to my spirit?'

Break the Habit of Being You

Breaking old habits and rewiring old thoughts and beliefs is messy before it's elegant! It's like cleaning out your closet. You have to get it all out on the floor: all the beliefs, thoughts, and patterns that are crammed down inside of you, keeping you blocked, numb, and in pain. You have to sit in the middle of this mess and start somewhere—*anywhere*—searching and rummaging through what fits, what's old, what you need to give away or burn. It's about being able to find yourself in every given moment.

When it comes to healing pain, we need to break the destructive patterns, throw out what no longer fits, and stop squeezing into tightly constricted personas with attitudes and ideas that are cutting off our life force.

Initially, change is challenging because our nervous system prefers familiarity, gravitating towards the easy, well-travelled path and favouring shortcuts.

Creating new neural pathways takes time, effort, and energy. We think that when we want to change, it should happen instantly, but this is not usually the case, and it's the number one reason people fail at diets, exercise programmes, and healing. Today's culture is all about instant gratification—we want something, click a button, and it turns up.

Firstly, we need to break old patterns and make room for the new. You have to have a solid foundation and grow deep roots, or else when the wind comes, you may become ungrounded, fall, and fail. Then, we must build new, health-enhancing neurological pathways and connections to make the lasting changes your body requires to thrive.

Breathe

Breathing is vital to healing the stress cycle—it's the one thing you can't live without. It is something we do automatically, yet most of us do it wrong.

Whichever pain, numbness, emotion, or stress you are struggling with, learning to use and harness the power of your life force (breath) is the vehicle of choice for any transformational health journey.

We're so programmed to avoid our pain, hold our breath, and struggle against it; we feel we simply have to live with it and fight against it. I teach women to breathe into the pain and 'put your hand in the fire.' Rather than burning you alive, this opens the door to your healing. Breathing life and aliveness into areas of pain and numbness is one of the most important things you can do to help yourself get out of pain and heal.

The divine lives within, so when we breathe, we connect deeply to the expansive mystery of the universe. Breathing enables us to explore our internal landscapes and opens the door to the magical world within.

Tip: Take 10 deep breaths, ground, and reset.

Begin by breathing into the pain. Take four deep inhales and four long exhales, eventually building up to 10. On the in-breath, visualise your breath carrying oxygen and nutrient-rich cleansing nutrients to the area, and on the out-breath, see your body releasing all the toxic stagnant energy and pain. I sometimes imagine that I'm breathing in white light and breathing out black-brown smoke, but you can use any colour your body wants.

Feel the pain leaving your body, surrender it back to the earth, thank it for protecting you, and send it out with love. Feel the magic that the breath *is*.

Case Study: Anne

Anne was a stressed-out mum of two. She worked part-time and found juggling home life with her stressful job overwhelming. She had pain in her ribs and lower back, and she suffered from headaches and shortness of breath. She was a typical struggler. She believed in 'no pain, no gain.' Whatever she did, she had to do it perfectly. Working with her was difficult at first because she tried to control the treatments and always fought against me.

One day, while struggling to connect her breath to her pelvis, she finally decided to release the struggle and allow the breath in and through her body. Before, she just couldn't allow the breath to flow into her yoni and womb space; she would tense her whole body in protest. The moment she stopped struggling and allowed the breath to move into the tightness and restrictions, her whole body opened up. That single visceral feeling changed everything for her. She started to shake and sob uncontrollably as all the pain and numbness began to be felt and released. She wept for all the times she had pushed away her feelings, all the pain and numbness that had been living within her body and in her sex life, all released. After a few more treatments, Anne's pain fell away as if it hadn't ever been there. She was able to breathe easier, sleep better, feel more relaxed and connected to her children, and surprisingly, she said her sex life had never been better. For years, she couldn't orgasm because she couldn't relax. She often didn't like pleasure from herself or her husband because she just didn't feel anything. Now, she was experiencing orgasms from sex that she thought were only for special people; all that time, she had believed that her body couldn't do it and she was broken in some way. Anne's symptom was pain, but underneath the pain was so much more waiting to be experienced and expressed.

⋙❧⋘

Pain is a portal into the body and its inherent wisdom.

Self-Trust and Commitment

It takes commitment to get out of pain, break a habit, and get healthy—it's work, and it all starts with a decision and a commitment to change. Ask yourself:

- Am I ready?
- Am I willing to break free of toxic patterns and build a healthier body, mind, and spirit?

Make yourself a vow, not just a promise. We make promises every day, but a vow is visceral. It's deeper, carries weight and consequences, and requires action. We make promises and commitments to ourselves around diet, exercise, and self-care. However, most of us can't even manage a 5-minute meditation or 10-minute walk without falling off the wagon.

We have the best intentions and want to do it, but we need more conviction, strength, and self-love. A vow is a soul pledge to God—the Universe—a promise you don't want to break. An unbreakable vow to yourself requires backbone, not a wishbone. This backbone will support you when you go deep and start digging and unearthing why and where you are stuck in pain and not living the life you know you were born to live.

Having Faith

When I hear the word 'faith,' I'm caught between the Sunday school teachings and George Michael's song, 'You gotta have faith.' I have struggled with faith, and perhaps you have, too. Ask yourself:

- Do you have faith in yourself?
- Can you keep your word to yourself and others?
- Where do you betray yourself, and why?

Spirituality, religion, and mysticism are all founded on the pillar of faith, and many of us lack faith in something greater than ourselves. How can we believe and have faith in a God or Universe and our healing when we can't trust and have faith in ourselves? We let ourselves down constantly. We make promises and goals that we never get around to doing or completing because something gets in the way—mostly ourselves.

Healing from any type of pain is a soul journey that begins with having faith in yourself.

Developing faith in yourself also develops trust and faith in others. When we lack faith in ourselves, it's harder to trust others. If we can't show up and care for ourselves, how can we trust others to have our best interests at heart? This leads to more disease and stress in the body as we develop hardness in our being, thinking it's 'us against the world.' Waiting for others to betray us or let us down keeps us feeling separate and is ultimately a projection of what we've been doing to ourselves our whole lives.

Transformation is built out of self-esteem, self-respect, and self-love. It's learning to trust yourself, your decisions, and your ability to change your life and health by making one choice, one action at a time.

As you develop faith and trust in yourself and your body heals, you can develop faith and awaken to something bigger than yourself—the Divine. This ultimately frees you and connects you to deeper spiritual and soul healing.

Building faith every day creates a bridge back to yourself, allowing you to walk home to yourself. When we break promises to ourselves, we burn our bridges and feel we can't return home. We feel distrust, self-loathing, and shame because betraying ourselves means we have let ourselves down again and are further off track than we intended.

Learning to commit and be empowered by your body, emotions, mind, and soul is your magic. We must stop giving it away or pushing it aside because we feel powerless, distracted, and fear-driven. We make promises to others and bend over backwards to keep them, but when it comes to ourselves, our health and life are so easy to give up that we end up putting our needs and dreams at the back of the line. What is it you're hiding from? What are you really afraid of?

Transformation and healing are in the small details. The little things we do daily build trust, self-respect, and a loving relationship with ourselves, creating a portal for change and miracles.

Every day, show up for yourself and take a baby step toward your desires. When you give yourself your word, show up for yourself. Your words have power, so start thinking about what you promise yourself and how that commitment feels inside you.

When you keep small promises, you start to feel good about yourself and see yourself differently. Your power begins to grow, and you develop a foundation of trust that ignites your intuition, gut instinct, and divine guidance. You feel more supported, enabling you to start trusting yourself more. Then, you begin to make bigger promises to yourself, trusting that you'll keep them. You no longer feel alone; you feel healed and trust the divine power that lives within—not the rational process we are taught, but a deep inner knowing. Suddenly, you know what to do. You're no longer shooting alone in the dark, tripping up and falling flat on your face. You can see the path ahead.

When we don't trust ourselves enough to act, we listen to voices outside of ourselves and give away our power. Now is the time to reclaim your inner knowing and honour your voice. Feel what is moving within and awakening in you, and know you have all the answers you ever need and the faith to take action from there. You have direct access to your inner guidance and how to heal in every situation.

Now it's time to make that vow, trusting that you can—and will—heal. To break free from the bondage of pain, I encourage you to try the following:

- **Make a vow to your higher self:** Write it down and commit to healing your pain.
- **Be a Detective:** Be aware and present when old behaviours come up. Pay close attention to habits that worsen your emotional or physical pain. To create a new behaviour, we must first recognise what we are doing. Where and how do you want to numb out? What thought or events preceded the pain? How does your body respond?

Start looking at possible causes. How you sleep, stand, lift, and sit can contribute to lower back and neck pain. For example, if you slump over a laptop, you'll get neck pain, headaches, a foggy brain, and radiating pain into your shoulders and arms. Are you able to turn your head fully without twisting your upper back? Can you bend down and pick things off the floor with ease?

Emotional pain is a bit trickier. It can show up physically but not always in the part of the body we think it should. Heartburn, for example, may be caused by a fight with a loved one. Pain between the shoulder blades may be caused by feeling betrayed or 'stabbed in the back.' Perhaps your neck is tight because you're scared to speak your truth and say what you really feel.

When you experience pain in the body, ask your body, 'What is it you're holding onto? What do I need to do to release this?'

Treat pain as your GPS that gives you directions on your journey to healing. It's not a time to go into the victim role or start asking, 'Why is this happening to me?' Instead, ask, 'Why is this happening for me?'

Listen to the answers that come and then take action.

- How do you react to stress in your life?
- Where does the stress response activate in your body? Is it increased heart rate, chest pain, shortness of breath, clenched fists, shoulder pain, or even a head-ache?

When we feel physical pain, we tend to contract and avoid it, which causes more restriction and reduced blood flow to the area. Bringing the breath into the body and the pain helps relieve tension and stress and allows the body to relax. When you're connected to the breath, ask your body what it needs. Is it a walk, a break, some water, a hug, 'She-Movement,' or a chiropractic adjustment? Listen in and follow your inner knowing.

Our habitual breathing and postural patterns tend to function on autopilot, creating a breeding ground for stress, tension, and pain. By breaking a pattern and changing our position and focus, we start to break bad habits. This positive turn affects how you walk through life and heal from the pain cycle. Once you've identified the source of your pain, you can keep an eye out for it, watch your reactions, and change the biography of your body, ultimately reducing your pain.

Forgive and Praise Yourself

Forgive yourself when you fail or forget and find yourself slumped over the desk, leaning to one side, crossing your legs. Be kind to yourself and stop using shame-based thinking and self-talk like, 'I'm so stupid. I'm so fat and flabby. Look at my bloated stomach. I suck at everything.'

Physical and emotional pain go hand-in-hand. So when you're feeling bad about yourself, you'll feel more pain as that part of your body's intelligence hears and understands you. It will start to mirror your thoughts by constricting and defending itself with more self-protecting mechanisms.

Ground, Re-centre, and Re-balance

Do not push yourself—all new habits take time, which is part of the healing process. Stop trying to be Miss Perfect and get it all right. This only creates more stress and pain. Be gentle, kind, and compassionate as you create new ways of being.

Replace negative self-talk with self-praise. Praise yourself for catching and breaking the patterns. It takes courage to catch yourself and turn your thoughts and behaviour around.

Reward yourself, but not with food, wine, or anything else that will harm you. Instead, go for a walk, have a lovely tea, buy flowers, or take a deep breath. Awaken to and feel the new experiences that are born when you start to break away from your own painful reactivity.

- What is it you are really feeling?
- What's rising and coming to the surface to be seen, heard, and expressed?

Every day, take one small step towards your healing. Remember, baby steps get big results. Your body took so long to get into this pain that it needs time to unravel and unwind its way out of the pain. Send your intention and breath into the pain, asking:

- Who or what am I carrying here?
- Where did this originate from?
- Where in my life am I also stuck?

Feel into your upper shoulders, a common place to feel tight and restricted. Where are you taking on too much responsibility or other people's responsibility? Where in your life are you carrying the weight of the world and others on top of your shoulders?

Inquire about what your body wants and needs. When we are fully present, it begins to communicate with us. Over time, it learns to unfold like a flower, revealing emotions that may have been suppressed or ignored for years—feelings we may not have wanted to acknowledge, such as 'ease up on work,' 'this relationship isn't right,' or 'learn to say no.'

Instead of heeding these messages, we often turn to distractions like a glass of wine or a biscuit. By altering how we treat our bodies and being present, we create a space for them to open up. Establishing trust is key, and it requires attentive listening and taking action when our bodies awaken and start speaking to us.

Tip: Communicate with Your Pain

When you have pain in your body, put your hands on the area. Take some breaths into the pain and ask, 'What do you need from me right now? What's the next step towards our healing?'

Listen and feel for the answers. At first, you might get nothing; trust and persist. After a few times, you might get a nudge to start sitting better, change a pillow or desk chair, work fewer hours, forgive a friend, or say what you mean at work. Keep asking for what you need and get curious about what wisdom lies within the pain. Every tree has roots, and those roots have other roots that attach to the network of other trees nourished by a mycelial network. You don't need to find all the roots, but you need to find the one that's not getting nourished or is cut off from the others. You need to find the root of your pain. Can you give your pain a voice? Does she have a colour or form? Write down what comes up, and let your feelings and thoughts connect and come to life together on the page. Learn what's living there, taking up space and giving you pain. What needs to happen so you can release and let it go?

Emotional Pain

When we hold onto any negative emotion, such as fear, anger, rage, jealousy, hate, or resentment, we leave ourselves open to the manifestation of pain in the body.

What is repressed must be expressed.

Expressing our feelings is how we allow our emotions to flow. When emotions become stuck, they stagnate and take up space within the body. Feeling and expressing our emotions fully stops them from getting stuck and leading to pain, disease, and chronic illness. Often, when we heal our emotional pain, our physical pain subsides. The two often go hand-in-hand, especially in the feminine body.

You've got to move your emotions, feel them, shake and breathe into them, scream and release them, but for the love of God, they can't stay stuck inside you like a ticking time bomb waiting to erupt. Releasing these emotions helps remove them from within our cell tissue. They depress our immune systems and leave us like sitting ducks waiting to be prey to illness.

The connection between emotional and physical pain is extremely important. As an illustration, grief is also an emotion that needs to be freed and expressed. When we lose someone we love, we also lose part of ourselves. The body starts to protect and compensate for the loss, and scar tissue builds up around the pain, especially around the heart. Dying with a broken heart is a real thing. Grief can also manifest in the lungs, such as shortness of breath or pain in the arms or ribs. Pain and headaches are also common manifestations. The grief needs to move so as not to consume you. It's a natural emotion, and grieving in a healthy way moves stuck emotions along with the tears, anger, and toxins stored throughout the grieving process.

In Western society, we tend to put on a brave face, carry on, and return to life quickly. We feel guilty if we overindulge our feelings, which can lead to shame. Even when we lose someone old who had a good life, it still takes time to process. Don't deny yourself this rite of passage and expression of your grief—it's there to heal you, not destroy you. Your life won't fall apart when you feel all of it, but it might if you bottle it all up inside and keep the lid on tight like a bottle of soda pop.

Bigger View

Imagine venturing into space and gazing upon Earth from afar. In this moment, you'd witness the planet in all its glory—a breathtaking, round, green, and blue sphere teeming with energy, light, and life. From this vantage point, the distinctions between countries and oceans become irrelevant, for the system is unified, with life flowing in and out seamlessly. The principle of 'As above, so below,' and 'As within, so without' comes to life.

This broader perspective, capable of perceiving an organism as a whole, is crucial for life and health, inherent in every human being and every living entity. When confronting our challenges, we must consider the entirety of our being, not just isolated parts. Ground-level observations of Earth may foster a perception of separation—different countries, seas, races, and mountains. However, this view stems from a limited perspective.

By adopting a bird's eye view and rising above the situations and issues surrounding us, we can recognise ourselves as integral parts of the whole, both within and outside ourselves.

What is in one is in the whole.

Believing in our separation from ourselves and each other is one of the primary reasons for falling ill. True healing occurs when we perceive ourselves as whole entities because sickness affects the entire being. In a physical context, addressing a heart problem involves more than just focusing on the heart; various other factors play a crucial role:

- Kidneys
- Veins
- Lungs
- Heart rate
- Blood pressure
- Arteriosclerosis
- Stress
- Exercise

This comprehensive approach is essential because the system is interconnected. A similar perspective can be applied to lower back pain. The pain itself is often not the root cause but rather a result of factors such as posture, compensations, thoughts, emotions, nervous system stress, trauma, and foot and knee problems. Merely addressing the pain is inadequate; the complete problem must be understood by considering the entirety of the person.

When delving into matters of the soul, it is necessary to cleanse and realign the physical, spiritual, emotional, and mental aspects to ascend to the root cause.

My Story

Every evening, I would come home from work feeling tired and wired. I'd been doing the job I love—helping people. I had amazing patients, and my life looked perfect from the outside. But I was lost, felt alone, and was searching for something. I had spent most of my life working hard to be a chiropractor. It had taken five years of my life, and it had been stressful as I had my first daughter in the first year. After my daughter was born, I was a student and single mother, and I felt lonely, scared, and overwhelmed. I sacrificed and pushed myself to the limit to achieve what I believed to be the pinnacle of my mountain. I believed that once I was at the top, I would feel satisfied and safe as if I had made it. All the people who had said I couldn't, or shouldn't, continue my study with a baby… the dumb blond jokes… all their expectations of me failing… pushed me to be the top of my class, whatever the cost. I was going to prove myself to all of them. I desperately wanted to feel loved and accepted. I wanted the feelings of inadequacy and smallness and of not being enough to go away—this was my fuel, this was my goal.

I did reach the top of that mountain. I won. I may have lost my partner, ended up a single mum, and become so thin I looked emaciated, but I'd made it. The euphoria lasted about half a day, a hot second compared to the hardship and sacrifice of the past five years. Doubt began to creep in. Maybe it was a fluke… I'm a bad mum; I've missed so much… was it really worth it? Am I going to be a good chiropractor? Nobody saw me differently, and I still felt the same. I turned around, and another mountain lay ahead of me, but this time, it was split into three. The first was one I had to climb to get the right job and build a practise; the second was to get off housing benefits, get a house and child support, and pay my student loan back, and the third was all the material things I needed to look like I'd made it.

I was 28 years old and felt the pressure of being materially behind in life. I needed it to look good and fancy on the outside because I wasn't feeling it on the inside. Overwhelmed and disheartened, I started to climb the mountains. My enthusiasm had worn thin this time, and I had less energy. So, I started to use wine to numb the feelings. My life consisted of working hard and then cooling down with red wine. I couldn't relax without it—I couldn't come back into my body without this crutch. I was exhausted in my search for my philosopher's stone and losing faith in myself every time I achieved my goals. I still felt empty.

When I had my awakening, or 'reawakening,' as I like to call it, I began my long journey into the divine feminine, spirituality, and sacred sexuality. That's when everything changed for me. I started working on ways to get in rather than out of my body. I started looking at how I could clean up my body and life and reconnect on a deeper level. I found my lost little girl inside; I held her and stroked her hair. We played and talked, and she guided me deeper into myself and showed me the treasure chest that had been discarded, awaiting my return. Every day, I would go there, and I still do now. I pray, meditate, and do my 'She' practises and movements to connect to my soul. I recharge and let Her guide my thoughts, actions, and life. I surrender and allow myself to be open to receive guidance and direction for my life. My health has never been better, and I've never been happier. This is what I want for you. The lie and misguidance you find outside of yourself is a distraction and keeps you powerless, disconnected, and in pain. The most valuable thing you possess is yourself—your essence—and I'm going to show you how to find Her again.

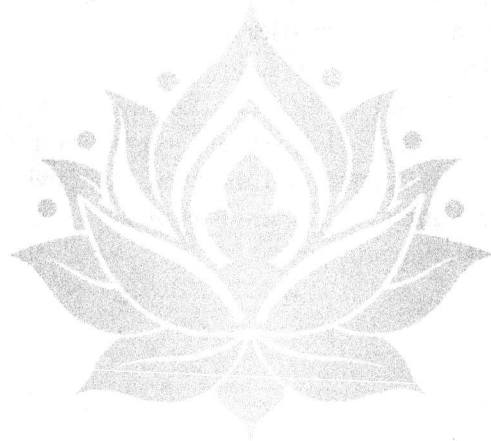

CHAPTER 4
ALIGNMENT

*'Though her soul requires seeing, the culture around her requires sightlessness.
Though her soul wishes to speak its truth, she is pressured to be silent.'*
—*Clarissa Pinkola Estes*

Your posture mirrors your soul, revealing a wealth of information about you, reflecting the life you've experienced and the kind of personality you possess. It discloses insights into your beliefs, self-worth, and approach (or avoidance) of emotions. Before delving into the profound impact of posture on emotional and spiritual well-being, let's explore the physical side effects and understand how stress contributes to them, creating a cycle that perpetuates stress itself.

Core Wounds

Pain is the universal language of the body, and it's the first way the body tries to tell us that something is out of alignment and that we need to pay attention.

Posture is how we see our core wounds reflected in us. Most of us have spent years trying to escape our core wounds or pretending they don't exist. We block emotions and feelings because we fear them and lock ourselves up in our bodies. These feelings get stored and contained within the cells of our body.

Our core beliefs are established during early childhood, forming the basis of our self-perception. We invest considerable energy in concealing these beliefs from others, driven by a desire to avoid the shame and humiliation we feel. These emotions are suppressed, and we have learned to dread them, as they ultimately exert control over us and influence decisions based on fear rather than genuine desires.

The six core wounds that can be trapped in the body:

1. Abandonment
2. Betrayal
3. Humiliation/Shame
4. Rejection
5. Grief
6. Trauma

Core wounds are formed when we perceive or experience a separation from love, which keeps us searching and trying to fill the emptiness inside.

Becoming conscious of what we are carrying and which core wound our posture is stuck in is the beginning of the journey back to you—back to love. Being able to face and feel the hole that is there from the lack or loss of love begins the healing process and allows the emotions to flow.

The Modern-Day Experience of Stress and Postural Changes

As we approach our late 30s, many of us find ourselves either having children or navigating the challenges of child-rearing, and the changes in our bodies can be surprising and disheartening. Extra weight may cling to us, shoulders may sag, and the emergence of a back hump becomes a reality, a feature we once associated with the elderly or fictional characters like the hunchback of Notre Dame. The sensation of bloating and a lack of energy permeate our daily lives, turning each day into an uphill struggle. Dealing with persistent aches and pains and diminished energy and motivation creates an ongoing battle with our bodies. Some may avoid mirrors, dress in the dark to shield themselves from a partner's or their own scrutiny, abandon once-confident sexual positions, and strictly control what images are shared on social media, seeking approval before anything is posted.

I understand, and many of us can resonate with that sentiment. My focus isn't on conforming to some societal notion of sexiness dictated by the patriarchy. Instead, it's about fostering a genuine love for your body, standing tall with pride, and being firmly rooted in the beauty of your authentic self. This involves embracing and owning your body regardless of its size or shape. One of the initial challenges I observe is poor posture—a common struggle for many. We've neglected the art of holding ourselves with grace, often caught in the cycle of survival and the relentless pace of our hectic lives.

Your posture mirrors your life and choices. Many of us need to learn how to move our bodies properly—whether sitting, standing, or sleeping—to regain control over our pain and avoid dependency on painkillers and other medicines.

Posture, often underestimated, plays a crucial role and serves as an indicator of the stress levels, pain, fertility, and hormone issues you might be grappling with. It even offers insights into heart health and can predict the onset of chronic diseases.

Just like your teeth, your spine requires love and attention. Consider what would happen if you neglected to brush and floss. Now, picture your poor posture and the prolonged hours of sitting each day like sugar for your spine. The solution? Move!

Postural changes are the first things to happen when we experience stress. The head drops forward, and the shoulders become hunched and ready for fight or flight. We tense our buttocks and hamstrings, and all our muscles get pumped and ready to run. Glucose is released into the blood to help. The digestive and immune systems become suppressed, and your whole body is fired up.

Yet the only thing we are doing is reading emails, going through our to-do list, or running late for the next appointment! This posture becomes the 'norm,' and because so many of us sit at computers all day, we perpetuate it further. Just as stress can cause a bad posture and pain, so can the bad posture cause more stress and pain. It's a vicious circle most of us find ourselves in. Posture, which goes hand in hand with the stress cycle, is the first part of what needs to be corrected to break the pain cycle. Understanding how sympathetic dominance shapes our body and life is key to unravelling the knot we find ourselves tied up in.

When our posture is good, messages can flow up and down the spine via the nervous system to every cell in your body. However, with poor posture, the messages get distorted, and the intrinsic feedback loop is broken.

Good posture is critical for our oxygen levels. When our shoulders are forward and rounded, we take short, shallow breaths. Our ribs become stuck, and our chest muscles tighten, leading to thoracic cage excursion, where the rib cage cannot expand and contract fully. The ribs are designed to move up and down when we breathe; they contain pressure receptors that send messages to the brain, which switch us to rest and digest mode. The parasympathetic side of our nervous system helps us calm down and relax. When we aren't breathing properly because of our posture, messages are sent that there is stress, and our biochemistry responds by pumping out more adrenaline, pushing us further into even more stress.

Every cell in our body needs oxygen to work.

When our shoulders are rounded and our head is forward, the spine's natural curve is altered, impeding functional efficiency. The body strives for balance, so it adjusts by changing the lumbar curve, leading to lower back pain. Consequently, addressing pain requires a holistic approach, recognising that everything in the body is interconnected. Improved posture and healing arise when viewing oneself as a complete, inherently intelligent human being.

Patients often present with lower back pain, yet the root cause may lie in the neck or vice versa. Addressing only the apparent pain in one area would be insufficient and fail to target the underlying issue.

The stress posture also gives rise to pain in the shoulders, arms, and hands, accompanied by sensations of tingling, itching, and numbness. This occurs when the space between the first rib and collarbone narrows, exerting pressure on the nerves and radiating discomfort into the arms. Additionally, tight chest muscles resulting from rounded shoulders contribute to nerve radiation into the arms and hands.

Beyond the physical, your alignment provides insight into emotional and spiritual alignment. It reveals areas of past hurt, fears, and places where you may have shut down or disconnected from yourself. The body encapsulates physical memories, storing trauma and pain within cells, and posture reflects this internal history. Your posture is a profound non-verbal communicator, speaking the language of your soul. It serves as a mirror, depicting aspects of yourself that may be confined, entangled, twisted, and stuck—often compensating for the burdens you carry, protect, and avoid. Therefore, posture isn't merely a correction to straighten; it is an opportunity to learn and gain insight into the unconscious dynamics within you, liberating not just the body but also the emotions, mind, and soul.

Throughout our lives, we often shut down and suppress certain emotions and experiences, leading to what can be described as emotional amnesia. While we may forget, our bodies do not; they retain these memories in our cells and tissues. The adage 'What is not expressed gets repressed' holds true, as the body locks away memories and emotions to shield us from pain, creating a barrier so we don't have to confront them directly.

To protect us from the potential agony, our bodies stash away memories and emotions, often behind and inside the spine, causing blockages in the nervous system and storing a range of negative emotions from rage to fear. This storage alters the functioning of our spine, transforming once-fluid and aligned curves into rigid and restrictive shapes. Kyphosis develops in the thoracic area, forward head carriage leads to the neck bump, and the lower spine and hips may thrust forward or backward, disrupting the lumbar curve's intended function. These changes lead to compensations, particularly in ligaments, sacrum, and hips, resulting in upper and lower cross syndromes.

The accumulation of unexpressed frustrations can lead to a protruding belly, affecting the liver's ability to detoxify and causing issues such as IBS, leaky gut, and potentially autoimmune problems. Hormonal imbalances arise, contributing to conditions like PMS, PCOS, and other reproductive problems in women. A compromised liver, strained by stress, particularly for those over forty, may result in a challenging perimenopausal and menopausal experience coupled with fatigue, burnout, and a rollercoaster of intense emotions.

Digestive functions are impacted, hindering the production of feel-good hormones like dopamine and serotonin and the synthesis of hormones necessary for balance. The stomach becomes a repository for things we wish to avoid, concealing and burying them deep within, causing blockages in the intestines. Repression of emotions is linked to conditions such as IBS, Crohn's, and ulcerative colitis.

The issue is in your tissue.

Stress and adrenal responses can result in increased pain and stiffness, placing us in a complex web of physical and chemical chaos intricately tied to our emotional and spiritual well-being. The consequence is a physical, emotional, and spiritual disconnection, leading to patterns that deviate from our true essence.

A well-aligned and healthy body, coupled with an optimally functioning nervous system, can effectively combat infections, promote wound healing, eliminate cancer cells, facilitate quick repairs, and mitigate ageing-related inflammation.

When postural changes and stress disrupt the proper functioning of the spine, messages between the brain and organs are compromised. This breakdown in communication hinders the body from receiving what it needs, creating obstacles and paving the way for illness and pain.

Often, we only focus on our bodies when pain arises, overlooking the gradual loss of function, poor posture, and muscle imbalances that stress can accumulate over months and years. Addressing physical issues necessitates understanding the root cause rather than merely treating the symptoms. Treating symptoms is akin to applying a plaster to a significant wound while hoping for the best; it doesn't address the underlying problems that persist. The spine, operating through the nervous system and brain, maintains an ongoing dialogue with muscles, internal organs, tissues, and hormones. It's crucial to remember that you are a complete and holistic being, and your body perpetually seeks balance and homeostasis—a balance often lacking in various aspects of our lives.

The nervous system's influence on both your posture and internal body is frequently underestimated, yet it holds significant implications for your overall health and longevity. The alignment of your spine serves as a silent messenger, revealing insights into what's transpiring within you, aspects that may not be immediately apparent. Postural shifts act as early warning signs, prompting a moment to become attentive, awaken, and nurture your body. It's an opportunity to pivot and delve into the root cause of your pain before it escalates into a more substantial issue demanding increased attention.

How does stress lead to postural problems?

Living with chronic stress puts us in a state of sympathetic dominance, significantly impacting our physical body over extended periods. It affects not only our posture but also the muscles, ligaments, tendons, and even our bones. It's crucial to consider the entire spine when assessing the physical body. The positioning of your feet, knees, hips, shoulders, and neck all play a role in influencing the spinal curves, altering muscle balance, and potentially causing issues if they are out of alignment.

The red nucleus, serving as the central motor nucleus for bilateral skeletal muscle tone, becomes activated in response to stress. It governs the muscles we flex and contract through the coordination of the brain, spinal cord, and peripheral nervous system. Common physical manifestations of stress include tense calf muscles, rounded shoulders, and a bent-over hump, often resulting in tightness and pain that may radiate to the head and arms. Prolonged exposure to this stressed state causes the muscles to harden progressively, contributing to stiffness and eventually leading to additional posture issues and alterations in bone structure and function.

Newton's law says that force equals mass and acceleration. This can also be applied to how we develop structural changes to our bones and posture over time. This is because every static and dynamic movement has a force. Muscles are the primary contractors that create a force on the body's levers (connective tissue and bone). When we apply this law to a static force such as forward head carriage, gravity and the weight of the head, which is around 5-6 kg, create an anterior and inferior force, commonly known nowadays as a text neck, or as I lovingly call it, a hump at the top of your spine.

In its continuous effort to assist and safeguard you, your body takes measures to prevent your head from feeling like it might snap off and roll away like a bowling ball. It engages the muscles in your upper back and neck to help balance the load, which, unfortunately, can result in shoulder issues as the stabilising muscles bear additional stress. This situation often leads to neck pain, headaches, and migraines. It's a sensation akin to carrying the weight of the world on your shoulders, both physically and metaphorically.

The body serves as a mirror, reflecting internal states outwardly—following the universal law 'So within, so without.' When stressed, anxious, or overwhelmed, these emotions manifest in our energy field. Lower vibrational energy affects our energetic state and lowers our physical vibration, creating density within the body that contributes to pain and discomfort. Energy has a tangible impact on matter, in this case, our physical body.

Observing people around you, from friends and colleagues to passing strangers, you can discern how they hold their shoulders and head, providing visual cues to their self-perception and stress levels. Individuals with slouched shoulders and a forward-leaning head often appear exhausted and lack vitality. In contrast, those standing tall with an open chest, shoulders back, and head aligned on top of the spine emit a different energy—one that is visible and palpable. They tend to be more approachable, open, and adept at giving and receiving in various aspects of life.

When we are stuck in a stress pattern, our biochemistry is affected. Stress lowers our energy and vibration, and because like attracts like, we start attracting more negative and lower-vibration thoughts and experiences into our lives, and we can become stuck physically and spiritually.

In conclusion, I want to emphasise the profound impact of posture on our physical, mental, and emotional well-being. Poor posture sends a clear message to others that we are closed off and prefer solitude. When we hunch over protecting our hearts and emotions, we inadvertently convey a desire for people to keep their distance, contributing to feelings of isolation.

Conversely, an open posture signifies receptivity, approachability, and an invitation for connection. With an open heart and the ability to breathe fully, we attract higher vibrational thoughts and experiences. An open posture alters our physical appearance and significantly influences our internal health. The constant communication between our spine, brain, and environment shapes our biochemistry, sending messages to relax and counteract the stress response.

If our posture is closed and bent over, our body interprets the surroundings as unsafe, triggering a stress response that tightens our muscles and heightens stress hormones. This creates a loop where stress causes poor posture, and poor posture, in turn, amplifies stress—a vicious cycle often unnoticed by many.

Understanding this connection is crucial, especially when seeking new friendships or romantic relationships. Taking a moment to check in and assess your body language can provide valuable insights into the signals you are sending and may be instrumental in fostering meaningful connections.

Upper Cross Syndrome

This is a pattern I observe in virtually everyone, including children. It stems from the stress response, which signals our brain and spine to prepare for the 'fight or flight' scenario by tensing, flexing, and getting ready to run. Additionally, our modern lifestyle, characterised by prolonged periods of sitting and extensive phone use, contributes to a lack of core stability awareness. Many of us struggle with maintaining core stability because we either don't know what to do or lack proper guidance.

Imagine this: you're under chronic stress, and your nervous system has been in 'fight or flight' mode for an extended period—potentially months or even years. This chronic problem results in muscle imbalances. If we divide the spine at T6 into upper and lower halves, everything above T6 is considered upper, and everything below is lower. Muscles in the upper region, especially those in the front of the body, have more muscle fibres and nerve supply—up to 70% more than the back. The forward-oriented movements of the spine, such as bending to pick something up or pushing, contribute to this muscle overactivation. Factor in activities like sitting at desks, using laptops, driving, and cycling, and our muscles become overworked, especially in stressful situations where the nervous system signals muscles to switch on even more. This imbalance weakens the upper back muscles, making sitting straight challenging and slouching the norm. Unfortunately, this stressed posture perpetuates the cycle by signalling to our nervous system that we are stressed, leading to the increased release of stress hormones.

Now, consider how bad posture affects breathing. Constantly hunching over compromises the diaphragm, leading to higher, shorter breaths that increase adrenaline and cortisol production. Breathing from the lower diaphragm slows down the breath, especially on the exhalation, activating the parasympathetic nervous system, reducing stress and pain. Another helpful tip is breathing in with the mouth closed, as many of us inhale with open mouths due to stress, which can contribute to tension, anxiety, and exhaustion.

The anterior muscles in the front of our bodies tighten while the deep neck flexors in the front of the neck weaken, often due to the 'text neck'. This occurs when we stop using our neck flexors to hold our heads upright, relying instead on posterior neck muscles and those turning our necks—an action they aren't designed for. This reliance leads to shoulder, neck, and arm pain and can contribute to headaches.

Furthermore, the tension and restriction in the upper body impact neck movement and function. Many people find it surprising that they cannot fully turn their heads or look over their shoulders without moving their bodies. This limitation is often a consequence of insufficient movement and excessive sitting.

Neck pain and restriction could mean that you are unable or unwilling to see things from both sides physically, mentally, and emotionally.

Lower Cross Syndrome

Now, let's shift our focus below the level of your spinal T6. In this region, the muscles at the back of the lower half of the body are naturally stronger than those in the front. These muscles are evolutionarily designed for activities such as squatting (in the absence of modern toilets), running, standing, and walking. However, they weren't intended for the prolonged sitting that has become prevalent in today's culture—whether behind a desk, at the wheel of a car, or on the sofa binge-watching Netflix.

When we are caught in the stress cycle and consistently stressed, these muscles tighten more than usual, primed for action as if preparing to flee from a bear. The body reacts to stressors like angry emails, looming deadlines, and endless appointments as if they were immediate threats, activating the body's stress response. Common manifestations include discomfort in the glutes, hamstrings, and calf muscles. Prolonged sitting can alter the natural curve in the spine, reducing lumbar lordosis and causing us to rely on ligaments rather than muscles, ultimately leading to pain.

For women, sitting with crossed legs can further exacerbate imbalances and pain, creating additional twists in the body. Leaning to one side while driving or using a mouse can induce functional scoliosis (an S-shaped curve) in the spine, resulting in more restriction and tension on one side of the body.

Extended periods of sitting also contribute to tightness in the hips and hip flexors. The psoas muscle, often affected by lower back issues, particularly in women who have had children, can be particularly sensitive. Furthermore, coccyx problems stem from the stress-induced flexed position. The coccyx, a small bone at the base of the spine, wasn't designed to bear the weight of the body while sitting. Instead, we should rely on the ischial bones (sit bones) in both buttocks. However, the stressed and flexed posture often causes the tailbone to tuck under, carrying the body's weight while perched on the edge of seats—creating a recipe for various problems.

Pregnancy

If you've birthed children, there are likely some ligament and muscle changes that occurred during and after pregnancy. Many women experience trauma from childbirth, leading to a sense of disconnection from their lower body and perpetuating tension, pushing them further into the stress cycle. Scarring from tears or cuts during childbirth is a common source of muscle imbalance in the lower back and pelvis. Scar tissue affects the fascia, influencing various aspects of the body that often go unnoticed. Unfortunately, not enough attention is given to this aspect of women's health.

Postpartum, women might perceive their pelvis as weak and attempt to strengthen it, but in reality, it's often too tense and numb. This tension contributes to pelvic floor problems, including urinary leakage, difficulty with bowel movements, painful periods, and discomfort or numbness during and after sex. These issues have unfortunately been normalised, but they are not inherent to being a woman, having children or a side effect of menopause.

Due to societal expectations or discomfort, many women may accept certain problems as normal and avoid discussing them with friends. Painful sex and numbness or pain after intercourse are common issues arising from unresolved trauma, stress, and tension in the pelvis. Your experience of sex and childbirth significantly impacts your overall physical and mental health, often representing a missing piece in the puzzle of chronic back pain. The tendency to compartmentalise prevents many of us from connecting the pieces of this intricate puzzle.

New Pains

As you initiate new changes, it's normal for additional pain to emerge. This typically indicates that you're on the right path. Muscles that have been inactive for a while are being reactivated, adapting to their intended functions. Just like experiencing muscle strain after returning to the gym, adjusting your sitting and walking habits may initially lead to discomfort. Seeking chiropractic care that considers you as a whole—rather than just focusing on a specific area of pain—can be beneficial.

Remember, pain is a signal that demands attention and a need for change. It doesn't necessarily indicate a life-threatening issue that requires cessation of activity. Instead, it suggests the necessity to breathe, balance your weight, readjust your posture, and move differently. Being afraid of pain and doing nothing can perpetuate fear and stress patterns, leading to increased pain. Movement is crucial; reduced movement limits blood flow to the area, causing the neurology to fire in an incohesive pattern, resulting in more pain and less mobility.

Approaching back pain from a different perspective, I aim to address the stiffness and protective response in the surrounding areas, encouraging movement and freeing up the affected area. The goal is to realign and reawaken your nervous system, allowing it to communicate effectively with your brain for optimal healing. Utilising your spine as it was designed, creating space through stretching or movement, and engaging in mindful breathing can alleviate pressure on the nervous system and bring harmony back to your spine. Embracing your entire body's capacity to breathe and move is essential, recognising that we often live too much in our heads.

Strengthen Your Core

Maintaining core stability is crucial. The core is a foundational support for your spine, yet many of us tend to collapse over our ribs, struggling to hold ourselves up. In my patients, core stability is often notably weak, emphasising its significance in preserving good posture and managing or preventing physical pain. Activating your core at around 30% capacity can protect your spine and reduce pain.

Harness the strength of your legs and feet to support your body effectively. This practise promotes healthy joints and disrupts unequal weight distribution, leaving you feeling more resilient in the face of life's challenges.

Challenge your mind and soul to expand, creating space within and releasing anything that no longer serves you. Breathe deeply, sit and stand without collapsing into your lower back, and envision your future self liberated from pain. Imagine how that future looks and feels.

Remember, pain doesn't have to be a constant companion, and it's not a burden you must endure indefinitely. Whether your pain is emotional, physical, or spiritual, you can break the cycle by perceiving and approaching things differently, starting with your posture. Cultivate a compassionate relationship with your body, tapping into its wisdom to emancipate yourself from the chronic suffering that may have become normalised in your life.

Moving Physical Pain

Learning how you live in your body means learning how to heal her. Begin by observing your sitting posture at your desk and assess the position of your shoulders. Counteract stiffness by stretching against a wall. Ensure a straightened spine, avoid crossing your legs, and distribute your weight evenly on both feet instead of favouring one hip. Taking charge of your body involves making thoughtful choices, starting with small adjustments and progressively building on them. Modifying our posture translates to a transformation and, ideally, an enhancement of the body and spine's functionality—akin to the impact of a chiropractic adjustment. Increased joint mobility often correlates with decreased pain. Breaking free from habitual poor posture patterns contributes to improved functionality, enabling us to step out of the cycle of discomfort.

Spiritual Alignment

Alignment serves as the bridge, reconnecting us with our authentic physical and spiritual selves.

A pivotal question is, 'What are you aligned with?' This inquiry carries significant weight and is essential for self-reflection. In my daily encounters, I frequently witness spines that have deviated from alignment, grappling with the physical challenges synonymous with a contemporary lifestyle. However, what captivates my interest is discerning how this physical alignment or misalignment manifests, influencing the health and life of my patients.

Alignment is the conduit that harmonises our energy with our intentions. If you find yourself questioning this concept, allow me to elaborate. The experiences unfolding in our lives, bodies, and relationships are intricately linked to what we align ourselves with. When I pose the question to many women, 'What are you aligned with? What do you desire, want, or need?' often, I'm met with blank stares or visible discomfort as they grapple with what seems like a complex inquiry.

More often than not, many of us aren't aligned with the life we're leading or the body we inhabit. This misalignment arises from a sense of limited choice as we conform to societal norms and expectations. We anticipate that adhering to the conventional path will bring us the happiness, bliss, and 'happily ever after' sensation we seek. However, a profound sense of loss and disillusionment sets in when the illusion shatters, and we realise we don't feel at home in our bodies or lives. We grapple with a pervasive feeling that something is amiss, accompanied by guilt for not experiencing fulfilment or love for the life we find ourselves living.

Most of us never asked, 'Am I aligned with this?' Instead, we asked questions such as:

- What will others think or say?
- Will this make me money?
- Will this bring me success?

- When I've achieved this, will my parents finally be proud?
- Will it keep me safe and secure?
- Will it bring me love?
- Will I have the family I always wanted?

We often gaze outward, aspiring to possess the elements we believe will bring us happiness and success, influenced by societal norms and ingrained habits. However, this may not be your true path.

Have you ever pursued a goal, achieved it, and found that it didn't bring the expected happiness or a sense of accomplishment? Perhaps attaining something you desired left you feeling empty, realising it wasn't what you truly wanted or needed.

Remember, you are the creator of your reality, shaping it with every thought, word, and action, whether consciously or unconsciously. Aligning with our bodies and minds and being mindful of what we manifest unconsciously is crucial.

Take a moment to reflect: What negative patterns persist in your life? What habits seem unbreakable? Which situations and patterns repeatedly resurface? The inclination to blame external factors, such as the past, parents, or ex-partners, often stems from the victim mentality within us. However, the truth is you hold the power to change any circumstance. It might be a wake-up call, and I apologise if it feels like a harsh truth, but recognising your role as a powerful creator is essential.

When we inquire about our alignment, we gain the ability to choose our manifestations consciously. Misalignments occur when our intentions deviate from our higher self, often stemming from wounded ego perspectives or compensating for perceived lack in our lives. Many of us seek to fill an internal void without clearly identifying what it entails. We embark on quests for the right person or thing to provide safety, love, appreciation, and acknowledgement. Creating from this place feels like something crucial is missing. Even for those who consistently strive to excel, it can be frustrating when efforts to get everything right fall short of the desired emotional fulfilment or the envisioned life.

> *When you're not aligned with your true self, your life looks, feels, and seems wrong—and you have no clue why.*

Clients often say, 'I have everything society says makes me successful, but I feel something is missing… I'm not happy, and it's driving me crazy! I need to know what it is!'

Throughout my life, my alignment was always with the desires of others—my parents, friends, and society's expectations. As the obedient and people-pleasing girl, I consistently aimed to fulfil what I believed would bring them happiness, pride, and greater affection for me. The notion of my own desires being important or holding significance never really crossed my mind since no one had ever inquired about them. My designated role was to ensure others' contentment and well-being. This worked well until I found myself grappling with illness and depression, awakening to the realisation that something was profoundly amiss. I had become dissatisfied with my life, disenchanted, and felt a part of me wilting away. A significant portion of my existence had been devoted to satisfying everyone else, neglecting my own needs and desires.

If I had carried on in that same ancestral pattern, putting everyone else before me at the cost of my health and happiness, I'm sure I would have ended up getting really sick. The resentment, frustration, and anger that was constantly bubbling under the surface was going to eat me up inside—it was just a matter of time.

Alignment is essential to your health and happiness and not some new age jargon. In fact, it's the first step in any healing or spiritual path. If you're not aligned with who you are, you can't heal or create what you want in your life.

When something feels aligned, it feels light and airy. You feel it within your heart and body. When you feel out of alignment, it gets stuck in your head, and there is a heaviness and a density that feels like you're dragging yourself through the mud.

Tools

Alignment requires pulling all the parts of you back to yourself, calling back your power, your voice, and the power of your desire and choice. You begin to connect with your soul and the parts of yourself that have been forgotten or lost. The journey is to bring all the pieces of who you are back into coherence and alignment and then create from this place.

We align with our culture's rules and belief systems until something shifts,
and we wake up to realise something's missing.

Begin by sitting upright and tuning into your physical body. Identify areas where you slump or feel misaligned. Note any blocks, aches, or pains. Later, during an energy cleanse, you can revisit these areas.

Imagine your spine as a transparent crystal tube extending from the tip of your sacrum to the crown of your head. Envision your body emptying out, like sand flowing from your head down through your spine and into the ground. In this emptied space, contemplate a desire or goal in your life. Feel into your body and inquire, 'Is this in alignment with who I am? Why do I want this, and is it for the highest good of all involved?' Clarify your intention, making it as pure, crystal-clear, and luminous as possible. Sit with these thoughts for 10 minutes, allowing the feelings to flow.

Listen to the truth resonating within your body. Journaling can facilitate an inner dialogue between your soul and the universe. The goal is to align yourself with the truth of your being and initiate a conversation that guides the soul into interaction with the ego. As the voice of your soul awakens, you'll learn to feel, rather than think, your way through desires. You may still need to discover what you truly want, so dedicating time to strengthen this aspect is crucial. Like any muscle, it requires regular use. Be patient with yourself; your soul and ego will harmonise over time, allowing you to experience magic in your physical life and tap into your divine insights.

Magic and miracles are just a shift in perception.

Our thinking and patterns often become rigid, making it challenging to perceive and manifest miracles, even though their potential always exists. Aligning and shifting our perception is crucial to healing and transforming our lives in miraculous ways.

When we maintain our intention in harmony with our essence and remain open to listening, we observe, almost magically, the joyful and harmonious order unfolding around us. As we recognise that we are the magic, we align ourselves with our innate and universal intelligence, and things effortlessly fall into place, accompanied by synchronicities that seem to appear as if by magic.

CHAPTER 5
STRESS AND THE NERVOUS SYSTEM

I'm so stressed... there's so much to do... I feel stressed... It's so stressful...
Can't you see I'm stressed?

I hear statements like these all too often in my practise. But unfortunately, stress is something that we can all identify with. Stress isn't necessarily always bad, but the chronic stress we are experiencing collectively and individually as women has become the norm and a day-to-day part of our existence. This chronic stress builds up in the body over time, creating havoc on health and vitality. Stress is one of the main contributors to the 'Modern Disease of the Modern Woman.'

Why are we so stressed?

Stress is one of the core issues we face in our day-to-day lives, and it comes down to our perception of stress and how we manage it or, in most cases, don't. Years ago, running from a tiger or not knowing where your next meal was coming from was stressful, and the stress response saved our lives on more than one occasion. If we're running from a tiger, we want all our energy and blood pumping towards our hearts and muscles so we can run as fast as we can to safety. When we don't know where our next meal is coming from, stress enables us to hold onto fat to protect ourselves. Stress has always been biologically about survival, and it still is. But we no longer chase after tigers and don't need to wait days or weeks to hunt for our next meal. We have moved on in time, but evolutionarily, our bodies have not, and herein lies the fundamental problem:

What was once there to save us is now slowly killing us.

Nowadays, stress involves worrying about deadlines and juggling everything and everyone. It has little to do with physical survival and is more about money and relationship worries.

Our stress today comes from the beliefs and conditioning we developed in childhood. We formed memories around past events and still avoid facing the pain from those experiences. This has turned us into people-pleasers with no boundaries, unable to say no, and constantly trying to prove our worth. We are in the grip of an unconscious fear that keeps us in the stress cycle, which negatively affects our hormones and our health. Some of us are stuck healing maternal and paternal wounds, which results in burnout and illness. Our role as women over the past 100 years, especially from the suffragette movement until today, has seen us fighting for the freedom of our body, our voice, and the right to choose who we are, what we do, who we love, and the person we came here to be. All the programming from our great-grandmothers and the women who came before us—and the stress they endured—are still present in our cellular DNA. Even though we are so lucky compared to past generations, we still live under self-imposed and unconscious stressors that have become normalised—but are NOT normal.

Case Study: Barbara

Barbara was thirty-eight when she was diagnosed with lung cancer. She was a single mum living with her ten-year-old daughter Laura. Barbara came from a working-class background and worked hard to get to the top of her profession. She saw working hard and proving herself as oxygen—it gave her self-worth and a sense of importance. She got a kick knowing she could do it all better than the men she worked with. But underneath the surface, she was angry that she had to work twice as hard for recognition, which she did despite being a single mum and a woman.

Barbara's mum died young. Her partner had left her when her daughter was a baby, so to get through the pain she was feeling, she threw herself into her work and raising her daughter. Her anger and need to prove her worth drove her to work long hours, thus blocking her feelings and keeping her pain at arm's length. Feeling it was too painful, she pushed it away and worked even harder. Barbara remembered when her mother had dreamed of having more choices. Barbara wanted the same for her daughter and was hell-bent on making her proud. She was always in a rush, working hard to give Laura the life she couldn't have and be an example.

When she was dying, I visited her, and she told me all of this and gave colour to the picture I already had in my head. She told me that she believed that the constant pushing, striving, and doing had led to her illness. She hadn't grieved her mother or dealt with her partner leaving her. She was holding on to an overwhelming amount of hatred, anger, and feelings of betrayal. Now, she couldn't breathe anymore. I will never forget her looking directly into my eyes. In that moment, I saw her, felt her soul, and knew that her words came from a place of true wisdom. 'Michelle, choose yourself, choose love, and don't miss life by trying to get or be somewhere else—it's not worth it. It's just running away from what you don't want to see. All the achievements—all of it—were me proving and protecting myself. I would gladly give it all away to see my little girl grow up.'

⟳৺৹

Barbara's story is dear to my heart, and I have seen many more women like her in my practise. Over the past 20 years, with mobile phones and constant emails, we have been constantly 'on.' We are always reachable and never completely turned off. We feel an urgency and overwhelming responsibility to respond to everything! Even when we decide not to respond, it still plays on our minds and messes with our stress levels.

But we only have so many hours in a day, and we need downtime to recharge and switch off. Just like our phones, after a few years, our battery is older and not functioning as well. To recharge, women need to replenish constantly—physically, mentally, and emotionally—otherwise, like your phone battery, you will stop working and burn out.

Which of these common stress symptoms resonate with you?

- When asked how you are, you answer, 'Stressed and busy.'
- Short-term memory loss.
- Brain Fog.
- Startle easily.
- Check repeatedly that things are locked.
- You love coffee and need it to get going in the morning. You believe it helps your brain wake up and focus and that it helps you move your bowels (bonus, flat stomach!)
- Feel like there aren't enough hours in the day.
- Constantly running late and feeling shame about it.
- Tired yet wired—it's difficult to fall asleep or stay asleep.
- Overreact easily but don't always outwardly display it in public.
- Quick to anger; angry and frustrated—let it loose at home.
- Can't relax, and you feel guilty if you do.
- Can't get to sleep or wake up around 2 a.m., unable to get back to sleep.
- Controlled by the never-ending to-do list.
- Feel panic and become anxious easily.
- Digestive problems, IBS, or a bloated stomach.
- Feel exhausted, especially around 3 p.m. when you crave something sugary or salty.
- Often reach for a glass of wine to relax or carbs to numb.
- Don't laugh much anymore, and don't feel happy.
- Feel like something is missing in your life.
- Find it hard to relax on holiday and feel tired after a holiday.
- Suffer from mum's guilt.
- Reoccurring thoughts and worry about what people think and say about you.
- Can't ask for help.
- Have a hard time saying no, but when you do, you feel guilty.
- Experience body shame and self-judgement.
- May feel jealous and judgemental towards others and compare yourself.
- Negative self-talk.
- Rarely feel like having sex, and when you do, you find it hard to relax and have orgasms.

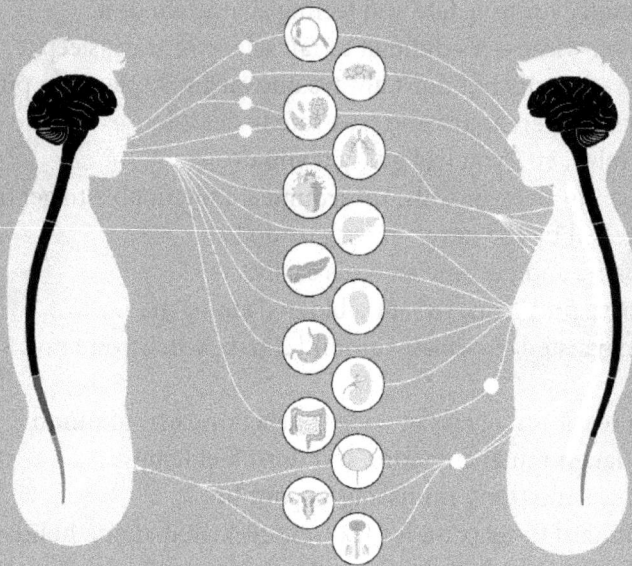

THE FUNCTIONS OF YOUR

Nervous System

PARA SYMPATHETIC

SYMPATHETIC

A Brief Overview of Your Nervous System

This intricate network facilitates communication between the brain, spinal cord, and every muscle, tissue, and organ in the body, affecting it physically, chemically, and mentally through various neural networks. The brain controls everything we do and how our bodies function. It is always sending electrical messages along the spinal cord and nerve fibres to all parts of the body and also receiving input from the body back to the brain.

The significance of spinal health cannot be overstated. Poor posture or limited spinal movement can interfere with your nervous system, impacting how you perceive pain and influence your body's healing processes in response to stress. In addition, between the meninges of the brain is cerebral spinal fluid (CSF). This CSF is made by tissues that line the brain's ventricles and circulates in and around the brain and spinal cord, protecting it from injury and stress whilst delivering vital nutrients. Movement of the spine is necessary to get this fluid pumping. Blockages or subluxations in the spine affect CSF flow, leading to more posture problems, pain, and stress, which are other reasons to get your spine adjusted!

The central nervous system registers every conscious and unconscious thought, orchestrating physical and chemical reactions to every cell in your body ceaselessly. Pain, generated in the brain, is mirrored in the body through sensory experiences. Chiropractic care offers a rapid means of altering input and output, positively influencing brain function, reducing stress, and interrupting the pain cycle.

In my experience, pain represents only 10% of the issue, encapsulating what you consciously feel. The remaining 90% comprises unconscious factors such as restrictions, blocked emotions, a dysregulated nervous system, and postural compensations, collectively called subluxations. Addressing subluxations is the key to resolving the root cause of spinal health dysfunction.

The Cerebral Cortex

This is the conscious brain, the command centre responsible for our thinking, actions, senses, and decision-making. The cerebral cortex is divided into four lobes: the frontal lobe, the parietal lobe, the temporal lobe, and the occipital lobe. Each of these lobes contains a left and right hemisphere. The left hemisphere controls the right side of the body, and the right hemisphere controls the left side of the body. The cortex is also divided into sensory, motor, and association areas that receive and give input via the spinal cord and nervous system, reaching every part of our body.

The Limbic System

The limbic brain is where we get entrenched in patterns and behaviours, making choices based on beliefs, emotions, and memories from the past. It shapes our responses and perceptions, whether through the filters of love, happiness, fear, or anger, rooted in our conditioned behaviours and past experiences.

When a person experiences a traumatic event, a memory is imprinted into the amygdala. The amygdala holds onto the emotional imprint of the event, including the emotion and stress that go with it. This can show up in day-to-day life as an emotional stress response when you think about something that might happen or an overreaction at work or home. The fear you feel is real, but it's not coming from present-moment reality but from your past and the memory that is ever so close to the surface running on repeat.

The Cerebellum

At the posterior part of the brain is the cerebellum. Our cerebellum controls our balance, posture, and coordination. It sends messages via the nervous system to the body to help adjust and coordinate movement, which requires multiple muscle groups. It times muscular movements so the body can move easily and smoothly, so we don't lose our balance. It uses proprioceptive and vestibular input via the nervous system. The cerebellum is also responsible for eye movements.

The Primal Brain

This part of the brain stem controls the autonomic functions that we don't usually think about. The primal brain operates at an unconscious level; it controls everything we do and how our body functions. It is the oldest part of our brain and is responsible for our most basic survival functions. It exerts control over us, often without our conscious awareness. Moreover, it oversees vital bodily functions such as heartbeat regulation, skin healing, hair growth, and lung expansion and contraction—essentially, the essentials that sustain life. Your unconscious beliefs and responses to perceived stress significantly influence the rhythm of your heart and the pattern of your breath. We will delve deeper into this aspect shortly when we talk about the autonomic nervous system.

The Middle of the Brain

This consists of the pituitary gland and pineal gland. The pituitary gland controls many hormone functions within our body. It controls the hormones needed for our menstrual cycle, whether we release an egg or not, and when we begin and end our periods. The pineal gland makes the hormone melatonin, which controls our sleep and waking cycles. I hope you can start to see how stress affects our nervous system, sleep, and hormones.

Examining these parts of our brain collectively, we need to recognise that addressing all parts is essential for healing—whether physical, emotional, or psychological. Our unconscious beliefs (primal) impact our emotions and feelings (limbic), influencing the decisions and actions we take (cortical). Therefore, when striving to change our health or life, it's crucial to understand who or what is steering the decisions underlying our life choices.

If unconscious childhood beliefs govern our emotions and feelings, our choices aren't conscious but rather repetitive patterns guided by a filtered perspective. This often results in health and life that diverge from our true selves, entangled in unconscious stress and pain patterns shaped by deep-seated emotions, thoughts, traumas, and ideas.

While much of psychology addresses the primal and cortical brain, the limbic system is frequently overlooked. The limbic system can be accessed and addressed by delving into the body to release stored, blocked emotions and feelings that hinder health and life. 'She-Movement,' which I'll introduce later, directly influences the limbic system, tapping into all three brain parts crucial for women's healing. It is the missing piece in the puzzle, particularly for women's health. When the limbic system is neglected or malfunctioning, suppressed emotions accumulate, leading to pain, disease, and a dysregulated nervous system. The inner voice and feelings of women, designed to rely on intuition, become stifled, causing the female body to lose alignment and become out of balance—a path toward pain and illness.

Case Study: Lisa

Lisa is a patient who lived on stress; it had become part of who she was. She worked hard and played hard. She controlled her body and emotions through exercise, often pushing herself to unhealthy limits to feel something and get rid of all the excess adrenaline she felt. Her spare time was spent running and doing HITT training. She had a six-pack and prided herself on being as strong as any man. To most people, Lisa had a perfect body, life, husband, and children. She seemed happy and was everyone's friend. But the cost of her life was taking its toll. She suffered from chronic neck and shoulder pain; her pectoral muscles were flexed, ready to run at any time, and her breathing was stuck high into her upper ribs. She was sweating a lot, felt anxious, and woke up with pain and tingling in her arms and shoulders at night.

She was tired, and the constant smile and picture-perfect life she was trying to maintain were taking their toll. She realised she was obsessed with her weight and weighed herself daily. She ate a strict calorie-controlled diet but couldn't lose the extra kg she perceived made her fat. She had built her self-worth around her appearance, especially how thin she was and how much she could achieve. The number she saw on the scale each morning dictated her happiness and moods and affected her communication with herself, her kids, and her husband, as well as how stressed she felt. Lisa sat in my chair saying, 'I'm doing everything perfectly. Why is this happening to me?' She was in pain, and this was stopping her from exercising. She felt like her life was spinning out of control. She wanted her body back again.

Lisa's story reflects the impact of stress on her body. Many women may not realise that stress tends to cling to fat. Our bodies are hardwired to store fat during stressful periods, a survival mechanism aimed at ensuring our survival. When the body senses stress, it redirects blood away from organs involved in rest and digestion, channelling it to muscles and the heart, preparing for a 'fight or flight' response. Over time, this can lead to issues like cortisol imbalance, high blood pressure, and oestrogen dominance, disrupting the body's ability to burn sugar, leading to fat storage, and making weight loss challenging. The perpetual stress cycle can escalate feelings of being out of control, compounding the challenge of understanding why the body isn't cooperating. For women juggling stress, motherhood, and the onset of their forties, the body signals that a shift in approach is necessary.

In Lisa's case, addressing physical stress through treatments, addressing biochemical factors, incorporating exercises, breathing techniques, She-Movement, and chiropractic adjustments helped her body unwind from the tightly constricted inhale it was stuck in, transitioning into a more relaxed and steady exhale. Our discussions delved into her approach to her body and exercise, introducing elements of yoga, pleasure, and posture work. Gradually, Lisa's body began to relax, mirroring the melting of ice, and her emotions started to surface. Through our work, she discovered that she had initially been concealing parts of herself to seek acceptance from others and later to accept herself. Lisa had suppressed her feminine aspects, perceiving them as inconvenient and weak. Throughout her upbringing and life, she equated strength, power, and dominance with success and happiness. Unconsciously, she labelled certain aspects of herself as unacceptable and burdensome, attaching deeper emotions and meaning to these beliefs. Fearing judgement, she rejected her true essence, convinced that revealing vulnerability would lead to disdain and punishment. In Lisa's case, this fear of judgement not only manifested in body shame but also in shame towards her authentic self.

Many of us strive to conform to certain expectations, seeking validation and acceptance from others. The idea is that through this external validation, we can cultivate love and acceptance for ourselves. However, what if we skip the elaborate process of proving ourselves and simply embrace who we are? Most people are preoccupied with their concerns, grappling with their core wounds, and navigating their individual journeys. Recognising this can spare us unnecessary pain and illness while liberating valuable energy and time. In my view, it's a victory. Attaining a sense of wholeness and illuminating the aspects of ourselves concealed in the shadows is crucial to breaking free from the cycle of stress and pain.

⟨∽❊∽⟩

The Autonomic Nervous System

Most women are deeply conditioned to stress, often without even recognising its impact on their health. Despite frequently proclaiming, 'I'm not stressed,' the body's truth cannot be denied. Stress is insidious, creeping in gradually until you find yourself entangled in its web. The body doesn't always signal stress overtly, as many have mastered the art of suppressing inconvenient or unpleasant feelings. Consequently, when the body eventually rebels—manifesting as fatigue, illness, hormonal upheaval, or pain—it often comes as a shock. We've become adept at silencing our feelings and devising seemingly foolproof methods to accomplish tasks at any cost.

Imbalances in hormones, pain, sickness, and fatigue are the body's desperate attempts to capture our attention as we've severed communication with it. Our intuition lies dormant, awaiting a mythical 'more time' that never materialises. While the autonomic nervous system initially copes admirably with the backlog of suppressed issues, persistent neglect leads to emerging problems.

I frequently emphasise, 'The body knows best,' firmly believing that our body's innate intelligence guides us. However, chronic stress impedes this inherent wisdom. Our thoughts, movements, breathing, and dietary choices contribute to this state. Many women I encounter grapple with the repercussions of a dysregulated nervous system. To delve deeper into this intricate system, let's explore how these issues arise.

The autonomic nervous system has two parts:

1. Parasympathetic—rest, digest, repair, and reproduction.
2. Sympathetic—fight and flight.

For good health, this system needs to be balanced. Remember, the body is always seeking balance. Think of the parasympathetic as the *yin/feminine* side and the sympathetic as the *yan/masculine* side. Both are vital for our survival. The problems begin when we get stuck in one side of the autonomic nervous system, which is usually the sympathetic side. When we sleep and relax, we digest our food, repair our body, and balance our hormones that signal to the body that it's safe to conceive, grow a baby, and burn fat.

On the other hand, when we get stuck in sympathetic dominance, our parasympathetic system can't do its job correctly, affecting our fertility, immune system, blood pressure, and whole body. We become tense, our muscles become short, our breathing gets shallow, and we experience pain and disease.

Both autonomic processes are primal and are not something we can simply control with conscious thought alone. Think about it: When we are stressed, unless we are comfort-eating, we lose our appetite and don't want to eat. This is because the nervous system doesn't have time to digest food; it's feeling stressed and is wired up to fight or flight. Its priorities are different, and eating, digesting, and keeping the immune system functioning well are not options right now. That's why we tend to get sick during or after a stressful period. It's why we fall ill on the first few days of a holiday when our body starts to slow down and reset.

What sympathetic dominance looks and feels like in your physical body:

- Your muscles are tense as your body prepares to run.
- Calf muscles, hands, and jaws become clenched.
- The head and shoulders get pushed forward, ready to run.
- Your breathing becomes short and high in your chest.
- Your ribs and chest muscles tighten.
- Your blood is pumped to your extremities away from your digestion and immune system.
- Your blood vessels contract, raising your blood pressure.

- Your heart rate quickens, and you may feel anxious and jumpy.
- Your adrenals are pumping adrenaline and cortisol throughout your body.
- Your senses of sound and light sharpen.
- You are more alert to the slightest noise.
- You're ready to run for your life.

Stress and busyness can also be numbing devices, so we don't have to feel and go deeper into our bodies and souls.

Imagine this scenario, especially if you're a mother: You return home from a stressful workday, burdened with pending emails that demand attention due to the perpetually insufficient hours in a day. After collecting your kids from an after-school club, you're running late despite daily promises to be early. As you enter the house, you're greeted by the morning's breakfast dishes still lying around. Frustration sets in, and you request assistance, but the kids are engrossed in a dispute over the TV, claiming unfairness based on their friends' privileges.

Glancing into the cupboard to prepare dinner, you discover essential ingredients have been eaten, with no time for a store run. Your partner will be home soon, expecting a meal before heading out for the evening. In a rush, you bring together a meal while tidying up from breakfast. Feeling famished, you scarf down a sandwich or grab a biscuit, washing it down with a large glass of wine to ease your nerves or a coffee to give you energy. Simultaneously, you embark on a multitasking frenzy—folding clothes, loading the washer, emptying the dishwasher, and organising the kids to do their homework. Your partner arrives, questioning your stress levels and wondering why you snap as soon as he walks through the door.

As you prepare food, the kids complain and leave half of it, arguing while you attempt to eat. Seeking relaxation, you drown out the noise and demands, feeling heartburn and indigestion intensify with every bite due to exhaustion. Eventually, you explode, shouting in response to rising emotions, witnessing your family's faces reflecting back at you. Your husband downplays it with a casual comment about your emotions and makes a shallow remark about your hormones, intensifying your anger, frustration, and humiliation. Familiar feelings of shame and guilt resurface, regretting the loss of temper.

Your kids often question your lack of smiles and perpetual anger, thoughts that linger as you lie in bed at night. After managing bedtime rituals, you pour another glass of wine, tackling the leftover work on your laptop while your kids interrupt. On different evenings, you numb out with a Netflix binge. Before bed, you check messages and emails, triggering your brain into overdrive, replaying conversations and scenarios. You collapse into bed, exhausted, hoping for a restful night without waking up at 2 am, staring at the clock until the alarm rings—an unsettling routine. The next day, the cycle repeats.

This pattern is a common experience for many women, and it doesn't even account for workplace stress and additional roles as a wife, daughter, and friend. This narrative encapsulates the modern-day disease of the modern woman—predictable, with a trajectory toward burnout, depression, chronic pain, hormonal chaos, and a one-way ticket to disease, far from a 'happy ever after' conclusion.

Chronic Stress and Headaches

Headaches and migraines are very common in my practise and are the second most common pain women experience, with lower back pain ranking number one. On my intake forms, 8/10 women say they have headaches, but it's not the main reason they come to see me. Usually, women think that having headaches a few times a week or month is normal and part of their life because that's what they know. They have no idea that this isn't normal and is usually part of the chronic stress and health problems that they are unconsciously dealing with.

Eliminating headaches is more complex than one would like to think. This is because the headache is the symptom of other physical, mental, and emotional imbalances. Earlier, I talked about the forward head position making muscles tight in the shoulder and back of the neck pain referring to the head, creating headaches. This is what I would call a straightforward or a referred headache, but stress and tension often come from something deeper.

Now, let's take a step back into your brain where your superior colliculus lives. You have two, one for each side of the body—one for each eye. They are responsible for your sight and the light that comes in and out of your eyes. They decide how your pupils dilate or constrict. When light comes into the eye, the thalamus part of the brain sends this information to the sight-seeing part of your brain.

This is important because our pupils dilate when our sympathetic nervous system gets activated and our stress hormones are turned on. This is an automatic response from your autonomic nervous system. When you hear a loud bang or are startled, your pupils will always dilate. It's a survival mechanism so you can take in what's happening around you and assess the situation. Again, it's all about survival and keeping you safe. It's also activated in the dark and at night so that we can see.

In moments of chronic stress, where tension and frustration prevail, your pupils tend to dilate more, potentially explaining heightened sensitivity to light. Instances where you find yourself wearing sunglasses in non-sunny conditions—using them to alleviate headaches—or noticing individuals fashionably sporting designer shades indoors might suggest stress-induced light sensitivity. This constant dilation of pupils, leading to heightened sensitivity, can contribute to persistent headaches and migraines. The impact may extend to nighttime, making driving challenging due to the glare from oncoming headlights. Even in dimly lit rooms, individuals with chronic stress might require darkness, finding even a digital alarm clock overly stimulating. In my experience, oestrogen dominance is a significant biochemical factor contributing to PMS and headaches.

Effects of Long-Term Chronic Stress on the Pupils

Earlier, I mentioned that during acute stress, our pupils dilate due to sympathetic dominance, particularly adrenaline. However, when stress persists for extended periods, and cortisol becomes the primary energy source (until it exhausts), we begin to experience narrowed, constricted pupils.

When I observe this constant pupil constriction in patients, it sets off alarm bells for me. Unless influenced by specific medications, it's a clear indication that they are undergoing chronic stress and it has persisted for an extended duration. On the other hand, if they exhibit signs of stress but with dilated larger pupils, it suggests they are in the early phases of stress.

The constriction of pupils during chronic stress is a response to heightened sensitivity to light. The body attempts to reduce this sensitivity while being deeply immersed in cortisol. It serves as a warning sign that burnout and chronic diseases may be imminent unless proactive changes are made to introduce more balance into our lives and bodies.

Headaches and Hormones

Headaches are a common side effect of menstruation and PMS, with some women only experiencing headaches around their period. When we are living with the effects of chronic cortisol and adrenaline pumping through our blood, our hormones are affected in a big way. Oestrogen-related headaches due to stress are a primary reason why women get PMS headaches.

Oestrogen dominance goes hand-in-hand with high cortisol, the hormone released when we are stressed, and is the most common hormonal imbalance I see in menstruating women. I see women and girls as young as thirteen suffering from oestrogen dominance due to stress, whether from home, school, or their peers, what they eat or do not eat. Girls as young as fourteen take the pill to relieve hormone imbalance and help with their headaches. I have nothing against the pill, which has liberated us and given us a choice. However, when it is given for PMS, depression, endometriosis, or any other female hormonal imbalance, I must take a stand. The pill is not a hormone balancer; it is a band-aid. Your hormones, like everything in your body, are seeking balance. When there is a problem with one hormone, the body tries to compensate to help out. When we are stressed, the body is so busy making and pumping cortisol around the body that it lets hormone production slip, so we become imbalanced. Your body needs you to correct this imbalance. It's saying, 'Help me out here; we have a problem.' Your body is innately intelligent and knows how to work properly when we give it what it needs and remove what it doesn't. When we don't get to the root cause of the problem and mask the symptoms with the pill, we are covering up a problem that will need fixing later down the road. Like all problems, when we leave or ignore them, they grow and become harder to tame.

Stress and Sound

Sensitivity to noise is a sign of stress and a struggling nervous system. Stress affects how we hear things. Have you ever been sitting at home or in the office and someone clicking their pen or tapping away at their computer keys really irritates you? It can be any background noise. It could be trying to have a conversation, but the radio is on, or being unable to talk or listen in a crowded place. You may need earplugs at night because the house is literally humming to you, or maybe it's your partner's snoring or the way he grinds his teeth or eats. Most people don't hear it, but if they do, it doesn't bother them. But when we are experiencing sympathetic dominance, it's too much to bear, and you may feel frustrated and annoyed.

The inferior colliculus in the brain is responsible for how we hear and perceive sound; its job is to receive as much sound as possible. It's another part of our survival system, developed so we can listen for predators. When you are stressed, the slightest noise makes you jumpy and on edge. This is because you can't relax, and your whole body and nervous system are fired up and tense. As a stressed-out mum coming home from work tired and wired, her kids arguing, the TV blaring, and the dog barking... it can all feel like too much. When the last straw comes, you can't even remember what it was, yet you react as if you just can't think straight anymore. The constant noise starts to bring on a headache, and a constant ringing in your ears at night has suddenly appeared.

Stress and Toxic Burden

Toxic stress is a major issue in our modern world. We know that some foods and products are harmful and can disrupt our hormones and nervous system. However, with so much conflicting information, it feels overwhelming and difficult to know where to start in changing our habits. Toxins are a big reason you feel stressed and overwhelmed and suffer from a handful of bizarre and completely unrelated complaints.

The expression of pain, stress, and anxiety are many, but the reasons are few.

Toxins create stress in your body, pushing you more into sympathetic dominance, the 'red zone' of your nervous system. They cause physiological and biochemical processes that burden your already struggling body.

Your mitochondria are organisms that live within your body's cells. Their job is to utilise energy from the food you eat. This energy is the main energy source for most of our physiological and biochemical processes. When our mitochondria are overloaded with environmental toxins from the air we breathe, the water we drink, the food we eat, and the makeup and lotions we use daily, they become sluggish and can't do their job properly. Their job is to produce energy. When they are overworked, we feel tired, anxious, over-whelmed, achy, and can't handle things like we used to. We basically feel like we have no energy. Many of us relate these feelings to insufficient or too much protein, carbs, or fats, but it is more complex than just the food we eat.

We are fed by our environment—by the sun, the water, and the air that we breathe. We used to spend a lot of time in nature; it's how we feel alive, replenished by spending time in her—we are nature! But the reality today is that not enough of us are supported by our environment, and instead of being fed by her, we are depleted because she, too, is struggling. We are a reflection of our environment. I don't know about you, but I do not like how this looks or feels.

We assume that we don't need to worry about 'all of this' because the government is taking care of us and keeping us safe, but unfortunately, that is not always the case. Even though we may live in a developed Western society, we are dealing with more sickness and disease than ever before. Food safety is our job (it shouldn't be, but it is.) It's the consumer's role to read labels and to prove a product isn't safe, not the company that made it!

Self-responsibility and taking ownership of your health, what you consume, and how you move is up to you.

Toxic overload is complex but simple when you break it down. Perhaps you feel unwell, are often tired, have hormonal challenges, suffer from digestive issues, sleep poorly, are anxious or depressed, or are overwhelmed and irritable. These are signs that you are suffering from a buildup of toxins in your body that make you feel like crap. When you remove the toxins, you will increase your resistance to stress and begin to feel better. There is no easy pill, and no one has your best interests at heart more than you. So be your own detective—you are your own healer and guru, and no one will save you but you.

Increase in Toxins and Low Resilience

We are replenished from the inside out, top-down, and bottom-up. When we aren't in alignment with our environment or body, we get sick. The soul energy transforms into the physical, and our physical body reflects our soul. When dealing with toxic overload, we struggle in every area of our lives—physically, emotionally, mentally, and spiritually.

Our exposure today is so different from that of our ancestors. We are dealing with more toxic overload now than ten years ago and are starting to hit real problems. We all want to live an amazing life and feel great in our bodies, but exposure means constant fundamental flaws, and we can't seem to feel well.

Our food has lost its nutrients due to processing, and the soil it's grown in lacks the micronutrients we need. These toxic burdens affect our emotions and resilience, making it harder to cope and leaving us feeling off balance. As our energy and resilience decrease, it becomes harder to release trauma and trapped emotions. If we weren't overwhelmed by toxins, we'd have more resilience to handle everything. By removing toxins from our bodies, healing becomes easier, turning big problems into manageable tasks.

The body is the vessel we have to experience this beautiful life. When we are full of toxins, it is often challenging to see the light, leaving us struggling and stuck in the dark. Your body is innately intelligent and can always heal; it's never too late. When we remove the disrupting blocks to the body and add support, she can thrive again and heal herself.

Toxic burden comes from makeup and skincare products:

- Shampoo and shower gel
- All the chemicals in our personal products and household cleaners
- Plastics
- Pesticides and chemicals in our food
- Toxins in our furniture and paint
- Medications
- Pollution in air and water
- Herbicides… and so much more!

You can't outsmart your body.

It's so important to me that women feel truly alive, understand why they feel the way they do, and know what they can do about it. When we start removing toxins and replacing them with safer alternatives while nourishing our bodies with nutritious foods and targeted supplements, we begin to thrive and feel more like ourselves. Clearing these blockages is essential for energy to flow freely! Toxins affect our stress levels, but more crucially, they impact our hormones, endocrine system, and gut health. Leaky gut, which we'll discuss shortly, is heavily influenced by environmental factors and is another source of stress. But before it all feels overwhelming, take a breath, grab a cup of tea, and trust that everything will fall into place as we explore your amazing body together.

The Endocrine System

The autonomic system consists of glands that secret hormones such as:

- Pituitary
- Thyroid
- Parathyroids

Your adrenals and ovaries aren't glands but organs with receptor sights that act like a lock and key. They are in constant communication with your endocrine system. The neuroendocrine system works together to coordinate all the functions your body needs. The nervous system maintains homeostasis and balance within your body by sending nerve impulses, whereas the hormone system uses chemical messengers.

The pituitary gland, housed within your brain, is often referred to as the master gland controlling the hormone system. It lets all the other glands know what hormones they need to make and how much. Every organ is in constant communication; we call it a 'feedback loop.' Messages are sent, received, and answered, and all your systems work together as a team; nothing works independently.

The Impact of Stress on the Endocrine System

Stage 1:

Adrenaline is the hormone that gets released first. It makes your heart race and gets you fired up to run from that tiger. It generates everything we need to get out of an acutely stressful situation. It puts our nervous system on guard, in the red zone, slowing down other functions such as digestion.

Sleep is often one of the first things to be affected by adrenaline because your body won't let you go into a deep sleep in case you have to jump up and run for your life. Breathing deeply and slowly can affect this response, altering vagal tone and activating the green zone—your parasympathetic nervous system.

Supplements and practises for Stage 1 stress:

- Vitamin C
- Vitamin B Complex
- Magnesium
- Rhodiola
- Withania
- Chamomile tea
- Lavender oil
- Diaphragmatic Breathing
- Restorative yoga

Stage 2:

The next stage initiated in the endocrine stress response is cortisol. Sleep is likely to be affected at this phase as well, but the difference is you can fall asleep quite well but wake up around 2-3 a.m. due to a rise in blood cortisol. Cortisol isn't all bad and can help us in the early stages of stress. Cortisol is anti-inflammatory and protects us from harmful inflammation that can be a side effect of too much adrenaline from Stage 1. It also regulates insulin levels, helping us burn fat as fuel and maintain blood sugar.

The problem happens when we stay under stress for long periods. Cortisol, during longer periods of chronic stress, breaks down your muscles to burn glucose. It suppresses your immune system, making you sick and craving carbs. Cortisol signals to your body that you need to store fat because there is a fear that there is not enough food, a biological survival process that comes from the days when we didn't know when or where our next meal would come from.

We become stuck in chronic stress patterns and high cortisol when our body feels that we must do everything faster and better but can't meet the demand anymore.

Cortisol levels vary throughout the day. By testing the levels at different times of the day, you can see what stage of cortisol or stress you are in. Over time, cortisol creates other changes in your body. Metabolic syndrome consists of high blood pressure and insulin resistance, leading to pre-diabetes, type 2 diabetes, and obesity due to slowed metabolism, meaning you don't burn fat like you used to.

Cortisol also breaks down our muscles, as it is catabolic. Our glands get the signal that we need to break down our muscles to release our proteins to survive. As a consequence of this breakdown of muscle tissue, the proteins get converted back into glucose and sugar because your body is trying to help you with all the stress it perceives you have. We aren't burning sugar when we are inactive, so we must make more insulin to balance our blood sugar levels. Over time, any glucose that can't be put back into the muscles and restored gets stored as body fat. Your body's primary concern is keeping your blood balanced, and it doesn't care how it gets the job done. Remember, it's all about survival. This leads to weight gain—those extra kilos or pounds you just can't seem to shift no matter how hard you try. Cortisol tends to settle around the tummy area, backs of the arms, and underneath your bra area.

It doesn't matter how much you exercise or how 'good' you eat; nothing will work when cortisol tells every cell in your body that there isn't enough food and you're in crisis. It will store everything as fat. Women tend to panic when they feel their clothes getting tighter and start to diet and exercise more than ever, which makes the problem worse because it's telling the body there isn't enough food (because you're not eating enough). There is stress because you are over-exercising, creating a vicious cycle. What is happening in your body is biochemical, and it's not your fault. Your body is actually doing its best to keep you safe based on its ancient hormonal feedback system.

Cortisol is a bully. When it's high, it impacts all the other hormones in your body.

Supplements and practises for Stage 2 stress:

All of the above (for adrenaline) can be taken, adding the following for high cortisol:

- Licorice
- Zinc
- Ginseng
- Fresh fruit and vegetables, limit unprocessed food (remember: no supplement is an excuse not to eat real, whole food)
- Dark chocolate 90% and above
- Spend time in nature
- Create a scared practise

Stage 3:

The next stage of biochemical stress that occurs is low cortisol. The seesaw effect goes from high to low. The stocks are empty; this is where we start to feel exhausted and when adrenal fatigue and burnout appear. Stiffness, pain, and tiredness in the body are common symptoms of low cortisol levels. Patients find it very challenging to get out of bed and need a lot of coffee to get going. By mid-afternoon, energy levels will be empty, and you will crave anything with sugar and or caffeine in it to help give you the energy you crave.

Autoimmune flare-ups can be common at this stage because stress creates inflammation, the main cause of autoimmune disease. Cortisol is normally the hormone the body uses to decrease inflammation. But when our body isn't making enough cortisol, there is nothing to help dampen down all the inflammation, creating a domino effect of other diseases within the body, such as MS, Arthritis, Crohn's, and many more. The first thing your doctor will prescribe is a corticosteroid to help reduce the inflammation—that is how powerful and essential cortisol is.

Signs of adrenal fatigue:

- Can't handle stress
- Unexplained tiredness and fatigue
- Sleeping problems
- Can't get out of bed in the morning
- Craving salt and sugar foods
- Over-eating
- Weak immune system—constant colds and infections
- Hormonal imbalances
- Depressive feelings
- Stiffness in the body
- Chronic pain in the shoulders and lower back.
- Headaches
- Feel worse after exercise—not better

Even though tiredness and fatigue are the most common presentations of burnout, some women can appear wired and can't relax at all. Cortisol also affects your serotonin and melatonin levels, leading to depression and low self-esteem. Serotonin, the hormone that makes us feel happy, safe, connected, and calm, and melatonin, the sleep hormone, work in a see-saw effect with one another.

When one is out of balance, it affects how we feel and function. Our feel-good hormones are often low because our melatonin levels are not optimal. This is because we spend too much time behind computers, phones, and artificial light. The natural rhythms of nature determine our circadian rhythms and how our body produces hormones. Serotonin is usually highest in the day, and as sunlight fades naturally declines and melatonin rises, melatonin is reduced by sunlight and artificial light.

Because we are still looking at our phones long after sundown, our melatonin production is affected, depleting our serotonin and leaving us feeling down, irritated, and like something is wrong.

Foods high in sugar and carbohydrates promote serotonin, leading us to reach into the fridge for a hit of happiness. But instead of happiness, we are left with guilt, body shame, and a sugar crash, making us even more tired and sick. Your hormones are more powerful than you think and are always trying to fix imbalances.

When trying to rebalance your hormones, getting up with the sun and winding down with it are great ways to get started. Spending time outside in nature, getting sun in your eyes, and turning off electronics after 7 p.m. will allow for the natural rise of melatonin, which can make a big difference.

Restorative yoga and breathwork, herbal chamomile tea, and lavender oil can make a difference in your sleep. Avoid caffeine drinks after 12 p.m. and limit alcohol to help rebalance your circadian rhythm. Eating nutritious foods balanced in protein and complex carbohydrates before 7 p.m. can help balance sugar cravings. When you mindlessly visit the fridge or cupboard in the evening looking for something to make you feel better, stop, get your journal out, and answer the question, 'What am I *really* hungry for?' When you let your soul write, I promise the answer won't be food.

Supplements and practises for Stage 3 stress:

All supplements already mentioned, plus:

- Foods rich in phytochemicals and nutrients
- Herbal tonic and Bach flower remedies for chronic stress and fatigue
- Rest!
- Sandalwood, Clary Sage
- Herbs in the ginseng family, alfalfa sprouts, vitex
- Melatonin taken at night promotes healthy sleep

Stress creates inflammation within your body and is one of the most significant contributing factors to disease. How we move, breathe, and eat can really affect the impact of stress on our bodies. Stress will always be there, but how we perceive and deal with it determines how our hormones and physiology are affected and, ultimately, our state of health. Chronic disease is killing more people than ever before! Yet even though most people think they have no control over their health, you are more powerful and have more control than they know.

Physical manifestations of stress:

- High blood pressure
- Increase in resting heart rate
- Insomnia

- Type 2 diabetes
- Tense, stiff, and painful shoulders and back
- Tingling in arms and legs
- Jaw pain
- Headaches
- Eye problems
- Anxiety and depression
- Shortness of breath
- Autoimmune disease
- Low immunity
- IBS and other digestive issues.
- PCOS
- PMS
- Infertility
- No interest in sex

Thoughts alone can't change the physiological response to stress. Apart from chiropractic adjustments, diaphragmatic breathing is an important way to directly and quickly influence the autonomic nervous system. Your diaphragm is a dome-shaped muscle that sits under your lower rib cage. Every inhalation and exhalation communicates, via your nervous system, how you feel.

If you are stressed, sit at a desk, and breathe high up into your chest, you are probably not using your diaphragm properly. This begins a cascade of subsequent stress hormone production, leading to more stress in your body. You begin to breathe more quickly and shallowly than before. Your pulse quickens, pupils dilate, and your body becomes tense, ready to run. Your body is getting the message that there is no time to chill and breathe properly. These symptoms lead to even more stress hormones being produced, and before you know it, you're stuck in a stress cycle of your own unconscious, making you unable to break free.

Slowing down your breathing to 6-8 breaths a minute will change your body's physiology and stress response, affecting your vagal tone.

Vagal Nerve

The vagus nerve is the longest nerve in the body. It is the main branch of the autonomic nervous system, affecting your heart rate, digestion, breath, and immune system, as well as connecting to all of your internal organs. When we are stressed, we have decreased vagal tone, also known as low heart rate variability (HRV). This is all the hype right now; we see it on smartwatches and rings. It gives us important information and shows how we can adapt and cope with stress, offering valuable clues to what's going on inside our body. In a nutshell, HRV shows us how we are able to adapt to stress by measuring how many times our blood vessels contract between heartbeats. It measures your adaptivity to daily stress and life.

For example, an old, brittle, and stiff water pipe can't handle an increase in or different water pressure fluctuations very well; it lacks adaptability to stress. In comparison, a more flexible water pipe can deal with more variability in water pressures and environmental stress. Our blood vessels are the same. A person with a higher vagal tone or HRV can deal with stress a lot better than someone with a lower vagal tone or low HRV.

I see HRV, or vagal tone, as how we adapt to stress and as a window into our nervous system and general health. The higher the vagal tone, the more we are in the green zone, or parasympathetic nervous system. This means that we react to stress well and can recover quickly. We will experience positive emotions and possibilities, have adequate energy and physical health, generally feel good, and function well. We also feel calm and can fall and stay asleep. When the vagal tone is low, we feel stressed, overwhelmed, depressed, tired, and wired.

Stress and Your Heart

Heart problems are on the rise, and more women are dying from heart attacks or strokes than ever before. Most women think that breast cancer is the number one killer of women, but statistics show that heart disease is far more deadly and claiming more of us every day. We must start addressing the stress we are carrying around the way we are pushing and not feeling, missing the signs of this silent yet deadly killer. Stress creates pain, tension, and constriction in your body and dysregulates your nervous system. This stress also affects your heart muscles, veins, arteries, and kidneys. The cardiovascular system is a closed system, and we need to be able to receive full, pure, oxygenated air into our lungs to filter the carbon dioxides and toxins that need to leave our bodies. The problem is most of us can't breathe or relax and aren't taking in enough air. We're so busy rushing around, surviving on shallow breaths, barely giving the body the vital nutrients and minerals it needs to survive and thrive. Our body craves more oxygen to keep us alkaline and able to fight diseases.

When we don't relax and breathe properly, this tension leads to problems we can't see or feel, and your pain may be just the icing on the cake, hiding a deeper sea of problems. When we start working with our breath and aliveness, we rewire the body. We learn to reconnect, relax, and slow down so we can heal. When we are stuck in sympathetic dominance run by adrenaline and cortisol, there is no time to rest and repair, and that's how we get sick. Prioritise your pleasure and health and begin to see how this starts to heal you from within.

Balance Your Nervous System

I invite you here to explore your perceptions of pressure, stress, and deadlines. What belief have you taken on that makes you feel you have to prove your worth to feel loved, liked, and respected? When we slow down and look at how we live our lives, choices, and actions, we can see things differently when we know what is driving us. How important is that deadline? Are you willing to sacrifice your health again and again? Sometimes, taking stock of what and who is important to us and having the courage to make small changes can save our lives and relationships with those we love.

Start keeping the promises you make to yourself. We are so good at being there for others, yet we always seem to let ourselves down and think nothing of it. Your health, nervous system, and hormones are vitally important. Your breath is your God-given right and an essential part of your physiology. We need to stop trying to make time for it and see it as a luxury self-care practise when it is essential to our well-being and life.

Breathe

Most of us breathe high up into our chest, sit with our mouths open, and don't breathe through our noses. We sit on the edge of our seats, forgetting we have a body, only breaking to eat something carbohydrate-based. We fuel up on coffee, which pushes us further into stress. We hold our breath, clench our jaw, and tighten our shoulders. We breathe approximately 17-20 breaths per minute and often feel fuzzy and can experience headaches and anxiety.

Begin by slowing the breath down to 8 breaths per minute. Breathe in slowly for 4 counts and exhale slowly for 4 counts. Feel the breath filling up your lungs and the diaphragm expanding. Try to let the breath enter your womb area, feeling your lower belly rise and fall with each breath. As you breathe out, don't just quickly let go. Make the exhale long, slow, and controlled, feeling it release slowly out of the body, touching all the organs it passes through.

As you empty your lungs, relax and drop your shoulders, roll them back, and let go of everything you perceive you are carrying. The inhale and exhale are both important, yet many of us don't realise that the exhale is even more important than the inhale. The exhale sends the message to the brain that you are safe; you can slow down and relax. Try this lying in bed when you wake up, sitting during your lunch break, before you sleep, or when you walk. Be patient with yourself. This seems easy, but it can take time for the breath to reach all the places it needs to go. Emotions can start to surface as we allow the breath to come in and free up parts of the body that we've shut down—the parts of ourselves that are restricted and tight. Try not to judge emotions or make them mean anything. Just witness the release. Emotion is neutral; it just needs to flow.

Laughter

We all know that having a good laugh feels amazing—the kind that after you've had kids, you're scared you might just pee your pants!

But seriously, laughter has so many health benefits. It releases powerful endorphins and alters our biochemistry for the better. It reduces stress hormones such as cortisol and adrenaline and has been shown to relieve physical pain. Orgasms are also a great way to change your body's biochemistry, releasing endorphins and feel-good hormones—but more about that later!

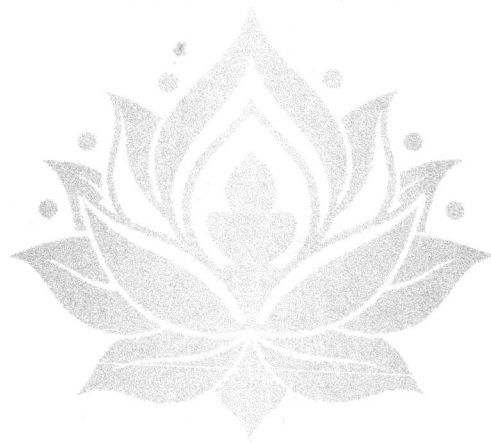

CHAPTER 6
HORMONAL DISTURBANCES

Balanced hormones can mean the difference between peacefully drinking a cup of tea versus wanting to throw it in someone's face.

In most women I see today, the current relationship between stress and sex hormones is in chaos. The impact of stress and its effect on our hormones is costing us our health, happiness, and fertility.

The Impact of Stress on Hormones

Hormones are an interlocking system where each hormone needs to find a specific receptor site and bind to it. When the receptors or the hormones aren't functioning properly, they don't fit together. Like a puzzle, all the pieces must be present for balance and health. When everything works optimally, our hormones give us energy, vitality, a sharp mind, and a sense of well-being. Our skin glows, we burn fat, we want to have sex and can get pregnant and keep it if we want to.

Oestrogen and progesterone are the main hormones that affect how we feel; when they are out of balance, the effects can be devastating. We should never underestimate the power of our hormones and how they can affect how we feel, think, and act.

Most commonly, I see women with high oestrogen and low progesterone levels. The key is to find out if you are suffering from oestrogen dominance, from either too much oestrogen in the body or because your body isn't producing enough progesterone.

Common signs of hormone dysregulation:

- Heavy, clotty periods.
- Painful menstruation that requires pain medication or the pill.
- Tender and itchy breasts before your period.
- PMS rage and unexplained outbursts of emotion.
- Feeling down or depressed a week before you bleed.
- Headaches or migraines before or in the first days of your bleed.
- Sugar and carbohydrate cravings.
- Irregular periods.
- Fluid retention and feels like you've gained 3 kg before your period.

- Can't get pregnant; suffer from miscarriages.
- Anxiety and panic attacks, feel more stressed out than normal.
- Feeling overwhelmed.
- Skin blemishes.
- Constipation and diarrhoea before your period.
- Weight gain around hips and bottom that you can't get rid of.
- Cold hands and feet and flu-like symptoms leading up to your period.
- Increased sensitivity to light and sound.

Oestrogen

Oestrogen can get a lot of bad press, but when it's working optimally, it protects our heart, brain and bone health, to mention a few, and it keeps us fertile in our childbearing years if we remember that our bodies are always seeking balance. Our hormones want us and the human species to survive. Our physiology is about this procreation survival feedback loop, which for us looks like an egg being released each month at ovulation and the egg being released when there is no embryo present, commonly known as your menstrual cycle. Each month, it wants or expects you to get pregnant. Oestrogen makes sure we have enough fat stored in our hips and thighs to support the growth of a foetus and enable us to carry and birth a child into this world successfully. It's this hormone that gives us our beautiful feminine curves and fertility.

Oestrogen dominance can happen in several ways, which include an overworked liver and nervous system; stress is also a major contributing factor. Increased exposure to oestrogens from our environment, pesticides in our food, medications, and toxins also leads to an overabundance of oestrogen. Body fat stores many of these excess toxins. At the same time, our fat also makes its own oestrogen, leading to a backlog in the detoxification process that the liver has to deal with. When our liver is overloaded, backed-up oestrogen often gets dumped back into the blood and fat cells. The liver is vital and should not be overlooked when regulating oestrogen. The liver decides whether it will get rid of or recycle oestrogen in your body. Because the liver makes oestrogen itself, ridding it from your body is not a high priority over the other harmful substances it has to deal with based on the modern world we live in and are exposed to.

Many women who are oestrogen dominant are walking around with months of built-up oestrogen circling around their system, leading to hormonal havoc. Over time, this can lead to an increased risk of feminine cancers such as breast and ovarian. Uterine cysts can also grow at rapid rates, fed by the dominant flow of oestrogen left unchecked by progesterone.

What to Do

- Love your liver. Detox her and feed her with nutrient-rich food, especially green cruciferous vegetables. Supplementing with herbs and specific vitamins is essential if you are struggling with oestrogen dominance.

- Milk-thistle, N-acetylcysteine (NAC) and turmeric are amazing supplements for your liver.
- Use a bioidentical progesterone cream. I prefer creams, as synthetic medicines can increase the liver's workload.
- Avoid plastic as it contains xeno-estrogens and releases toxins from food and drink into your body. Avoid pesticides and go organic where possible.
- Check your cosmetics for toxins.
- Supplement with a multivitamin that fits your age and lifestyle.
- Zinc helps to remove oestrogen from the body and activate progesterone.
- Magnesium is essential for any woman suffering from sympathetic dominance. It also removes excess oestrogen from your body, helping relax muscles, relieve restless legs, and take the edge off PMS symptoms.
- Take a B complex, in particular B6, especially if you take the pill, as this contraceptive naturally eats up your Vitamin B. B6 is beneficial for PMS and has been shown to decrease oestrogen access and their related female cancers.
- Starflower oil or evening primrose oil is a beautiful supplement that helps regulate oestrogen and soothe painful breasts.
- Eat real food, and eat a rainbow, filling yourself up on healthy, life-giving, phytonutrient-rich food we were made to eat.
- Create rest moments before and during your menstruation. Sleep and dreaming help ease the effects of PMS. Try not to push yourself too hard during this time.
- Move mindfully and breathe!

Who's running the show?

Often, our inner child takes charge of our life. She makes our decisions and keeps us small because she fears getting hurt and is busy trying to prove her worth. Can you relate?

A few years back, I had a revelation that I was making decisions and choices through the eyes of my 8-year-old self. If I had to work out, my inner child didn't want to. If I had to do some work or go somewhere, my inner child would come up and show resistance. And my 8-year-old self loves all things sweet and hates veg! So, sticking to a healthy lifestyle was challenging!

When I started working with my inner child, it was life-changing. I realised I was stuck because I wasn't making choices like the adult woman I had become. I was still dealing with fears such as:

- They won't like me.
- They will talk about me behind my back.
- What if I get into trouble?
- What if I try and fail?
- What if I look stupid?

I mean, seriously! I was truly living with the same fears I had when I was eight years old. I don't want you to suffer the same! Take a look at some behaviours that keep coming up for you and ask yourself, 'Who is running the show?'

Sometimes, we just need to tell our inner child, 'It's okay. You can relax. I've got this. I'm going to take care of you. Go and play. Be a child, and let me deal with this grown-up stuff. I love you, and thank you for looking out for me.'

The Hormonal Benefits of Orgasms

Finding time to self-pleasure or have sex gets your juices flowing and your hormones pumping. This alone can help reduce your stress levels.

When we have an orgasm, our body is flooded with beneficial hormones, and our metabolism is woken up and invigorated in exciting ways. Here are some of the health benefits:

- Supports healthy tissue growth.
- Balances hormones.
- Increases absorption of vital nutrients.
- Regular and less painful periods.
- Increases fertility.
- Natural pain reliever.
- Makes your skin glow and helps with the ageing process by stimulating the hypothalamus, which helps calm food cravings and balance blood sugar.
- Helps the lymphatic system get rid of toxins.

I recommend having regular orgasms at least once a week (but I'm hoping it's a lot more than that!) Self-pleasure should be part of your health regime, like brushing your teeth or going to the gym.

Progesterone

Progesterone helps us maintain a healthy pregnancy. It also maintains the lining of our womb until the end of our cycle. If we don't conceive, then progesterone levels drop during your monthly menstruation. In an ideal world, progesterone is more dominant towards the mid-cycle up until your menstruation.

Progesterone is our 'feel good' hormone, and when we have enough of it, it counteracts the negative side effects of our period. Progesterone is:

- Anti-anxiety
- Anti-depressive
- A diuretic that helps with fluid retention
- Helps us burn fat as energy
- Anti-clotting

When this hormone is low, we tend to experience more PMS and negative side effects because there's not enough progesterone to counterbalance the oestrogen. Feelings of depression, low mood, irritability, fluid retention, foggy brain, and fatigue around your periods are red flags, telling you that your progesterone levels need some help.

The feelings of anxiety and unhappiness caused by low progesterone can lead us to feel guilty and think there is something wrong with us. We often get prescribed anti-depressants or the contraceptive pill to help with these feelings when often our progesterone levels are never checked. By optimising our progesterone levels, we can feel better without prescription drugs. There are times when we need medications, and I have been there. When we are treating women, we are often missing the cause of the problem and just routinely treating a symptom. Low progesterone is very common, and a lot of women I see are on the pill or a mild depressive medicine for symptoms of low progesterone. None of them knew how they felt could be connected to stress, their nervous system, and hormone production.

Progesterone is made by our ovaries and adrenals. When our adrenals are burnt out or under stress, they produce high amounts of cortisol to help us survive, and progesterone production often falls. When your body is under stress, the last thing it needs to do is conceive a child. Progesterone production starts to slow and, in some cases, stops altogether. Cortisol uses the body's cholesterol, which is the main ingredient in hormones, so there's not enough to go around. Therefore, not enough progesterone is produced to oppose oestrogen. In this situation, oestrogen and cortisol dominate, and nothing can put the fire out. It's like a kid is throwing a party, and there are no responsible parents at home to supervise when things get out of control.

This affects how many women feel. We lose the 'feel good' hormone that helps us feel happy. We stop ovulating and experience debilitating symptoms. Our biochemistry gets completely disrupted, creating negative side effects in our bodies and lives. It makes us feel more stressed and rushed, and the feeling that we have so much to do becomes magnified. The mix of low progesterone coupled with high oestrogen and cortisol is most women's worst nightmare, one that they are already living and aren't even aware of.

Case Study: Anna

Anna was 42 when she came to me; she had two children in primary school and was working 40 hours a week as a psychiatric nurse. She was full of life, funny, and intelligent. She had always suffered from PMS, but in the past year, it had spiralled out of control, and she felt like she was losing herself. For ten days each month, she felt like she was carrying a black cloud around with her, swinging from rage and aggression to uncontrollable floods of emotions, followed by self-loathing, depression, and fatigue that made her want to stay in bed all day.

Her husband had been diagnosed with burnout and had been off work for the past year. He couldn't handle a lot, so Anna was left to work, cook, clean and be the best mum she could be. She loved her husband and didn't blame him but felt resentful and struggled to keep it all together. She became snappy with her kids, obsessed with the way the house had to look and how her children did at school. She wanted everything done perfectly, and even when her husband tried to help, it wasn't fast enough or good enough, and she thought, 'I just need to do it myself.'

Since she was a little girl, Anna had always had to care for others. Her parents were mild alcoholics, and her mum suffered from depression, often unable to get out of bed. Anna became the mum and carried this role throughout her life, believing that to receive love, she had to do everything for everyone else, neglecting her needs.

We began by resetting her gut, changing her diet, and adding the right supplements and lifestyle changes. Her oestrogen and progesterone ratio was off—she had too much oestrogen and not enough progesterone, so she started taking natural progesterone and started to make progress.

Making all these changes didn't fully heal Anna of her problems but helped her deal with the underlying cause of her PMS, which wasn't only physical. Beneath her PMS and anger, she discovered wisdom and truth. By feeling and accepting her anger instead of fighting it, she could see where it came from. She realised she had unspoken words and unshed tears.

⁓❦⁓

Women who suffer from particularly severe PMS have usually become disconnected and cut off from their feelings. The relationship between PMS and negating your life and putting others before your own shouldn't be overlooked as there is a clear relationship between the two. Ancestral wounds in the mother line are stored in the womb, and our monthly bleed can be part of the purge that needs to be moved. Every month is an opportunity to access the ancient wisdom held in your menstrual cycle.

When there is a history of codependency, self-neglect, and self-sacrifice, it can become a familiar pattern passed down from mother to daughter. Healing these deep wounds helps with PMS and clears your lineage.

When you reach the edge, that point where you feel like you are losing yourself to rage, take a deep breath, step back, and ask yourself: 'What is the pain I'm running from? What is the fear? What am I feeling at this moment? What's real right now?' You will always get the answer you need.

Hormones and Breast Health

Due to the number of hormone receptors present in the breasts, they are extremely sensitive to both oestrogen and progesterone. The connection between stress, breast cancer, a toxic liver, and PMS is undeniable.

Breast sensitivity can be one of the first things we experience when oestrogen-dominant. When the liver becomes too busy to detox, the excess oestrogen gets dumped back into our blood and breasts, and they can feel sore, itchy, and painful to touch—especially right before our period. Benign and malignant cysts and tumours, as well as fibrocystic breast disease, can manifest.

Progesterone can protect us against these problems, but when we're stressed out and not getting enough of this valuable hormone, we are more susceptible to breast disease and cancer.

TIP: *Healthy Breasts and Balanced Hormones*

- Reduce alcohol and caffeine, which have been shown to negatively affect our breast tissue and, in some cases, lead to a higher risk of breast cancer.
- Drink green tea, which contains a powerful antioxidant that maintains and supports healthy breast tissue.
- Eat a plant-based diet of fruits, vegetables, and foods containing beta-carotene and iodine.
- Sulforaphane, found in broccoli, kale, sprouts, and cauliflower, helps prevent oestrogen from attaching to breast tissue and stimulating cancer cell growth.
- Increase your consumption of essential fatty acids (EFA). You can supplement with fish oil or flax seed oil and eat oily fish, chia seeds, and walnuts.
- Take selenium as a supplement; it can also be found in Brazil nuts.
- Ensure you're getting enough vitamin C. Stress rapidly depletes vitamin C, which is water-soluble, so the body can't store it. Take it at least twice daily and eat vitamin C-rich foods.
- Vitamin B6 is a must for healthy breast tissue.
- Evening primrose oil or starflower oil is helpful when trying to balance the hormones that affect breast tissue. I love this oil because it's a great way to boost progesterone levels. By the time we hit 35, our progesterone slowly starts to decline, and this can make us oestrogen dominate. When we are deficient in progesterone, we can feel like a 'crazy hormonal bitch.' We can swing from weepy one minute to angry the next, leaving our loved ones in total confusion and despair! Physically, we experience water retention, especially around the stomach, painful periods, and hot flushes.
- Detox your liver and supplement with milk thistle. Remember, your liver is the dumping ground for everything, and it needs your love and support to work efficiently.
- Use a good quality probiotic, not the kind you find in yoghurt drinks at your local supermarket. At the moment, I use Nature's Best and Solgar.
- We're made up of 90% bacteria, so we need good bacteria for our whole system to be healthy and balanced. Processed food, meditation, and even the makeup on our skin all affect our gut-friendly bacteria. Increasing good bacteria helps to keep oestrogen levels in check, which reduces your risk of breast cancer and other female reproductive growths.

- Meditate to lower your stress levels. Meditation puts you back into a parasympathetic state and shifts you out of the sympathetic dominance you find yourself stuck in. In Western culture, we live in constant stress and find it difficult to relax. Stress is the biggest hormone disruptor, and reducing it starts with you and your choices.
- Take magnesium. If you are a woman who is still menstruating, you need this supplement. I prefer magnesium citrate taken orally, but if you struggle with diarrhoea, use chelated magnesium. Did you know that 90% of the population is now deficient in magnesium? This is due to our increased intake of processed foods, our reduced intake of greens and soil degradation. Magnesium is also primarily found in dark, leafy greens.

Fun Fact:

- For every molecule of sugar you eat, you need 54 molecules of magnesium to process it! No wonder we are all deficient. Primarily a muscle relaxer and depressing mineral, it also helps us deal with chronic stress. Take a good quality magnesium citrate (at least 200mg) before bed.
- Take fish oils.
- Check your breasts regularly, and get to know how they feel at different times of your cycle.

TIP: Reduce Your Consumption of Caffeine

Just one cup of coffee a day can significantly impact your hormones, especially if you have PCOS, ovarian cysts, fibroids, or any female reproductive disease. It's highly inflammatory and adds to the depletion of our friendly bacteria and magnesium. Usually, women who are wired and tired rely on coffee to wake up and go to the toilet. They believe they can't function without it. I suggest cutting back and being honest with yourself about how much you're drinking, especially if your hormones are out of balance.

I also recommend natural progesterone for women who don't respond to diet and lifestyle changes and who often tell me they are struggling with rage and emotional meltdowns. Natural progesterone also works wonders if you have hormone-induced migraines or headaches. Natural progesterone is not the same as synthetic progesterone. Don't be fooled when a practitioner tells you it's the same.

Synthetic progesterone has known side effects such as bloating, nausea, headaches, and weight gain and can actually increase PMS symptoms whilst decreasing our body's natural supply. Natural progesterone can be prescribed by your doctor and is usually applied a few days before the start of your symptoms on the soft areas of your skin, such as the tummy and inner thigh. I advise keeping a diary to track and understand your cycle and how it affects you. Using natural progesterone helps to rebalance oestrogen and progesterone; eventually, you may be able to lower their dose. Always work with your primary health care practitioner. When in doubt, ask!

TIP: *Reflect*

Take a moment and think about your life. Are you happy? Do your relationship and job light you up or deplete you? It's not about blaming yourself or making someone else wrong. It's about being honest with yourself. Often, we're too busy, and we keep busy because, deep down, we don't want to listen to the nagging voice of our soul. We know something has to change, but we resist it. Also, we are taught to avoid the unknown and not rock the boat.

When did you last *really* laugh or experience joy? Are you taking time to do the things you love? What is it you love? How is your perception of pressure and urgency in your life? Can you deal with stress, or is stress dictating your life and health? How often are you amping up with coffee and sugar?

Taking time to reflect on your life and getting honest about how you feel can show you where things need to change. Your truth and inner voice need to be felt and heard without judgement. Then, you can decide what, how, and if changes need to happen.

Remember, the truth will always set you free.

Stress and Your Thyroid

There are many types and causes of thyroid disease. For this book, I am concentrating on the impact of stress, cortisol, and oestrogen on the thyroid, particularly hypothyroidism.

This butterfly gland found in the front of your neck is affected by the Modern Disease of the Modern Woman. The thyroid gland makes hormones that regulate our temperature, metabolic rate, and energy. Many women I see in my practise have 'normal thyroid' blood test results but are experiencing early signs of low thyroid disease, commonly known as hypothyroidism.

The hypothalamus, the control centre in your brain, signals to the pituitary gland to make thyroid stimulating hormones (TSH), which then signals to the thyroid to make T4 (thyroxin). T4 is found in the blood in two forms:

1. T4
2. Free T4 (FT4)

Both T4 and FT4 are inactive hormones that must be converted into T3 (triiodothyronine). T3 enables your body to regulate metabolism, temperature, and energy.

Selenium and iodine are minerals needed for the conversion of T4 to T3. They are trace minerals that used to be found in abundance in the soil where our food is grown. Due to industrialisation and the mass production of farming, these minerals are no longer available in our food in the quantities our thyroid needs to function optimally.

Symptoms of an underactive thyroid include:

- Constipation
- Unexplained weight gain
- Feeling cold most of the time
- Hair loss
- PMS
- Dry skin
- Chronically stressed
- Frequent headaches
- Brittle hair and nails
- Difficulty getting pregnant
- Fluid retention
- Forgetfulness
- Bloated face and swelling in hands and feet
- Muscle pain and stiffness
- High cholesterol levels
- Swollen joints
- Depression
- Husky voice
- Exhaustion
- Reliance on coffee to get you going
- Using chocolate to get through the day

Thyroid function can be suppressed when oestrogen and progesterone levels are out of balance as oestrogen suppresses thyroid function and progesterone supports it. Stress and high cortisol levels also interfere with the production of T3, slowing your metabolic rate and breaking down your muscles to use the glucose stored there for your brain.

When overworked, your adrenal glands interfere with thyroid function. Stress affects your HPA axis (hypothalamus, pituitary, and adrenal). When a woman is suffering from constant stress and the HPA axis is under too much stress, this interferes with the function of her thyroid. Adrenal stress can also lead to thyroid problems by hormone resistance and reduces the conversion of T4 into T3.

The innate feedback system sends chemical messages to your hypothalamus, saying, 'There isn't enough thyroid hormone. Please send more.' Then, your pituitary gland keeps pumping out more thyroid hormone because your adrenals are exhausted. Your thyroid can't access and follow the instructions it's given because it doesn't have the essential nutrients to do its job anymore. The thyroid gets bigger, eventually leading to a goiter in the anterior neck.

In the case of the Modern Disease of the Modern Woman, most women are experiencing thyroid problems due to stress on the HPA axis and the sympathetic dominance that is running their life—and eventually their health—into the ground.

Testing Your Thyroid

Thyroid testing can be a very grey area. Everyone is different, and a result for one person can mean something else for another. This is especially true when we're looking at thyroid hormone levels.

Currently, the 'normal range' for TSH is 0.4 - 4. If you have your thyroid tested and fall in this range, you will likely be told there is nothing wrong with your thyroid. The tests don't always consider someone's lifestyle, age, weight, and individuality.

TSH can be 2 or more, yet the body is desperate for the thyroid to make FT4, but the thyroid can't convert it into T3, so it can use it. Testing FT4 is also important because we can see if the body is producing enough and where the problem is. Often, women are told they have a normal functioning thyroid gland when they are exhausted, constipated, cold, depressed, and can't lose weight. These women often intuitively feel that there is something wrong with them. As a first step, I recommend using selenium and iodine for thyroid support. Boosting the adrenals and rebalancing oestrogen helps to alleviate the symptoms and restore thyroid function. There are times when thyroid medication is needed, and I suggest working with a functional women's medicine practitioner who can help you get more sensitive thyroid testing done.

What to Do

Don't give up! Getting a proper thyroid diagnosis through the traditional route can take years. Get your thyroid tested, take your results to a functional medicine practitioner, and have more sensitive tests done if needed.

Support Your Adrenal Glands

Supplement with:

- Iodine is found in seaweed such as kombu. You can add it to the water when you cook rice or pasta or to soups and sauces. Celtic sea salt also contains trace amounts of this mineral.
- Selenium can be taken in supplements or found in Brazil nuts, seafood, and organ meats.
- Increase your iron. If using a supplement, ensure it's non-constipating and take it with vitamin C. Meat, eggs, spinach, and dates are all good sources of iron. If you are a woman of menstruating age and you have heavy periods, it is essential to make sure you are getting enough iron.

Most blood tests only test the level of iron in your blood. The ferritin levels within your liver are often low and aren't picked up on a routine blood test. Low iron can make you feel anxious, have low energy, and mimic the symptoms of a low thyroid.

Use your voice and speak your truth. Metaphysically, this gland can be blocked when we cannot express our feelings. To free up any blocked energy, try singing when no one is listening or making noise when you exhale.

Humiliation and Resentment

Thyroid problems can represent repressed feelings and beliefs we have around humiliation and resentment. As busy women, often sacrificing ourselves for others, we can secretly feel unseen and unheard, never doing the things we love because we are so busy prioritising everyone else. Everyone comes before us on the list of priorities. Secretly, we crave time and space for ourselves. We feel weighed down by our duty and everything we need to do. We feel guilty for feeling this way and rarely voice it out loud. We often get jealous of others who can choose for themselves, especially our partners. No one is stopping us from living or speaking our truth. Our perceptions and beliefs about being a 'good' mum, friend, daughter or partner often restrict us.

Ask yourself, 'What could I say now? How can I see this differently?' Grab a pen and start writing, remembering your biology is your biography, and you are the creator, the author of your own story—no one else. You get to decide how the story of your reality plays out.

Menopause

In a nutshell, menopause is when your ovaries stop producing hormones. As we discussed earlier, progesterone is made in the adrenals, and when all hormone production ceases in the ovaries, we rely on these glands for our progesterone supply. Now, if you are over-stressed and dealing with the Modern Disease of the Modern Woman, then your adrenals are probably not making enough progesterone. They are too busy trying to make enough cortisol to deal with all the body's stress. Have you noticed that some women seem to float through menopause as if on a cloud while others struggle with every negative side effect possible? I believe stress plays a big part. When women are supporting their adrenals and can deal with stress, their bodies can make progesterone, and this counterbalances some of the nasty side effects of menopause. The problem is most women enter perimenopause stressed out and overloaded with cortisol and oestrogen. Even if these women were able to produce progesterone, it would be drowned out by the other dominating hormones, leaving them struggling with the debilitating side effects of menopause.

Menopause is a time to reflect on who you are and where you're going. It's a chance to pause and make different choices. Heart problems, cancers, and autoimmune diseases are some of the ways life grabs us, kicking and screaming to slow down, and your symptoms are asking you to slow down and do things differently. Your body knows what to do—she's been running the show your whole life! She has so much wisdom to share. It's time to wake up and pay attention.

Addressing your adrenal health, changing your diet, and diaphragmatic breathing are important during this time, as well as lifestyle changes. Rituals, She-Practises, and connecting to your soul also help and support you when so much is ending. You can't solve a hormone problem with medication alone. You may take medication and feel good for a moment, but it won't last or give you the full relief you need. Remember, we need to heal the whole of you, not just attack the symptoms. You are more than just a symptom.

There are three phases a hormone has to go through to be used in your body and cells.

1. You need to be able to produce the hormone in your body. Your endocrine and nervous systems must be communicating optimally.
2. You have to be able to metabolise your hormones, which means having an optimally healthy gut and liver as well as all the essential vitamins and minerals.
3. Your cells must be able to receive the hormone so your body can use it.

When dealing with a hormone issue requiring Hormone Replacement Therapy (HRT), thyroid medication, or any other hormone therapy, it's crucial to concurrently address lifestyle and health choices to maximise effectiveness and ensure long-term benefits. Relying solely on medication, in my opinion, does a great disservice to a woman, preventing her from reaching her optimal health potential. Women require comprehensive lifestyle tools.

Integrate

1. Slow Down and Enjoy the Ride

Whether your goal is to have more energy, lose weight, feel more connected to your body, resolve a health concern, or be the best version of yourself daily, enjoy every part of that journey. The lows have as much to teach us as the highs. Get to know yourself on an intimate level. We expect others to treat us well, but we are so hard on ourselves, often showing ourselves loathing rather than the compassion and love we deserve.

When we start taking better care of ourselves and making better decisions for our lives, especially our health, we stop playing small, self-hating, and repressing. We reduce and stop medicating ourselves, unconsciously using food and alcohol as mood-altering drugs. Taking care of your health and filling your body with love and healthy foods allows you to become naturally still. In this stillness, you can see and feel snippets of who you really are and your life's potential. This stillness offers physical benefits, as well. Your body won't have to work so hard to maintain homeostasis, and your blood sugar, cortisol, temperature, and heartbeat all operate optimally.

When our bodies slow down, we slow down.

2. What do you really want?

Whatever you dream of is possible. The universe wants you to fulfil your dreams and have everything you desire, but many people don't know what they want or what will make them happy as they've always been on auto-pilot or followed the crowd. When you learn to nurture your health and well-being, space will open up for you to dream and create your future. Things that seemed impossible will start to fall into your lap, and your life will change because you have, but faith and perseverance are required! Start by letting go of old belief systems holding you back and clarifying what you want. If you feel stuck or are unsure, I suggest recruiting a coach to help guide you through this process.

Allow yourself the time, energy, and space to decide how you want your life to look and feel. What is it that you would like to achieve or accomplish? Where would you like to go? With whom do you want to spend your precious life? The more facts you have and the more time you take to get to know yourself, the clearer your intentions and the easier it will be to fulfil them. It's a bit like trying on a dress. You need to see if it fits. You don't just buy it and wear it out to a special event, but you see how it feels and looks on your body. Dig deep. What do you want to achieve in this lifetime? What person do you want to be? Reach for the stars!

CHAPTER 7
DIGESTION AND THE GUT

'You are not what you eat. You are what you digest and absorb.'
—*Ashley Koff*

I see the impact of stress on digestion in every woman I treat. Many of my patients have had symptoms for years and just accepted them as normal. Women suffering from hormonal issues can reset their digestive tracts and relieve their symptoms. Hormone imbalances are the by-product of stress, a classic symptom of the Modern Disease of the Modern Woman, leading to poor digestion and gut problems. Getting to the root cause of these issues has never been more critical. The most common digestive issues I see are:

- Bloated stomach
- Mucus and occasional blood in stools
- Intermittent constipation and/or diarrhoea
- Incomplete elimination of bowels
- Undigested food is visible in stools
- Bad breath or a bad taste in the mouth
- Noisy stomach
- Belching
- Acid reflux and indigestion
- Feeling tired or depressed after eating
- Overeating and loss of appetite
- Fatigue and tiredness, even when you sleep well
- Feeling stressed
- Sensitivity to certain food groups
- Diagnosed with depression
- Dry skin congestion and breakouts

The digestive system comprises numerous organs, including your stomach, small intestine, large intestine, liver, gallbladder, and pancreas. Digestion begins with chewing, then enters the oesophagus, and then the stomach. Because most of us are rushing around, we tend not to chew our food properly. This is the start of many digestive issues.

Chewing releases digestive enzymes in the stomach and prepares it for the food that will enter. Because of high adrenaline, cortisol, and unbalanced hormones, our stomach is already getting the message that it's time to run, not the time to eat. As a result, the nervous system is not activated for rest and digestion, bringing a cascade of digestive issues.

Mindful Eating

When eating, slow down, turn off your computer, chew your food really well, and pause between each mouthful. Pay attention to your eating—it can tell you so much about your digestion.

After masticated food leaves your mouth, it enters the oesophagus and then passes through a valve where it enters the stomach. Your empty stomach is about the size of your fist. Think about how much food you're eating at a time and how much you're asking your stomach to distend. The stomach takes around 30 minutes to break down the food so the digestive tract can absorb the nutrients. Perhaps you can see how this may make you feel bloated and tired when you overeat. Overeating also stretches the stomach receptors, meaning you need to eat more food to feel full, leading to weight gain and disease.

Stomach Acid is Good

Your stomach acid must work properly to ensure sufficient digestion. The sensations that happen as you eat—smell, taste, and chewing—get the 'juices' flowing so your stomach is ready and waiting to do its job. Stomach acid's job is to break down the chewed food into smaller, more digestible pieces for optimal absorption of nutrients.

Most women have a lower than desirable PH level, and this leads to digestive issues. The ideal PH level for the stomach is 1.9.

Indigestion or reflux is another common side effect of poor digestion and stress. When stomach acid isn't high enough, food stays in the stomach for extended periods, causing the body to regurgitate. This results in a burning sensation that leaves you running for the antacid medicines. The burn you feel is the stomach acid coming through the valve from the stomach into the oesophagus. Even though the acid is not strong enough to break down the food particles sufficiently in the stomach, it is acidic enough to cause pain in the tissue outside the stomach.

Long-term use of antacid medicines makes this problem worse because they make the stomach acid less acidic. Stomach acid needs to be higher to support good digestion. Although antacid medicines temporarily relieve the burn, they can actually add to the long-term problem.

Stimulate Stomach Acid

Combine a tablespoon each of lemon juice and apple cider vinegar in a little warm water. Drinking this ten minutes before you eat can help the digestive enzymes to break down your food more readily.

Stop drinking water during meals. Water has a PH of 7, depending on where you live and the mineral content, whereas the ideal PH for stomach acid is around 1.9. When we drink with our meals, the essential stomach acid needed for digestion gets diluted, resulting in a bloated, uncomfortable belly. So drink water between meals, around 30 minutes before and after.

Identify foods your body reacts badly to and stop eating them. Pay attention to how your body feels after eating, and keep a note in your phone or diary. Two common culprits are dairy (due to the casein) and wheat/gluten. While food is in your stomach, the pancreas secretes Sodium bicarbonate, which, unlike stomach acid, is alkaline. There is something known as the PH gradient, where PH levels begin very high (acidic) in the stomach and reduce as we go further along the digestive tract. As I mentioned earlier, if the stomach acid isn't strong enough (acidic enough), this creates problems such as bloating, gas, and abdominal pain. Digestion-related pain under the rib cage can be due to insufficient sodium bicarbonate production or a gallbladder issue.

After food leaves your stomach, it travels through the pyloric valve and enters the small intestine. The small intestine is where your body absorbs all the nutrients needed to keep you healthy. Nutrients are absorbed into your bloodstream and sent around your body to all your cells and tissues.

Just because we eat something, it's wrong to assume that we can absorb what the body needs from it. Many of my patients eat a vitamin-rich diet and cannot sufficiently absorb these nutrients. Friendly gut bacteria are critical to high nutrient absorption throughout the digestion process.

Gut Bacteria—You Need More!

After food leaves the small intestine, it enters the large intestine, travelling from the right lower abdomen up and across the mid-abdomen and descending down the left side until it comes out as waste in the descending colon and rectum.

Within your large intestine are trillions of bacteria. On average, adults will have around 1.5-2 kg of bacteria in their gut. Bacteria can be good or bad, and we want more good bacteria. The good bacteria ferment the food that enters the large intestine. Day in and day out, they love turning your food into poop! When your colon receives partially digested food from the stomach and small intestine, it tries its best to ferment it. When these pieces are too large, we get more gas than usual. This can sometimes be the painful, embarrassing kind that stinks and we can't control. Bloating and pain in the stomach are very common side effects when the colon receives bigger pieces of undigested food. This leads to Irritable Bowel Syndrome (IBS), which is an umbrella term given to everything that isn't going right in the gut, and 9 out of 10 times is related to stress.

A bloated stomach can create a deep psychological wound in women who try to eat well, yet by the end of the day, they can feel and look three months pregnant or more. Poor digestion is often the culprit, which all begins with stress and our perceptions—because that governs how, when, and what we eat.

Get to the Root Cause

One reason you have digestive issues may be that you can't 'stomach' something or someone in your life and are having difficulties digesting your problems. Perhaps you have to recognise or resolve a fear or underlying feeling. Observe how you feel before you eat with certain people and in different situations and how those feelings impact your digestion. You might get some insights into what may be hiding in your stomach.

Stress and Digestion

As you can imagine, stress is a major contributing factor to poor digestion and gut problems. If you've been under stress for more than a few months, you will start to have symptoms of IBS, which, in my experience, is always stress-related, and this stress can come from many things: how you feel, think, eat, move, and your environment. All of these factors contribute to sympathetic dominance and low resilience. I talked earlier about the stress response and how it switches all of your physiological and chemical processes into the red zone to keep you safe when optimal digestion happens in the green zone. When your body feels stressed and imagines it has to run from tigers, your blood and energy are pumped to your muscles, particularly your arms and legs. When you eat food in this state, your body doesn't have all the resources or time it needs to digest it, which leads to painful gas, bloating, and other symptoms, classic IBS. When your stomach and intestines are irritated and inflamed, your body says, 'Wake up! We need you to pay attention. You need to do things differently. Otherwise, something bad is going to happen.'

I see many women who ignore their gut feelings—both physical and emotional—and they all have symptoms of IBS. All the pushed-down emotions, loss of intuition, and stressful conditions leave them living in their heads, cut off below the neck, surviving, dragging their body around with them like a piece of meat. At the same time, they focus on doing, moving from activity to activity, and trying to be perfect while ignoring the body's intuitive voice and signals.

Women who have experienced sexual abuse as girls are significantly more likely to have chronic somatic health problems, for example, IBS, chronic fatigue syndrome, or anxiety. And one in four women has experienced some level of sexual abuse. We hide and tuck all the shame and humiliation away, especially in our intestines, hiding it away from the world and ourselves. Poor gut health also leads to a greater increase in anxiety and depression. There is an undeniable link between our gut and brain health, commonly known as the 'Gut brain brain axis'. This means that what you eat and how healthy your gut is directly impacts your emotional and mental health.

How your body functions is your business and has to start being a priority for you. Without this body, we can't do or be anything in this world. The body is intrinsically connected to how we feel. Most women think that their soul is disconnected from their body, that being spiritual isn't experienced in the body but in the head or higher chakras. But that's bypassing the truth of who we are physically and metaphysically. We can't get into and feel all the places we want or need to when we aren't fully rooted and embodied in our sacred vessel.

Your life and soul are not separate from your body. Many women believe that if they can just push through or get over their bodies, everything will be okay. The truth is you are your body! The idea that the body is seen as bad or unimportant originated from patriarchal indoctrination, namely the church. They spread the belief that 'the flesh and body is sinful,' especially stigmatising female anatomy as inherently bad. For at least two thousand years, we've been taught to transcend the body, that it's something to escape or tame, to feel humiliated or shameful about. This lie lurks beneath the surface of our consciousness, imprisoning us and making us sick.

Case Study: Dana

Dana was always ambitious. She excelled in school and university, actively participating in all the right groups and social scenes. As she entered the workforce, she effortlessly ascended the corporate ladder, easily achieving success. Dana took pride in her image—successful, thin, and fit—the life and body many women coveted.

However, since her early twenties, Dana battled digestive issues that manifested as painful gas, constipation, intermittent diarrhoea, a bloated stomach, and indigestion. To manage these symptoms, she resorted to self-medication with over-the-counter drugs and altered her eating habits. She was also struggling with a mild case of bulimia from her teen years.

Despite her health struggles, Dana continued to achieve, maintaining a slender physique that garnered admiration. This pattern persisted for 15 years until her late 30s, when the toll on her well-being became undeniable. Anxiety set in, and Dana found herself unable to ignore the mounting stress. Weight gain ensued, accompanied by persistent stomach pains, heartburn, hives, and inflammation inside and outside her body. A diagnosis of fibromyalgia left her feeling scared, lost, and alone.

The severity of her symptoms forced Dana to work from home, seeking solace near a toilet and her bed. Anxiety attacks and dark thoughts overwhelmed her, and she felt as if her body was turning against her.

Desperate for a solution, Dana explored various medical avenues without success. It was at the recommendation of a friend that chiropractic care, specifically working with me, became a last resort. Initially skeptical, Dana's perspective shifted as she began to experience subtle improvements after chiropractic adjustments. Her energy levels increased, her focus sharpened, and her body felt less stiff. Though the pain persisted, she could now sleep without relying on constant painkillers.

As weeks passed, Dana and I addressed her physical symptoms and delved into healing her gut and digestion. The journey toward improved health was slow but steady. With my guidance, Dana learned that stress had been a significant contributor to her illness. Her nervous system underwent a transformative process, rewiring and regulating.

Reflecting on her life, Dana realised that stress had been a constant since childhood, triggered by a traumatic event that set off a cascade of nervous system deregulation. Her coping mechanism involved avoiding feelings and burying herself in achievement, a distraction from her true self. Dana recognised this as a form of self-protection driven by fear and survival.

⁂

Breaking the ingrained stress patterns and neurological wiring proved to be one of Dana's most challenging yet crucial decisions. By incorporating She-Practises, Dana reconnected with her body for the first time since childhood. Unforeseen healing occurred, and challenging preconceived notions about her limitations became conscious and rewired. Most importantly, Dana gained a profound understanding of the pervasive impact of stress on every aspect of her life.

The path to everything you want to be, feel, and do is through the body. The journey is from your head to your heart and womb. It's time to stop chasing and running and remember that you are not your beliefs, past, stories, or circumstances. Nothing can hurt you unless you let it. It's time to re-honour your gut feelings and intuition, the voice of your soul. It starts with changing how you think, perceive, believe, eat, move, breathe, and drink—and you have the power to change it all.

Leaky Gut

Many women come into my practise suffering from a leaky gut. Our gut is vital for our immune system, and when we have a leaky gut, our immune function can often be compromised. This is why it is essential to balance digestive health and reset before throwing every test, supplement, and therapy at our bodies.

A leaky gut occurs when the lining of the intestinal wall becomes 'hyperpermeable.' The gut lining acts as a barrier to protect the body. When this barrier is compromised, and the normally tight junctions are wider, particles of undigested food, toxins, and waste products can pass through the cell lining into your bloodstream, creating inflammation, disease, pain, and autoimmune disorders.

When these foreign substances are released into the blood, our amazing body goes on high alert and mounts an attack on the invaders. This defense response triggers the immune system to release inflammatory proteins called cytokines, which attack any potential threat. Autoimmune disease happens when the cytokines travelling in the bloodstream begin attacking parts of the body. Other common symptoms include:

102

- Allergies, running nose, and itchy eyes
- ADD, ADHD, problems concentrating
- Multiple Sclerosis
- Arthritis
- Psoriasis
- Joint pain
- Asthma
- Eczema, acne, rashes
- Food intolerance
- Chronic diarrhoea or constipation
- Bloating and flatulence
- Nutritional deficiencies
- Fatigue
- Headache
- Confusion
- Brain fog
- Inflamed and or itchy skin
- Acne

Often, medications such as corticosteroids are prescribed to help deal with pain and inflammation. These do not treat the underlying cause and can add more damage, enhancing the problem and causing more gut challenges. When we add in anti-depression medication, birth control pills, pain medications, and everything else the average woman may be taking, it takes its toll and starts attacking and inflaming our gut lining. Where we may be trying to cure ourselves, we may actually aggravate the problem. I'm not saying don't take your medicines; instead, we need to look at everything you're taking and see how we can support and repair the gut to help you feel better and live a healthier life.

Gut bacteria are vital for a functioning immune system. These bacteria create an immune response against viruses and bacteria that affect not just the gut but the lungs and other areas of the body, as well. Taking care of your gut can improve recurrent bouts of the flu, yearly lung infections, heavy colds, and upper respiratory diseases.

The gut microbiome is not only one of our major lines of defense but also provides around 90% of the serotonin the body needs.

Your brain is inextricably connected to your gut. We hear 'the gut is your second brain' a lot these days, yet some of us are still not connecting the dots and how that may influence depression and anxiety. As I mentioned earlier, your gut and brain constantly communicate via neurotransmitters and hormones called the 'gut-brain axis.' That gut feeling you get when things don't feel good is your brain communicating with your gut and vice versa.

Approximately 90-95% of our serotonin, which is responsible for our emotional feelings, is made in the gut. When serotonin is low, we feel anxious, depressed, and a bit off. In addition, low serotonin levels cause a marked deterioration in the gut's lining, slowing down the movement of waste through the bowels, leading to constipation and bloating. It also affects nutrient absorption and digestion. Therefore, if you are suffering from IBS, leaky gut, yeast overgrowths, sibo, or any other digestive complaints, there is a high chance you have low serotonin levels.

Everyone is uniquely individual and has different genetics and epigenetics. If you are suffering from a leaky gut, a few known culprits are a problem when your body is stressed. The truth is you may not be allergic to a particular food; you may be sensitive. In earlier life, when you had less stress, your body could deal with this food, but now, when it is over-stressed and inflamed, it just can't process that food anymore. Eating that one extra thing our body is sensitive to creates symptoms, 'the bucket is full,' so to speak.

Wheat and cow's milk are two likely culprits that may be affecting you, as well as coffee and alcohol. These are too acidic for our bodies' optimal slightly alkaline PH of around 7.4, and when consumed too often will begin to cause negative side effects. Cow's milk is meant for baby cows, not humans. Would you be so eager to drink puppy or pig milk? We've been brainwashed and sold the marketing image that cow's milk is good for us and where we can get most of our vitamin D. This is not true. Cow's milk actually takes calcium from our bones. Have you ever wondered why most Western populations have so much osteoporosis compared to other countries? Excellent sources of calcium are leafy greens, almonds, butternut squash, sardines, and tofu. All of these can contain more calcium than a glass of processed milk.

Another reason not to drink milk is it's full of oestrogen that upsets your hormones. Most cows have had a cocktail of antibiotics because of the environment and conditions in which they are kept. They are pumped full of hormones to keep producing milk because a cow, like a human, only produces milk when she has a baby. It's not on tap for life! Cows are regularly treated with steroids to help with the swelling and painful ulcers from the constant milk that gets pumped from their udders day after day. When we drink in all of that, is it any wonder our hormones are out of balance? If you want to drink cow's milk, buy organic, local, and unpasteurised milk.

As children, we lose the enzyme lactase, which breaks down the sugars in lactose found in milk. Because we no longer have this enzyme, we develop problems in the gut. Stomach cramps, pain, and diarrhoea all are common symptoms of lactose intolerance. I see it in kids who drink their bottle or cup of milk before bed. Asthma, eczema, and chronic ear infections can all be symptoms of a leaky gut and intolerance to milk-based products, especially in children. Instead of loading our kids up with antibiotics and having tubes repeatedly inserted in their ears (as the procedure usually doesn't work!), we should look at what our kids are consuming and examine their gut health, getting to the root cause rather than just chasing symptoms.

Casein is a protein also found in cow's milk. In fact, milk consists of 80% casein. It's what gives milk that lovely white colour. It's also found in all milk products, such as baby milk, cow cheese, and yoghurt. Casein has been shown to induce an inflammatory response in the gut. In other words, it causes gut lining inflammation, making it weak and leaky.

Casein has also been linked to depression, ADD, autism, bipolar disorders, and anxiety because of the elevated inflammatory and immune response it creates. Caesin may aggravate and make the symptoms worse. Remember, your brain is your second gut.

The next big culprit is wheat. I live in the Netherlands, and most people here eat a lot of bread! Since the 1980s, wheat production has changed dramatically, and the image we are given by marketers showing us romantic pictures of farmers harvesting the field on a sunny day is not the mainstream reality. Hybridisation has mostly replaced the old ways of farming wheat, which means more quantity but less quality. Hybridisation works by producing dwarf varieties of wheat, which are achieved by cross-breeding two genetically different varieties of wheat. This process increases mass production and improves the crop's strength, which means it lasts longer than nature intended. What is this Frankenstein wheat doing to our food? The fact is our wheat today, due to modern-day farming, contains more gluten than years ago. Gluten is a protein found in wheat that our bodies can't digest easily. Although today's farming process makes farming more efficient, it has little nutritional benefit and can harm our gut and brain.

Our body and innate immune system mistake this gluten as a foreign invader. It creates antibodies and an immune response, leading to autoimmune disease and other negative processing in the body. Coeliac disease is the most known form of wheat intolerance; however, you don't have to have coeliac disease to suffer from the adverse effects of wheat and gluten.

Reducing or eliminating milk and wheat products from your diet will help you see which foods irritate your gut. I have an elimination protocol available on my website, and you can also sign up for our next round of the MDMW protocol.

While not everyone is intolerant to wheat, many find that consuming too much of it can irritate the gut. Many women who cut it from their diet report feeling less bloated, sluggish, and tired.

If you think you are wheat or lactose intolerant, I suggest an igG (food sensitivity) test. Again, more information about this is on my website. Please remember that you are uniquely individual, and not one diagnosis fits all. Reviewing all your symptoms, culture, epigenetics, genetics, and lifestyle are all important factors that should not be overlooked.

How to Help Heal the Gut Lining

Using functional medicine, I follow the following protocol:

1. Remove
2. Replace
3. Reinocculate
4. Repair

1. Remove:

- For the next 21 days, eat clean, whole foods that are unprocessed and unpackaged, with no hidden sugars, sweeteners, or artificial additives.
- Eat organic food when possible, lean proteins, and a plate full of vegetables. Avoid caffeine, alcohol, and chewing gum. In addition, eliminate all dairy and wheat-based products.
- Pay attention to food combinations. Don't eat protein with a carbohydrate. Eat potato or rice with vegetables, but not with protein. Protein can be eaten alone or with vegetables. Don't eat or mix fruit with any other food.
- Begin eating your vegetables first and add fermented vegetables to the mix.
- Drink water at least half an hour before and after you eat to keep the stomach PH acidic.
- Chew your food and breathe as you eat. Make sure you are having a bowel movement each day.
- Don't skip meals unless you are following a 'She-fast.'
- Add a smoothie for breakfast. This allows the gut extra time to relax and repair as a smoothie takes little effort for your body to digest.

Example smoothie:

- 1 tablespoon of plant-based protein powder
- 1 tablespoon of flaxseed
- 1 frozen banana
- 1 tablespoon of almond butter or coconut oil
- 1 cup of baby spinach
- 1 teaspoon each of cacao and maca powder
- 1 teaspoon of lemon juice or finely grated ginger root
- Water or coconut water

Place ingredients in a blender in the order listed. Blitz and bottoms up!

2. Replace

This step is where we add supplements that help support your body during digestion. Digestive enzymes taken at the start of each meal help boost stomach acid, which can help with bloating, gas, and a painful stomach after eating.

- Boost stomach acid with digestive bitters, such as two tablespoons of apple cider vinegar before you eat or Betaine HCL (around 650mg per day), taking 1-3 at each meal. You can reduce the dose as your body produces more stomach acid. If you have a stomach ulcer, talk to your primary healthcare provider before starting this regimen, and always listen to your body—she knows best.

- Liquorice and zinc are also great supplements for inflammation of the gut.

3. Reinoculate

After removing and replacing, we need to start adding healthy bacteria, which can be done with fibre, lacto-fermented foods, and probiotics.

- Eat dark leafy greens, at least two cups with each meal.
- Eat more fibre. You can supplement with psyllium husks but try to get it from your diet. You're looking to get 30-35 grams of fibre daily. Fibre is also an excellent way for toxins and excess oestrogen to exit the body more efficiently. In addition, fibre nourishes the gut flora. If the gut flora doesn't get fed, it begins to eat away at the protective mucosal layer of the intestines, causing inflammation and, yes, a leaky gut.
- I add flax seeds to my food to help increase fibre. Try adding two ground tablespoons daily.
- Take a good quality probiotic that contains around 10 billion CFUs with a variety of lactobacillus and Bifidobacterium. To help restore gut function, take these daily for a few months, then drop them down to a few times a week.
- Supplement with 4-10 mg a day of prebiotics. These are starches in garlic, onions, asparagus, fermented foods and oats. They contain fructooligosaccharides, which create health and vitality in your gut.

Additional supplements that help heal the gut:

- Turmeric, marshmallow root, and liquorice root—help heal the gut lining.
- Zinc—is integral for maintaining the intestinal wall, stopping inflammation, and healing stomach ulcers.
- Glutathione—helps rebuild tissue and repairs bodily functions.
- Resveratrol slippery elm—helps ease the symptoms of gut-related problems.
- Vitamin D3—supports the immune system.
- Antioxidants A, C, and E, as well as the minerals selenium, zinc, and copper help protect cells from oxidation and damage. They also help mend membranes, particularly the gut membrane. Most good-quality multivitamins include this.
- Omega 3—reduces inflammation in the body.
- Magnesium citrate is also wonderful for naturally relieving constipation and restoring regular bowel movements.

As with anything I recommend, if you are breastfeeding or pregnant, you should consult with a primary health practitioner before starting this regimen.

4. Repair

Repairing and regulating immunity is at the heart of healing from the effects of stress and the impact this has on your gut. When we are stressed, our immune system can't function and do its job well. Inflammatory signals get turned on, and we get to a stage when we can't just turn them off anymore. We are inflamed with an immune system that starts attacking the body. Confused, tired, and overworked, the immune system is low. We need our immune system to protect us and help us heal. It needs to be working for us, not against us. Regulating immunity is, therefore, key to healing, which begins by taking care of our stress levels. Getting your cortisol levels back on track is vital for the gut, immune system, and longevity. The idea is to calm down the inflammation.

I recommend taking the following:

- Green tea extract is an antioxidant that helps boost immune system inflammation and promote healthy gut flora.
- Ginger can act as an NSAID by relieving pain and inflammation in the body.
- Omega 3 reduces and removes oxidative stress and protects against inflammatory conditions.
- N-acetylcysteine (NAC) works by boosting glutathione, which is depleted by inflammation, chronic stress, and oxidative stress that damages cells.
- Curcumin is an anti-inflammatory extract from turmeric that is specifically used to treat stress-related depression. It relieves pain and gut inflammation, reduces DNA damage from oxidative stress, and is simply amazing!

Take one or a combination of the above recommendations, and you will begin to see aches and pains ease, menstrual symptoms reduce, and depression begin to lift. Again, these must be taken with lifestyle changes and a whole, plant-based diet for the best results.

Remember, trauma and stress stored in the body need to be identified. While changing your diet, microbiome, and digestion can make a huge difference, IBS and other gut problems can be rooted in something deeper and shouldn't be overlooked. As we journey further, we will dive deeper into why and how we can rebalance the whole of you.

The Gut Factor

When our Gut instinct isn't working with us, it starts working against us, and we become sick. The gut is where our second brain is housed. It's where all our hormones are made, our immune system begins, and the feel-good neurotransmitters are produced. This is why the physical consequence of a blocked Chakra 2 can affect our hormones and give us PMS, creating chronic illness, depression, and anxiety.

Digestive System

Stress and anxiety are felt in the gut, showing up as indigestion, gas, bloating, abdominal pain, and piles. Everyone feels stress in their digestion in one way or another. Some feel it as acid reflux; you may experience diarrhoea or constipation or both and perhaps a hard, gassy, and painful bloated stomach. Whatever your experience, it all points to you losing power through stress. It's your body's way of telling you something is wrong, whether that's the food you are eating, how you feel, or both.

Constipation can be a sign that you're not eating enough fibre and you're mentally and physically constipated. Mental constipation can be seen when you resist change in your life. We feel stuck but usually don't want to change things because we fear discomfort. When we suffer from constipation, it can also indicate that we are holding on to everyone's crap, including our own. Just like spring cleaning your closet, spring cleaning your friends, relationships, and old belief systems helps you let go of what is blocking your flow. You get to recycle and keep all the nutrients, but you are letting go of the build-up of waste that's been weighing you down.

Diarrhoea can mean that we are scared and anxious to hold onto something or someone but are unable to. We may have patterns that mean we are self-sabotaging, anxious, and over-controlling to the point where we just can't hold it anymore. Our over-controlling nature is a protective mechanism because we can't let anything fall apart, because what would that mean? In truth, it doesn't mean the end of the world, but to the over-controlling perfectionist in us, keeping those walls up equals letting everyone else and our ego think we have everything together. Being scared of the unknown and change is normal—it's all about the cycle of birth, life, death, and rebirth.

Tension can also build up physically in this area, which is the most common cause of sciatica and lower back pain. Stress causes tension, which ultimately leads to lower back pain.

Remember: You are a whole being, and one area that's out of alignment can have the ability to affect and infect your entire system.

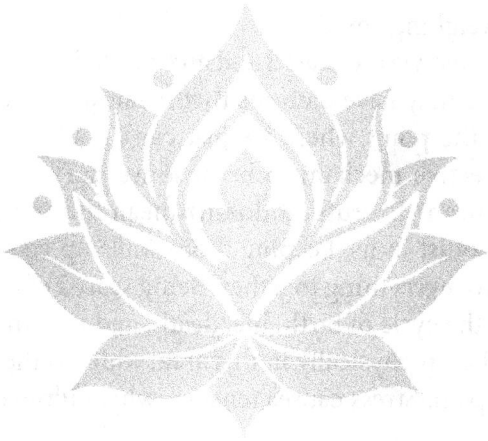

CHAPTER 8
YOUR FEMININE LANDSCAPE–OVARIES, WOMB, & BREASTS

'If you want to know where your true power lies, go to those places you have been taught to fear the most. Your orgasm, your period, labour and birth, menopause… this is where your real power lies. In the sacred temple of your womb.'
—Dr. Christiane Northup, MD

Within your feminine organs, tissues, and cells lies ancient, encoded wisdom. These are unexplored, blocked, and forgotten places inside you; this dormant wisdom patiently awaits your awakening. Imagine your external body as the tower, and you, like Sleeping Beauty, are just discovering the magic within. Coming back home into your feminine body is often the missing piece and is crucial to this inner journey. Coming into the body allows you to tune into the feminine codes of energy, intuition, and magic you possess. All the vitality and aliveness you seek are already within, waiting for you to awaken to your power. As a priestess whose sacred gifts are kundalini and tantric awakening, I have worked with hundreds of women, helping them awaken and reconnect to the fire and aliveness of their sacred sexuality locked within their womb and lower chakra centres. This reconnection, this work, changes everything.

The Feminine Energy of the Womb

The womb serves as your creative core, birthing all aspects of life. It's a potent portal that transforms the nonexistent into existence. This centre of wisdom holds the creative energy flowing through your body and life, yet many of us tap into only a fraction of our potential. The energy and wisdom in this sacred space connect us to spirit, bridging the divine and human within us—the sacred union that leads to wholeness.

Unfortunately, we often live separated from this power by societal expectations and roles, forfeiting our birthright to our creative life force. We confine ourselves to small ideas, reactions, and chosen shapes, carrying the weight of unprocessed traumas, betrayals, and grief. This emotional baggage, nestled in the womb, silently influences our decisions and actions, hindering our ability to heal, create, and live joyfully.

Remaining stuck manifests in our energy field and physical body, resulting in issues like cysts, growths, PMS, infertility, and pain. To remedy this, we must honour the sacredness of our wombs, recognising their voice as our own. Returning to our womb's wisdom helps us reclaim our bodies as sacred vessels. We are powerful creators shaping our universe from within, and true vitality emanates from this internal source. Many of us feel off because we've neglected this internal connection, seeking external solutions for an internal issue.

We are intricately linked to the cosmic womb that birthed Gaia Sophia Earth, and in turn, Earth birthed us. We are integral to her cell body, never truly separated, and our bodies serve as a potent portal for all life. Our monthly cycle mirrors the rhythm of birth, death, and rebirth. Observing it through our menstrual cycle, syncing with the moon and seasons, we resemble a snake shedding its skin, constantly renewing and ushering in new life and projects. Now is the moment to be mindful of what we are birthing and giving life to.

What is dying or dead that we are still trying to breathe life into?
What needs to die so something new can take its place?

Picture yourself standing on a threshold, empowered to shape who and what you become. You are the one you've been waiting for, and it's time to stop waiting, channelling your energy inward. True healing and alignment arise from embracing vertical consciousness in kairos time rather than getting trapped in the horizontal Chronos time. When we linger in the horizontal, burdened by beliefs and unresolved emotions, the psychic weight takes on a lower vibration, transforming it into physical matter within our tissues and cells, ultimately paving the way for disease.

Your issues live in your tissues.

Creation is unfolding, whether you're aware of it or not. Taking control and self-authority back into your body and life means creating and healing from a place of alignment. You become lighter and more fulfilled. The world you live in, your future, days, months, and years are being birthed through you in every moment, shaped by every thought, feeling, and choice you make. When you become conscious of your power, your entire world changes. You transition from being a participant in life, where things happen to you, to the creatrix of your life, giving you control over what you birth and the reality you create.

The Red Thread

A red thread connects you to every woman who came before you—an ethereal umbilical cord winding and pulsating through time and space, connecting you through your mother line all the way back through your blood lineage.

It connects you to their physical DNA, traits, and genes, as well as to their stories, beliefs, traumas, and events in their lifetime. Everything gets remembered in our DNA, whether physical or crystalline, and is passed down from woman to woman, mother to daughter, and womb to womb throughout time, all the way back to primordial eve. So, not only are you carrying your own wounds from your life, childhood, and past lives, but you also carry theirs.

Releasing the baggage, the heaviness and weight of what you carry for yourself and past generations will free up your vital life force within your womb. Here, we release the pain, fears, limitations, control, and lack thereof. We take back our power and refuse to numb the pain and shadow. Here at this centre, we come home and reclaim this sacred part of ourselves. Having a regular 'She-Movement' practise is vital for women as they awaken to the energy in the womb.

Waking up to yourself can feel quite challenging, especially if you've experienced trauma in this area. Engaging in deep-releasing work to clear your womb from past violations, betrayals, lies, and self-abandonment can significantly transform the energy in this centre. When stuck in past trauma, you're essentially feeding that history every waking moment. It drains your energy and life force, leaving you depleted and making it difficult to make decisions or move forward in life.

Ovarian and womb energy is where your shakti life force and sexual energy originate. It's like a powerful stove residing in your second chakra that heats up your energy, allowing you to manifest your desires. The ovaries play a crucial role in revitalising the womb space and nourishing the female body, and their health influences your happiness and radiance. Many women have depleted energy in their ovaries as if their fire is dying out. This depletion often leads to burnout, PMS, and challenging menopausal symptoms because the fire has been used up on all the stress and cortisol accumulated over the past years.

When you reconnect with your ovaries and Sacred Sexuality, you rediscover lost parts of yourself that light you up—the parts that love to dance and belly laugh. This energy fuels a craving to express yourself and create something wildly expressive; its power is your power. Yet, many of us aren't aware that there's a light down there or where the switch is because it's been turned off for as long as we can remember.

This potent force has been controlled and kept quiet for centuries due to its immense power. It's a taboo, rarely discussed and often feared. This is usually the part of us where we have turned down the volume. This wild, untamed aspect gets hung up or packed away while we try to be and do all the things we think will make us feel safe, happy and fulfilled; it's the 'good girl' archetype on steroids. We trade our aliveness and soul for security, acceptance, and compromise, relinquishing control even when no one is asking us to. We don't realise its value, and we crave the safety of codependency until our inner fire starts to dim, until there is nothing but ash where once was a radiant blazing inner furnace.

We tone ourselves down to become more palatable, respectable, and serious. We wear sensible clothing, make correct choices, and play it safe. Soon, dampness sets in where there was once fire. We no longer desire sex, lack drive and energy in many areas of our lives, and are tired all the time. We feel down but don't know why, put on weight, and become physically and emotionally stiff. Overstressed and overworked, we grow bored and dissatisfied with our privileged lives. One day, we wake up and think, 'What happened?' Our relationships suffer, and we argue over the smallest things, but the real issues are money, power/control, and sex. You over-control every detail because deep down, you feel everything will fall apart if you let go for even an inch. When the walls come down and cracks appear, light filters in, and slowly, you wake up and remember who you are.

Case Study: Freya

Freya came in with lower back pain that extended down her right leg. During the examination, it was clear she had asymmetry, with the muscles on one side of her body being too tight and short. She also had a significant kyphosis and anterior head carriage from sitting slouched over and twisted at her computer most days. Freya had battled breast cancer the previous year, and the tension in her upper spine indicated how she had hidden her soul and protected her heart. Her body was expressing emotions through disease and pain.

As she began to talk, Freya shared that she was the oldest of eight children and had taken on the responsibility of caring for them. Her strict father made saying no impossible, leading her to compromise and neglect her own needs to please others. Despite feeling many emotions, she had learned to suppress them over the years, believing that showing emotions was a sign of weakness. Freya felt stuck, acknowledging that unexpressed rage was eating her up inside, and her body was sacrificing itself to protect others.

After months of chiropractic care, sacred sexuality, and She-Movement practises to address the blocked womb and ovarian energy, Freya experienced relief. She could express the built-up anger in her pelvis and womb, regulate her nervous system, and forgive herself and others. She felt more integrated, emotionally fluid, calm, and able to openly express herself without fear or shame. Freya no longer lived in her head, afraid of feeling, and started to appreciate moving into her feelings, breathing, and releasing them. She recognised her body as a powerful vessel and finally felt at home and safe in her body again.

⚜

The Feminine Energy of Your Ovaries

'All the bliss I'm chasing is there waiting, in the listening.'
—Marya Stark

Your ovaries are one of your most potent feminine resources, containing the energy and light that empowers you. When in balance, they nourish and inspire all your creations, health, and life. While we commonly associate ovaries with releasing eggs during menstruation, they play a much broader role. They not only house eggs for creating life but also contain your creative potential and the energy needed to manifest your desires.

Imbalances often occur in the ovaries, leading to underachievement or overactivity, impacting our bodies and how we feel. Even if one or both ovaries are removed, we can still tap into the energetic flow stored and generated within this chakra. Ovary imbalances are common, and we may not realise them until we feel pain, cysts, or other female health-related issues. The effects of unbalanced ovarian energy become apparent in our outer lives before experiencing symptoms within the body.

The challenge lies in not being taught how to harness this transformative life force within us, resulting in stagnant or depleted energy in our feminine core. Over time, this leads to pain, disease, and burnout, contributing to painful periods and debilitating menstrual and menopausal symptoms.

Blocked Ovarian Energy

This leads to a build-up of stagnant energy because there's no flow. Think of a stream that has clean running water running through it. When a stream becomes blocked over time, the water builds up and stagnates. New fresh water can't filter through, and the biochemistry and ecology of the environment change to that of a pond. For us, this can show up as pelvic congestion and pain, usually around the blocked ovary. Learned protective mechanisms that shut down our feminine essence and emotions, combined with feelings of unmet desires and rejection of the feminine, are the root cause of a blocked ovary. A blocked ovary can feel dense, heavy, and small, preventing you from receiving your gifts and power. You experience scarcity and are overwhelmed as you cannot replenish this energy.

Another way we can block ovarian energy is by turning off and becoming numb to the energy flow. In this scenario, the energy flows, but we cannot receive it. We then have an outpouring and leakage in our ovaries. It's like having a bucket with a hole in the bottom that you keep filling but cannot hold. This can make a woman feel powerless; she can't hold onto or feel powerful in her own life. We become victims, overwhelmed and confused because nothing we do seems to work. We then start an endless search outside of ourselves for answers, as we've lost trust and connection with our bodies.

Overactive Ovarian Energy

Many women are familiar with this one. It's when we're overworked, overloaded with tasks, and constantly over-committed—can you relate? We struggle to say no, needing to continually prove our worth. Excessive doing and overcompensating quickly drain our vitality and energy, leading to depression, low energy, fatigue, and burnout. This tends to affect nurturers, caregivers, and those who struggle to prioritise themselves over others. It's like people-pleasing on steroids, a constant effort to be everything for everyone, driven by the desire to pacify our feelings of unworthiness and the good-girl complex. The result is feeling drained, depressed, and disconnected from our true selves.

This stress and overcommitment often manifest as tension and pain in the body, including pelvic tension and distortions. Eventually, it can lead to ovarian cysts and polyps as we push our ovaries to burnout. We might find ourselves overly active in our work life, being a workaholic, and feeling blocked in our intimate and personal relationships. Acknowledging and supporting our ovaries is crucial in creating a more balanced outer life that aligns with our inner well-being.

Left Ovary Manifestations

Let's dive into the left and right ovaries because even though they're both ovaries doing similar things, they're quite different physically and energetically.

The left ovary is all about receiving, allowing, replenishing, abundance, and embracing our desires. It embodies flow energy, letting us stand still and be present—the essence of femininity. Unfortunately, culturally, we've been taught not to value this, and many women lean more towards the masculine energy of constant doing. This imbalance blocks intuition and guidance from the feminine, turning the vibrant, playful energy of the masculine into a punishing force that eats away at our energy, causing power leakage and burnout.

Apart from undervaluing feminine energies, we've also learned to reject our feminine identity—our body, femininity, and sexuality. We relate to an external feminine identity instead of our soul's feminine essence, affecting how we talk, act, dress, and express ourselves. Forgetting who we truly are in our feminine power can lead to wrong choices, relationships, and career paths, making us live as a shadow instead of the light we were born to be.

The left ovary invites us to take long walks, enjoy luxurious baths, daydream, and be creative, all of which replenish our feminine identity.

True protection is aligning with the truth of who you are.

The common imbalance I see is an underachieving left ovary with an overactive right ovary. Blocking feminine energy cuts off all the creative force available to us. There's no filter to let in only the good stuff and keep out the bad. Conversely, blocking negative energies threatening the feminine can also lead to a blockage, creating a paradox. Holding these blocks takes a lot of energy, leaving us open to receiving others' negative energy.

Blocking emotional and physical pain also hinders feminine intuition and creation, making decisions difficult and leaving us stuck and lacking energy and motivation. Growing up, many of us learned that femininity and sensuality don't align with success, so we rejected this part and chose the safe, strong, and valued masculine traits. We hid our vulnerability, compassion, and dreams because they seemed to work against us.

The left ovary can affect left muscles, leading to pelvic distortions, PMS, lower back and pelvic pain, PCOS, and ovarian cysts. Realigning with your true self is true protection. Remember, your left ovary is here to align and embody your radiant feminine self.

Reclaim your feminine nature by choosing beliefs that resonate with your lineage, following your gut feelings and intuition, and discovering your feminine gifts. It's time to dump old, outdated beliefs and realign with your truth.

Overactive Left Ovary

As women, we often take on more energy than we can handle, usually from caring for and overgiving to others. We frequently feel compelled to overcare for others while dismissing our own needs as unimportant or a luxury, reinforcing the belief that our worth in this world is tied to our actions.

As mothers, we might believe our worth is solely derived from how well we care for our children and others. We may have been conditioned to think that being a mum or caring for others is our primary purpose, with everything else coming second. We're expected to excel in various roles, from being a great cook and businesswoman to maintaining a perfect appearance and excelling in bed, all while managing a spotless house and coordinating everyone's schedules. The demands are endless, from school runs to family obligations, leaving little time for self-care, and most are self-inflicted.

Even if you don't have children, different stresses may place you at the end of your to-do list. The to-do list is never-ending, and taking care of your own needs often falls by the wayside. As a mum of four, I understand the struggle. The resentment and anger I harboured daily were becoming toxic to my health, marriage, and kids.

Changing our perspective on self-care is transformative, not just for ourselves but for everyone around us. Just like a car can't run on empty and needs regular attention, service, and fuel, we, too, require care and time away from life's demands. We need feminine nourishment and time to savour beautiful food, whilst moving our body in ways that are pleasurable and fill our energy body up. When our left ovary becomes overactive and burns out, it mirrors an underachieving ovary, depleting our feminine energy and leading to illness. It's crucial to prioritise self-care for our well-being and those we care for.

Right Ovary Manifestations

The right ovary is your powerhouse for projecting feminine energy into the world. Its role is to actively put your essence out there, driving visibility and projection. It shapes how you utilise your femininity, impacting your career, feminine roles, identity, power, and control. A balanced right ovary empowers you to step boldly into the world, manifest your desires, and fulfil your life's purpose. It fuels the energy needed for creation, work, healing, and the courage to be seen as the unique individual you were born to be.

When the right ovary is balanced, you effortlessly embody and project your feminine essence in all aspects of life. There's enough energy to both be and do everything you desire. However, imbalances arise when the left ovary lacks the reset and replenishment it needs. This disconnection from your feminine identity leads to projecting and working on things misaligned with your true self, resulting in frustration and feeling stuck in undesirable situations.

I often witness this misalignment in women who exert immense effort but don't experience the fulfilment they seek. The constant pursuit of achievements without true alignment leaves them feeling empty, driving them to quickly move on to the next goal in search of that elusive solution. It's like searching for that pot of gold at the end of the rainbow. The work environment, often designed in a linear, masculine way, adds complexity to this struggle. As cyclic feminine beings, the relentless pace and goal-oriented nature of work don't align with our natural rhythms—it's like forcefully pressing the gas pedal, depleting fuel, ruining the engine, and risking a breakdown.

In this frantic pace, it's easy to ignore warning signs, pushing the body to its limits. The body, mind, and soul become exhausted, leading to resentment, numbing out, and neglecting the inner whispers of the soul. The Modern Disease of the Modern Woman, marked by rushing and denial of the feminine, underlies many health-related problems. Simply addressing symptoms won't resolve this issue; true healing comes when you re-connect with your body, embrace the feminine, and restore balance to your energy, inner ecology, and body chemistry.

This might resonate with you if you find yourself creatively and expressively blocked. There's a deep, intuitive feeling of misalignment with who you are and your life's direction. When not in sync with the soul, everything feels off. We fear being seen and expressing ourselves, often resorting to our egoic persona, using fake masks and smiles to hide the feeling of being a fraud. Vulnerability is daunting, and we avoid eye contact to escape the discomfort. The masks we wear conceal our true emotions, and we strive to appear put together even when falling apart inside.

Many settle for less due to a lack of self-worth, believing they can't manifest their desires. This compromises personal power, leading to unexpressed rage and projecting blame onto others. Taking back our power involves acknowledging our role in giving it away, dispelling victimhood, and accepting responsibility. Relationships involve an energetic exchange, and balance is achieved when both partners fully contribute, avoiding dependency, projection and power loss.

Like a bird born to fly, we crave the wildness within, yearning for freedom from self-imposed limitations. Our 'cage' comprises societal roles, routines, and fears of the unknown. Reinventing ourselves, relationships, and routines keeps the inner fire burning. Underachieving right ovaries may lead to self-sabotage, avoiding the spotlight, and downplaying success due to feelings of failure. Dimming our light becomes a coping mechanism, resulting in stored anger and frustration.

We often wear practical, unremarkable clothing, seeking validation through safety rather than expressing our creative essence. Jealousy and comparison arise, hindering self-acceptance. Our health and relationships suffer when our feminine identity stems from obligation rather than essence. Disconnected from our desires, we may stifle our children and relationships, seeking external validation.

Reconnecting with our deep desires and embracing the feminine essence revives our vitality. It's like waking up to the beauty around us that we were too busy to notice. Our flourishing becomes a model for our children, impacting the decisions they make in their lives. Remember, children follow actions more than words; they do what we do, not what we say. Creating space for your dreams fulfils you and sets an example for your kids to do the same.

Overactive Right Ovary

When our right ovary is in overdrive, it's like boarding a fast train headed straight for burnout or a health crisis. Our modern lives, commitments, and routines are draining our vitality. Many of us are trapped in patterns of overachievement, goal setting, and constant doing without truly aligning with our needs, desires, and the essential practise of rest, replenishment, and repair.

Living on an empty tank and pushing hard for those extra miles harms our well-being. The relentless cycle of overextension, overwork, and undervaluing ourselves—what we mistakenly label as 'normal life'—must stop. Stopping, slowing down, and facing resistance are crucial steps. Fear of the unknown often keeps many women pushing themselves to the brink before acknowledging the need for change.

Taking an eagle view of our lives allows us to recognise self-destructive patterns. Aligning with our true feminine essence acts as our internal GPS, our north star, providing a roadmap to what we truly want and where we need to go. If we don't choose to stop willingly, life and our bodies have an innate way of making us stop. Too often, it's through pain or illness that could have been prevented and ultimately avoided.

Identifying women dominated by their right ovary is observable in their rushed, multitasking demeanour. Physically, they exhibit right-body dominance, with elevated neck, shoulder, and lower back tension. The constant state of readiness to run, wired adrenals, reliance on cortisol, and disrupted sleep patterns become evident. The pursuit of productivity, purpose, and an overly busy life drains energy, fuelled by a belief that being indispensable to others at work and home is the key to personal worth.

A core belief that we are not enough pushes many women to constantly seek something more, deeply fearing feeling irrelevant and invisible. Society's pressures to stay young and avoid blending into the background perpetuate this fear. The relentless quest for a particular purpose can make us lose touch with our authentic selves, leading to a constant struggle to prove our worth when, in truth, we are already enough.

Returning to the sacred womb within us, embracing the feminine aspects of ourselves, allows for the release of what holds us captive. Whether through menstruation or the lunar cycle, letting go physically and spiritually becomes a powerful practise. Realigning with the cyclic feminine soul, capable of seeding, growing, releasing, and renewing in every cycle, daily, monthly, and seasonally, empowers our transformative journey.

As the ovaries reawaken, you may feel some twinges or aches. She-Movement practises can be valuable for activating and unlocking stagnant ovarian and womb energy.

The Feminine and Spiritual Connection Between Your Sexual Organs, Womb, and Throat Chakra

Let's discuss the profound link between your throat and sexual organs—something deeply rooted in the physical, emotional, and spiritual aspects of your being. Chakra 2 (representing the sacral) and Chakra 5 (the throat) are intricately connected. While many chakras usually operate in pairs, my experience underscores the need to address these two simultaneously. It's no coincidence that the larynx lives in the CERVICAL spine and mirrors the anatomy of the CERVIX. During embryonic development, the larynx, mouth and jaw develop from the same embryonic membrane known as the ectoderm. The jaw and pelvis are also connected via deep fascial networks, which means that tension in the jaw can cause tension in the pelvis and vice versa.

In my work with the womb, I find that every woman harbours stuck energy in her pelvis, sexual organs, and throat. This accumulation, shaped over a lifetime, demands release. We rely on breath, movement, and, most importantly, sound to unlock this energy. Your voice becomes the vehicle for expelling deep-seated wounds from the womb. When we struggle to vocalise pain and guide it out, there's a limitation in clearing and a lack of emotional fluidity, which means we remain blocked. Alongside sexual repression lies the suppression of self-expression and your voice. Instances of self-deception, unspoken feelings, and withheld truths accumulate in your throat chakra, longing for release.

Case Study: Laura

Meet Laura, whose throat chakra was notably blocked, manifesting in persistent neck and jaw discomfort, leading to radiating shoulder pain and headaches.

Laura is a dedicated people-pleaser who cherishes maintaining harmony and helping others. However, over the past year, she sensed the need to assert herself by saying no. The fear of judgement and the worry about others' opinions held her back. Laura's inclination to feel needed can be traced back to her childhood when she took care of her mother, who was grappling with chronic depression. Her sense of love and worthiness became intertwined with doing for others.

As Laura endeavoured to reconnect with her truth and liberate years of self-denial, an unexpected surge of anger emerged. Buried rage and frustration from a lifetime of repression surfaced. She directed this anger towards her mother, resentful for not being the nurturing figure Laura needed and for burdening her with premature responsibilities. Laura grappled with mothering herself and her own mother, a role she shouldered throughout her life.

Upon releasing this pent-up pain and authentically expressing her truth, Laura underwent a transformative journey. The revelation of her ability to say no allowed her to rediscover herself. With a newfound sense of empowerment, Laura awakened to her desires, and there was no turning back.

Mouth of the Goddess

A lesser-known but highly significant aspect of our female anatomy and chakra system is 'the mouth of the Goddess,' also known as the atlas major chakra. This often-overlooked area plays a crucial role in unlocking transformation and profound healing, particularly for women. Activating the Shakti energy through this sacred portal can awaken intuition and sacred wisdom.

As a chiropractor, I've come to appreciate the importance of the atlas bone, situated at the top of your neck, where your head rests. Over my chiropractic career, I've observed that this bone tends to be stuck in most individuals I work with. Physically, a blocked atlas can manifest as neck pain, headaches, poor posture, and, interestingly, for some, lower back pain, dizziness, and tinnitus. Misalignment of the atlas bone can lead to low energy levels and persistent fatigue, as its nerves are closely connected to the lower brain stem and the vagus nerve.

From a spiritual perspective, when the atlas is misaligned, it restricts the amount of light the chakra in this area receives, impacting the overall energy flow throughout the body. While claims about it being a portal to other worlds lack scientific evidence, in my experience, aligning the atlas bone often corresponds to a holistic transformation—physically, emotionally, chemically, and spiritually. The benefits vary based on an individual's placement on their spiritual journey, but the tangible physical improvements alone make realigning the atlas a worthwhile pursuit.

The Feminine Alchemical Power of your Heart and Breasts

Let's explore the profound connection between the breasts, heart, and Chakra 4—the primary power centre for women. The energy flowing through this area influences our sense of aliveness and empowerment. Many of us have experienced heartbreak, leading to the shutting down of this vital region. As a result, physical manifestations such as neck pain, headaches, and poor posture often emerge, signalling unresolved traumas and the struggle to forgive.

It is essential to tackle emotional blockages to mend the energy in the heart and breasts and rejuvenate the life force confined within. Stagnation in this area may contribute to physical issues, including breast cancer, cysts, heart disease, and lung problems. Even with a healthy lifestyle, a blocked heart energy centre can pose a risk to overall well-being.

Closed hearts typically result from past hurts, prompting the construction of emotional walls that hinder trust and openness. The problem is that we are blocking both positive and negative experiences, numbing our feelings and relegating us to living in our heads to avoid pain. A dysregulated nervous system, dominated by cortisol, leads to feelings of numbness, coldness, and distance from ourselves and others.

When Chakra 4 is open, love flows freely without attachment, just like in our early experiences before we learned that hearts could break. However, maintaining a consistently open heart in the modern world is impractical. This is where a robust Chakra 3 becomes crucial, acting as the gatekeeper for Chakra 4. A weak Chakra 3 results in poor boundaries, leading to overgiving, overcaring, and burnout.

Striking a balance between over-giving and withholding requires cultivating a strong Chakra 3. For many women raised to be 'good girls,' prioritising others' needs over their own becomes a habitual pattern. This adherence to societal expectations stifles intuition and instincts, trapping them in a cycle of seeking external validation for self-worth.

A closed Chakra 3 leads to exhaustion, resentment, and projection of blame onto others. Recognising and acknowledging these patterns is crucial to breaking free from victimhood. You can redirect your energy toward positive change by making conscious choices and embracing self-responsibility.

Persistent resentment, judgements, and negative beliefs contribute to bitterness, impacting physical and spiritual health. An imbalanced heart centre can cause conditions such as osteoarthritis, osteoporosis, a hunched back, breast cancer, heart problems, and more. Achieving balance and homeostasis requires releasing negative thoughts and emotions that pollute the body, mind, and spirit.

The heart and breasts are about giving and receiving love and pursuing one's passions and dreams. Incorporating activities you love into your life is essential for soul nourishment. Despite common excuses like being too busy or lacking time and money, being fully present in the moment is a conscious decision that can lead to greater happiness.

Resistance and fear often obstruct our path to happiness, but breaking through these barriers can elevate us to a more joyful state. Embracing change starts with saying yes and engaging in activities that align with your true desires. Remember, happiness is an inside job.

Heartbreak over unfulfilled dreams is a common struggle, but confronting the broken dreams from your childhood can bring clarity. Acknowledge and release your feelings through journaling, self-expression, and She-Movement practises. Make it a mission to break free from the chains of resentment and bitterness that have held you captive in this lifetime. Being radically truthful with yourself and addressing the truth is essential for healing—after all, we can't heal what we are unconscious of.

Your Beautiful Breasts

Let's rethink the power of breasts beyond societal norms—they're not just objects for pleasure or nurturing babies. Throughout history, we've relinquished the rightful power of our breasts, and now it's time to reclaim that innate strength for self-nurturing.

The breasts embody feminine energy and hold the incredible power of healing. They possess the unique ability to transform negative emotions into positive ones.

Our breasts often store negative thoughts and stagnant emotions, impacting lymph and blood circulation in this delicate, hormonally active tissue. The use of tight underwire bras and poor posture further disrupt the energy circuit within the breasts. Is it any wonder we face so many breast-related issues?

Breasts are composed mainly of lymphatic tissue and have the transformative power to detoxify by turning negativity into positivity and releasing old wounds. Your breasts are truly magical forces of nature, and tuning into them will reveal this profound connection.

Many women have become disconnected from their breasts, influenced by societal expectations of size and appearance. This disconnection often begins at an early age during puberty, leading to shame and attempts to hide their changing bodies. Mixed messages from the media about breast appearance contribute to self-consciousness, shame, and humiliation, intensifying with age and after having children.

Fear surrounds discussions about breasts, especially concerning breast cancer. Some women avoid touching their breasts due to the fear of finding a lump. This fear-driven disconnect leads to numbness, preventing us from truly feeling and trusting our breasts.

Your breasts are more than society tells you. They possess a highly sensory nature, extending beyond sensuality and sexuality to a kind of sixth sense. They sense the environment around them, communicating directly with your hormones. The breasts can produce milk based on chemical changes, ensuring the right amount, consistency, and nutrient content for your baby.

In Taoism, we learn about six meridians running through breast tissue. Blocked meridians increase the risk of breast cancer, and they are influenced by emotions like anger, negativity, worry, unforgiveness, chronic stress, and overwhelm. Waking up to your aliveness, clearing energetic blocks, and improving lymphatic drainage can significantly benefit you and your breasts.

Consider avoiding restrictive bras that impede blood and lymph drainage, potentially linked to cysts and breast cancer. Bras, often viewed as a patriarchal invention, mentally and psychologically restrain women. Opting for supportive crop tops, bralettes, or going braless can offer freedom.

Regular breast massage and stimulation aid blood and lymph circulation, reducing toxins and hormone accumulation. Skin-friendly oils like lavender and rose can enhance this practise. Avoid toxic cleaning products and household items containing chemicals and oestrogens which directly impact hormone-receptive breast tissue.

What you give attention to grows, and this applies to your breasts. Women who regularly massage their breasts often experience visible changes—less pain, increased firmness, bounce, and even a rounder and lifted appearance. The crucial aspect is developing a relationship with your breasts and learning to love them just as they are.

Breasts reside in the energy centre of Chakra 4, offering a way to open our hearts and release physical and emotional blockages. Your breasts and heart are interconnected, necessitating simultaneous healing. If your heart is closed, it affects your breast tissue, making it limp and lifeless. Initiating a regular breast massage practise may release built-up emotions, and guidance from a trained sexual teacher can be invaluable for navigating these emotions, especially if carrying unprocessed trauma.

As you engage with your shakti and sexual energy, you'll discover how to channel the flow of aliveness into your breasts and heart. Ensuring these energy centres are open allows you to fully receive all the transformative benefits. Your shakti will naturally clear energy blocks in your body, and focusing on your breasts provides a head start, fostering even more profound healing and transformation.

Physiological Reasons for Breast Massage

A regular breast massage routine not only awakens oxytocin but also plays a crucial role in regulating the nervous system and boosting feel-good hormones throughout your body. This practise is a powerful tool to re-establish the mind-body-spirit connections that might have become disrupted over time. Moreover, it revitalises your senses, making you more attuned and alive, heightening sensitivity in your breasts and nipples, and alleviating numbness and pain. Stimulation of blood circulation and lymphatic drainage work together to reduce fibrocystic tissue and cysts that tend to accumulate in our breasts.

It's essential to acknowledge that every woman's sensitivity to breast tissue varies. Factors such as past surgeries, cyst removals, previous experiences with cancer, biological distinctions, trauma, and emotional blockages can influence this sensitivity.

In addition to housing six meridian pathways, the breasts are intricately connected to numerous nerves, particularly the vagus nerve. Regular breast massage can serve as a holistic practise, promoting overall well-being by nurturing both the physical and energetic aspects of your body.

Benefits of Breast Massage

- Increased sensitisation
- Increases milk flow while breastfeeding
- Clears emotional blocks
- Helps with lymphatic drainage and toxin buildup
- Increases circulation
- Regulates nervous system
- Releases oxytocin, the feel-good hormone
- Opens the heart
- Prepares the sexual organs for sex
- Stimulates your 'turn-on'
- Nipple orgasms (yes, there is such a thing)

Breast Massage Practise

Breast massage is the first thing I focus on when teaching sacred sexuality. I love to use breast massage to accompany jade egg practises, but I also use it for clients who need to reopen their hearts.

Sacred breast massage should be taught in a sacred circle or container because this work is ancient and powerful and, when used properly, is highly transformational. So, to honour the Sacred Rose Lineage and all the teachers who came before me, I will teach a basic lymphatic drainage massage in this book.

In this exercise, I want you to change the relationship you have with your breasts and heart, developing more profound love and communication between your body and soul essence.

You can do this massage with your clothes on or with bare breasts using a skin-friendly oil. I use jojoba oil.

Let's Begin...

Sit in a chair or on the edge of a bed. Slow your breathing and start rubbing your hands together to create heat.

Place your hands on your breasts, breathe, and feel their weight, the softness, and the contours of them. Release any anxiety or negative feelings that come up. You can journal about them later.

Start by touching your nipples slowly and softly, rubbing them between your thumbs and forefingers, being mindful of how they feel. Breathe into any numbness or pain.

From the nipple, begin stroking the breast in a clockwise direction. This direction helps to clear any negativity or stagnation in your body and breasts. Feelings of shame, unworthiness, and deep sorrow can be released here. You can do this up to 36 times. Remember to breathe, and relax, and be gentle.

In your mind's eye, imagine that you are clearing negative feelings, energy, and blood out of the breasts. You can visualise a colour if this helps and see it leaving your breast tissue. On a physical level, this direction and movement helps to release built-up toxins, increases lymphatic drainage, and increases the circulation in the breast tissue. If you do not have breast cancer, repeat this in a counterclockwise direction. Now, as you breathe in, imagine your breasts filled with a bright white light, full of vitality and love—clean and sparkly. As you exhale, visualise any negative emotions or feelings leaving your body, allowing the exhale to help you surrender and melt into the heart.

*PLEASE NOTE: If you have breast cancer, avoid this counterclockwise massage of the breasts. After the clockwise direction, simply hold your breasts and visualise health, vitality, and healing, filling up your breast tissue.

Hold the breasts on either side of the nipples, inhale and exhale, and be in the present moment, letting go of the past and the need to be anything more than what you are right now in this moment. Feel your heart and breasts open, full of love, innocence, and a sense of wonder. Cup the breasts and whisper beautiful things to them, to you.

CHAPTER 9
THE PATRIARCHY

'Women whose wisdom is in dreams,
Where do I go to find images of women, women made?
Our wisdom cannot be lost and our spirit cannot be broken
Awaken to your power.'
—*Marya Stark, 'Awaken to your Power'*

I invite you to take a breath and bring your awareness down into your womb space. Tune into the energy here. Bringing our energy into our womb area can bring up a lot of discomfort, shame, and feelings of fear and lack of safety that we want to push away. I invite you to breathe into these feelings, be with them, and tell your body that she is safe.

You are safe to remember your history from this lifetime and others—from your ancestors that live within your DNA. There have been centuries of not feeling safe, hiding who we truly are, and it's time to bring this into the light so we can heal it individually and collectively. Moving forward into the future, we need to understand where we've come from and what we are carrying physically, emotionally, and spiritually.

Close your eyes—feel into this space, and the memories curled up in your DNA, tissues, and cells. Breathe in light and allow them to unfurl. It is safe. You are safe.

My lineage is Celtic. My roots come from Wales and Ireland. Understanding my lineage through past life regressions has led me to free up energy that had been trapped in other lifetimes where fear, suppression, and control of the feminine were normal. Often, fear in the body now can be a symptom of unresolved issues from your motherline or a past life. This may seem too far for your mind to stretch and grasp, but receive this chapter with your womb and with your heart. The mind wants to understand things through logic and order, and the feminine is none of that. She is the unknown—flowing, unpredictable, dark, chaotic, and sometimes a bit angry because she has been forgotten. I invite you to listen to her—She, of a thousand names, voices, and forms that live within you.

The way to make dreams come true is to wake up.

We all come from different lineages and levels of privilege based on where we live right now. We need to respect each other, honour our various stories, and acknowledge that many women are still not physically and culturally free of patriarchal oppression.

As females, we all share the same wound—our femininity has been bound, owned, betrayed, and violated throughout time. We all have fragments of the feminine wound deep within us. This chapter is here to awaken an understanding and deep gnosis within, offering a foundation in patriarchal culture and how it has and still causes fear and stress.

When I use the word *patriarchy*, I'm not talking about men. This isn't a 'feminist women-against-men' party. This is about a system that affects both men and women. Patriarchy represents a societal framework marked by oppression and characterised by the dominance of a small group wielding power and establishing norms that shape our community. Historically, this system has permeated various facets of life, including religion, politics, education, healthcare, and governance, often operating beneath our conscious awareness yet influencing our thoughts, emotions, and behaviours to this day.

History, or 'HIS-STORY,' has traditionally been narrated from a male perspective, and the female counterpart, 'HER-STORY,' is often overlooked. The historical accounts we've been exposed to were predominantly written by men, leaving women without a voice—or at least one that was permitted to be documented. It's crucial to recognise that the history we encounter is often monolithic, probably patriarchal, and lacking the dualistic nature that encompasses the feminine truth.

Our voices and stories, relegated to the shadows, were concealed and transmitted through myth, legend, and symbols. Unravelling this mystery is a lifelong endeavour, and it's your responsibility to embark on this treasure hunt, discovering the hidden narratives that exist in plain sight, living and breathing within and around you. My aim is to show you how I believe the patriarchy was born, how it affected history, and how we are still dealing with its effects today.

I invite you to become aware of how your body is holding on to internalised patriarchal systems. If you are a woman alive today, you will have beliefs that you didn't consciously make about your body, femininity, sexuality, and your role in the world. These blueprints were passed on from generation to generation, from DNA to DNA, and from lifetime to lifetime. I believe we are living in times when all of it is ready to be healed. Most female illnesses come from the suppression and repression of our unconscious beliefs and stories. We haven't been able to fully express who we are, and some of us don't even know who we are or that there is anything wrong. Your body wants you to wake up and venture inside. She wants to show you herself. It's about coming home to her, to you, and to all the women who came before you.

Women have been conditioned to be excessive givers, often neglecting their boundaries and self-care. Each of us harbours our unique version of a victim mentality, blending elements of overachiever complexes and a pervasive feeling of inadequacy. The perpetual quest to validate our worthiness, both in the eyes of others and ourselves, drives us. From an early age, we were instilled with the idea of being 'good girls,' emphasising politeness and discouraging any disturbance. Societal norms often present conflicting messages, shaming women for their choices in ways not applied to men. This internalised shame and judgement become imprinted in us, affecting how we perceive ourselves and how we view and criticise other females. Consequently, this emotional wound intensifies, leading to a sense of disconnection from our true selves, our inner truth, and each other.

In today's world, we navigate the delicate balance of cultural archetypes, choosing between roles such as the good girl, mother, virgin, martyr, the servant, or the slut. Society often imposes labels like selfish, vain, or vixen, creating a spectrum of characters typically viewed negatively.

I recall the time when I was expecting my first daughter, Olivia. My mother-in-law was devastated by the news of having a girl. She actually said, 'Oh no, a boy's life is so much easier, poor thing. A boy would have been better.' The rage of injustice and maternal fury mixed with a good dose of hormones made me rip into her about how narrow-minded and selfish she was to say that. However, over the years, I now see this scenario differently and can resonate with her words and empathise with her pain.

My ex-mother-in-law's reality was different from mine. Born in the 1950s, it was hard for a woman; there were fewer choices. I understand how she was projecting her pain and suffering, not wanting that for her grandchild. Our mothers, grandmothers, and other women we know and love have all suffered at the hands of the patriarchy. They had fewer choices, no voice, less pay, and fewer work opportunities. Their roles were defined for them from an early age. Just look at how 1950s advertising reveals a woman's role as taking care of her husband's every need, with little concern for herself. A woman was portrayed as the cook, cleaner, mother, and wife—all done with a pristine, lipsticked smile. She was seen as never complaining and eternally grateful for being married to her perfect husband, completing her entire existence because she was incomplete and unworthy without him. The women of our past were treated as second-class citizens and were taught to bind, push, squeeze, and diet their bodies into the patriarchal fashions and ideologies of the moment. Our worth was defined by our appearance and how many babies we could have.

Times have changed; we have the vote, great jobs, and the potential to have it all. However, this also comes at a cost. Now, we are expected to do it all perfectly, just like men, yet we still, in some areas, earn less and have to keep up with all the household and kids while appearing as if we are doing it perfectly. It's like being stuck between a rock and a hard place, the ultimate classic catch-22. We have been taught to wear our achievements and struggles with honour, constantly pushing and proving ourselves.

When we're busy running around like headless chickens, disconnected from our bodies and feelings, focused on our future and others, never in the present moment, we can be easily controlled. How many of us say, 'When I lose weight, I will be happy,' or 'When I get that job or that man, I will feel complete'? We are constantly distracted by things that we are told will make us happy, loved, and worthy because we are shown and taught that we aren't lovable, beautiful, or enough just as we are. We spend our lives pushing, searching, and looking for the thing that will make us feel completely whole. We are distracted with everything 'out there' when the actual gold and all the answers lie inside us.

You are the philosopher's stone; you are everything you are searching for right now in this moment exactly as you are.

The true alchemist's journey is discovering who you *really* are, born perfect, divine, and whole; you have just been programmed not to see it. This is not a complete retelling of the patriarchal story, but it's a way to get you thinking and feeling and ultimately understanding where your beliefs have come from and why you act as you do. Discovering your own culture and indigenous lineages is so healing. In all of our ancient heritage lines, there was and is a remembrance of the sacred feminine. She still lives in you, and following your root system back through your lineage helps you uncover who you are.

A Journey Back In Time...

Once upon a time, a long time ago, the feminine was worshipped and adored. She was sacred—seen as the giver of all life. Her body was voluptuous, her hips and thighs bountiful, and she glowed with radiance and health. People worshipped the goddess, recognising her as the powerful Creatrix she is. Women's bodies were sacred; they lived and breathed in time with the moon and seasons. Intuition, feeling, and the feminine arts were sought after and respected as a way of life. The goddess manifested in various forms—fertility, creation, love, sensuality, healing, and the wise crone woman. She kept us in tune with the earth's rhythm, connected through the umbilical cord of the earth's heartbeat. We respected the earth and each other; we thrived.

Tribal life flourished before the Bronze Age in 4,000 BC; we lived in groups, not separately. Women's bodies were seen as powerful, magical vessels and were treated and respected accordingly. It was a time when our bodies would swell and grow with life, revealing the magical creation of the female body. All life came from her; there would be no life without women's wombs, which is powerful and magical in itself, yet many have forgotten or medicalised it. We have forgotten the magic that the body knew—how to make, grow, and deliver babies long before sterilisation and patriarchal control. We held that power, and we still do. Just like Mother Nature provides sun, water, and food, our bodies produce the life-giving milk with everything our baby needs to grow and flourish.

Nowadays, we lack confidence in our bodies and in nature. We often feel powerless and look to doctors for answers, afraid to trust our inner knowing. I understand technology has moved on, and for some women, it is the only way to have a baby. I praise the medical system for that and would be first in line if I needed their help. But the majority of women are giving away their magic and their power. Your body never needed to be monitored or controlled; it has always known. It is us who have forgotten.

Early depictions of goddesses that were worshipped show the fertility goddess as full and voluptuous, with heavy breasts, a beautiful booty, and a soft, expanding stomach. Over the years, our bodies have been corseted, covered, bound, restrained, pushed, and squeezed into a shape deemed acceptable and desirable by the patriarchy and powers that be. I also think this restraint had other advantages; it meant women literally couldn't move; hence, a restricted body leads to a restricted mind. We were shamed and looked down upon in society if we didn't wear the approved attire. If we showed an ankle or wrist out of context, our whole self-honour would be destroyed, and no one would want us.

Our body was seen as evil, an object to tempt and turn men to sin, just as Eve had 'supposedly' done in the Garden of Eden. Man's fall from Eden was 'her' fault (and ultimately, the fault of every woman who came after her). She had lured and tempted him with her body. Subconsciously, women have been paying the price for it ever since.

Ancient civilisations were home to priestesses, the revered women of sacred temples. These women were the guardians of profound wisdom and the custodians of women's rites of passage, embodying the essence of love and spiritual knowledge. Skilled in anointing, midwifery, healing, and the observance of seasonal customs, they honoured and worked with the cycles of the moon, the rhythms of the seasons, and the power of oracles and intuition. Their expertise extended to the use of herbs and natural remedies. As the spiritual backbone of their communities, these priestesses wove together the fabric of communal life. Knowledge was carefully passed down through generations, fostering a culture of love, peace, and a deep reverence for nature and its sacred laws.

For thousands of years, we worshipped the mother goddess, the Great Mother—she of many names like 'Gaia' and 'Sophia.' She was known as the creator and gave life to all things; we treated her Earth with respect. She was nature, nurture, birth, death, and rebirth; the seasons, the elements, the sun, the moon—she was the giver of life itself. When we respected the laws of nature and her mystical truths, all was good; everything, including humans, flourished. She was the embodiment of the feminine and masculine, and we were all connected to each other through her. When the patriarchy came in and took this away, both men and women became disconnected from who they really were, and we've all been searching for what we lost ever since.

Our sacred way of life—how we flourished, healed, and lived in harmony—was torn away by the patriarchy. Capitalism and the pursuit of power have kept us disconnected from ourselves and each other. Control and money became the driving forces, replacing wisdom and love. The church, wealthy landowners, governments, and the elite seized control, erasing the goddess and her priestesses. Our communities were shattered, and the values of greed, ego, and dominance took over.

They stole our spiritual practises, severing us from the power and magic within our bodies. We became obsessed with power, money, and status, driven by a need to fill an emptiness that only deepened. We turned against each other, always chasing the next paycheck, outfit, car, or home, thinking it would fill the void inside. This wound has been with us for centuries, passed down through generations, embedded in our very DNA.

The patriarchy has built firm foundations and structures in our world. Take a look around… How have you become compliant? Where have you given away your voice, power, and inner knowing?

Without the input of feminine perspectives, men and women alike are stuck in the routine of daily tasks, just a cog on the endless hamster wheel of the systems made to oppress us. We aim to be compliant citizens, avoiding questioning, minimising influence, and steering clear of controversy due to unspoken but palpable fear. We've come a long way in the last half a century, but it's the tip of the iceberg.

Here are a few ways we find ourselves trapped in this system with the patriarchy still controlling the feminine body:

- Lower pay than a man for the same job
- Hair removal
- Magazine and photo filtering
- Plastic surgery
- Anti-aging industry
- Porn
- Control and ownership of women
- Rape
- Stereotyping gender
- Erasing of the feminine landscape

Connecting to Our Sensuality

In many religious institutions, anything related to the female body is considered dirty or sinful. Our sensuality and menstruation have been labelled as wrong and unclean. Consider how we are programmed to need to purchase 'feminine hygiene products' to make our yoni smell better, as our natural odour is deemed disgusting and unclean. We've all bought into these beliefs at some point in our lives.

Our culture is confusing; we're expected to be sexy but also know when not to be. It can drive you crazy trying to wear all the masks to fit into the patriarchal norm. Sensuality is marketed as both dangerous *and* desirable. When we embrace our sensuality, we're accused of tempting men, and if anything happens to us, we're blamed for it. Many women who have experienced rape or sexual assault carry guilt, thinking that if they had dressed differently or not been so friendly, they wouldn't have given the wrong message. This mindset is nonsense, and deep down, we know it. We should be free to be ourselves without fearing for our bodies and safety.

Connecting to our sensuality empowers us; it links us to a source through our bodies. However, we've been conditioned not to explore this, keeping us away from our life force, power, and soul. It's a crucial piece of the puzzle missing in many of us. When we believe our sensuality is dangerous or untrustworthy, fearing judgement or loss of control, it's no wonder many of us live in our heads, disconnected from our bodies.

Mary Magdalene, long misrepresented as the repentant prostitute and sinful woman forgiven by Jesus, was distorted by patriarchal interpretations. She was not the repentant whore we were led to believe. Evidence now suggests that she was an original disciple and even authored a gospel, rediscovered in the last century along with other lost Gnostic texts. The true story of Mary Magdalene, as presented in the New Testament, was incomplete. After centuries of neglect and distortion, she is finally reclaiming her rightful place in Christianity. In France, July 22 is Magdalene Feast Day—a day dedicated to her, commemorating her death and serving as a national occasion to correct the record, honour women who have been unfairly accused, judged, and shamed, and address the pain passed down through generations due to these false narratives.

Can you imagine if we had been told the truth about Mary Magdalene as a disciple, not as a whore? As a woman of equal importance to the male disciples, fully accepted by Jesus? How would this have changed the narrative and the lives of the women who followed? The implications for us as women are profound.

You might wonder why and how this happened. It's another classic case of HER-STO-RY not being told. I encourage you to delve deeper into this topic and the distorted HIS-STORY we have been fed. This story has affected us all, fostering hate and distrust in ourselves and the feminine based on misinformation rather than truth.

The Witch Hunts

'The connections between and among women are the most feared, problematic,
and potentially transforming force on the planet.'
—Adrienne Rich

Let's talk about the word 'witch.' The patriarchy has twisted and weaponised this term to create fear, superstition, and distrust towards the feminine. Witches were depicted as devil worshippers, casting evil spells with dark animals, wearing pointy hats, and having old, warty skin. This distorted image was designed to discourage girls from embracing their natural magic and connection to the earth. As a result, we suppressed our magical instincts, stopped talking to trees, flowers, and stars, and dismissed our imaginary friends. We tucked these experiences away, buried them deep within, and never spoke of them again. Over time, we forgot our true selves and conformed to a patriarchal world for the sake of safety.

Growing up, many of us turned to Disney films, which often portrayed a narrow, submissive version of femininity—the beautiful princess waiting for a prince to rescue her and fulfil her dreams, as if we were powerless to do so ourselves. Can you relate? While modern Disney characters now feature more empowered female leads, today's young girls face even stronger influences, often getting lost in social media's expectations for appearance and behaviour to gain love and acceptance. The early conditioning of our girls is a worrying trend, and it's our responsibility to guide them once we recognise what's really happening.

In 1484, the pope ordered the church to find and execute all witches, often denying them the right to a fair trial. If I had lived then, I would have likely been the first on the stake. As a chiropractor, I heal with my hands, not to mention other energy-healing practises that might be considered a bit witchy.

Any of the following could have led to you being burnt at the stake:

- Healer
- Midwife
- Herbalist
- Potion-maker
- Intuitive
- Accusations of infidelity
- Palm reader
- A physical threat to men or other women
- Too sexy or sensual
- Outspoken
- Truth-teller
- Basically, any strong woman

Contrary to the negative portrayal, a witch is a wise woman connected to nature, the elements, seasons, cycles, plants, and her own body. She uses intuition to heal and help others, and she emphasises the importance of healing and protecting the earth.

Some of us might be feeling the pressure—literally. If you have crystals, tarot cards, or spiritual books at home, you might feel judged. Anyone—a spiteful neighbour, a jealous lover, or a vengeful friend—could point a finger and accuse you of being a witch. We once lived in constant fear for our lives, unable to trust anyone, especially other women who might betray us to save themselves. The pain, mistrust, and betrayal from that time still linger in our blood and DNA.

Back then, the punishments for women accused of witchcraft were severe, as this crime against the church was seen as the most sinful. The agenda was clear: divide and conquer. They broke us down, making us renounce our beliefs, our bodies, and each other. They wanted us to live in fear, giving them control over the feminine—our bodies, our creativity, and our lives. This left us lost, afraid, and distrusting of ourselves and each other, treated as property to be owned, sold, or bartered for.

Our fathers, brothers, and husbands owned us. We were traded for land, status, money—you name it. We had no voice, no say. Our voices were silenced, buried, and kept safe until a time—like now—when it's finally safe to be heard and to speak our truth.

While not applicable to every woman in today's modern world, some cultures still witness women enduring oppression and repression. We are responsible for reclaiming our voice and power, recognising that empowering one woman benefits the entire collective.

Throughout history, the patriarchy crafted a new, more palatable but less empowered image of femininity. This model became a societal obligation for all women aspiring to be socially acceptable, safe, and alive. A woman's existence was considered devoid of gender unless her husband needed an heir. Sexual activity for women was solely for reproduction;

any enjoyment was deemed sinful. The expectation was to remain a virgin until marriage and to embody submission. Women's bodies and menstruation were labelled as sinful and shameful. They were regarded as property first by their families and then by their husbands. In this framework, women had no rights. Women distrusted one another and turned against each other, giving rise to the sister wound. This wound persists in many of us today, leading to a sense of isolation. Even now, we can all recall instances where we've been wronged by fellow women—slut-shamed, judged, outcast, or looked down upon for being perceived as smarter, prettier, or a threat.

We carry the weight of feeling that if we were our authentic selves, no one would like us, and we wouldn't fit in. Consequently, we wear masks to be liked, seeking safety and acceptance while withholding our true feelings and keeping our hearts closed. I believe this behaviour stems from the collective consciousness shaped by the historical context of that time.

How is this showing up now?

I refer to this as the 'something's missing' dilemma. Nine times out of ten, women tell me, 'I have everything I thought should and would make me happy: a great partner, healthy kids, I'm comfortable... I should be fulfilled and happy, but there is just this thing that's missing, and I just can't put my finger on it. I've tried therapy, pills, talking about it... it all helps for a short while, but there is this dull ache, a hole inside that I just can't seem to fill.'

I respond, 'Yes, of course, you thought your primary reason for coming to this earth was just to be a wife and a mother, bring home the bacon, and do it with a smile!' This indoctrination that we are here to fulfil our roles as mothers and wives is what trips us up and has kept us bound for centuries. Yes, we can be loving wives, mothers, daughters, and friends, but that is not your soul's purpose and reason for your existence. Is it any wonder you feel like something is missing? Your soul is screaming out for you to wake up to who you really are, to this brainwashing that is still controlling us. We need to remember that our worth is not solely based on our ability to mother and be a good wife. Your role is not just to bring babies into this world for the capitalist society to create the workforce for the elite few who control everything.

I see this in women who are confused about whether they want to have kids; they feel pressured, judged, and less worthy because they choose not to be a mother. It is deeply ingrained into our psyche that a woman's worth comes from her ability to produce off-spring. Your worth, my worth, every woman's worth is not based on her having kids; we've just been programmed to believe this. I have four children whom I love dearly, and they are my world, but they are not my sole purpose for being here on this planet.

Wandering Womb

It was only in the last century that women were locked away in institutions for being hysterical or not obeying their husbands. If they deviated from societal expectations, they were deemed insane and locked up. The term 'wandering womb' was used to describe women experiencing severe premenstrual syndrome (PMS) and menopausal symptoms.

Upon moving to the Netherlands, I was surprised to learn that the pubic bone is referred to as the 'shame bone.' Women told me they experienced pain in their shame bone, and the sublingual energy surrounding this issue speaks for itself. It serves as a subconscious reminder that we are meant to feel shame and our sexuality is viewed negatively. The fact that this term is still in use highlights how far we still have to go.

Past Life Regression

I was hesitant about delving into past life regression work. The idea of exploring things that truly terrified me made me avoid it, but deep down, I knew there were unresolved issues that needed clearing. Our souls and energy systems carry the weight of lifetimes, creating invisible cords that bind us to the past. Past life regression is a powerful tool to remove these blocks, allowing us to move forward in life unburdened, free from the lingering ties to our history.

Clearing past lives helps release a multitude of blocked emotions and beliefs. Personally, I had to clear seven past lives before fully embracing and practising this work. Overcoming my fears, a deep-seated anxiety that even made me fear for my life at times, was transformative. The key lies in soul-changing experiences, freeing fragments of our soul trapped in lifetimes of trauma, often unknown to us.

I look around the room; it's a small cottage with one room where someone sleeps, cooks, and lives. It's set in the Middle Ages. A small window in one corner lets in a feeble light, but the rest is filled with smoke from the dying fire. The darkness makes it difficult to discern who is in the room with me, but I sense the presence of another. My eyes gradually adjust to the light, and I see her—I see myself. I step back in horror; there, in the corner of the room, is my body attached to the wheel of a cart. My arms and legs are spread, and I am bound and gagged. Dried blood runs from my wrists and ankles, starting around my ripped skirt. My blouse is torn and dirty, my hair mangled, my eyes dead, yet I am still alive. I want to run away, but I'm paralysed in fear of who might come and catch me. I step towards her, knowing I can't leave her like this. Our eyes meet, and instantly, I realise this is a fragment of my soul stuck here on the Earth plane. This is a part of me that I need to retrieve. To become whole again, I must set free this part of my soul. We both need to be set free.

As I walk over to her, her story starts flowing through me. She had been given the gift to help women birth their babies; a secret passed on from mother to mother. She had been at a birth assisting a young mother when someone had reported her. Her husband, furious with shame and disobedience, kept her here, barely alive, as punishment. She knew it was a matter of time before she was turned over to the authorities and executed for her crime of midwifery. She feels broken inside and bound physically and spiritually. She feels betrayed by her friends, the community, and her husband.

Words come to me, and I hear myself saying, 'I'm going to free you; together, we are going to get out of here.' She looks at me, and her face starts to change. I see hope, love, and recognition. She sees me, realises that she is me, and says, 'I have been waiting so very long for you to come for me.' Suddenly, a beautiful white light appears above her head. I see her transform before my eyes. The light envelops her, evaporates her, and she is free—I am free. I see her before me, surrounded and encased in the white light. I see the woman she was and is—strong, beautiful, wise. We lock eyes one last time, and I feel the part of me that was trapped leave my body. A fragment of my soul has returned to me. I feel lighter and more free.

The history of witch hunts attempted to erase the untold story of the persecution of women. These women weren't witches; they were individuals like you and me, perceived as threats. I urge you to recognise your own power deep within and reclaim the magic that is your birthright. It's time to awaken and embrace your healing.

Let the memories awaken within. Let them come to the surface to be healed.

Our Place in Christianity

I'm bringing up Christianity because it's a story we all know, and it has been the backbone of every rule, belief, and action made for women in the Western world. I think it's important to briefly examine how this has affected us. Also, I'm a geek, and I did theology A level 25 years ago, which taught me to question and dig deeper. I want to express that I respect your beliefs, and I'm not trying to change the way you think. All I'm doing is planting a seed, and if that wants to grow, then you can go with it, or you can just skip this bit.

Around 400 AD, the first widespread version of the Bible was compiled, including all 39 books of the Old Testament and the 27 books of the New Testament. Constantine, a Roman Emperor, chose these books, and his influence greatly affected Christianity as we know it today. The books were selected as a tool for power. The authorities didn't appreciate Jesus teaching that one could find God within. Constantine decreed that to get close to God, one had to go to a church and go through a priest or a king, taking all the power away from the individual and placing it in a church system. It became an effective way to get people to fall in line and conform. God became a big white, angry, punishing Man in the sky, and women were blamed for the fall of men. The New Testament provided rules on how to keep women in their place, controlling and owning them. It gave man the power over whether one went to heaven or hell and justified taking taxes and land. The Bible was used to invade, destroy, and kill, all in the name of religion. The feminine was lost, and the masculine was left out of balance.

Important Parallels Between Paganism and Christianity

The birth story of Jesus was chosen to be celebrated at the same time as the long-held pagan celebration of light. For years, we celebrated the winter solstice, the darkest and longest day of the year. Placing the birth of Jesus here made it more acceptable to welcome the 'light of the world' because we had been doing it for thousands of years. However, what happened was a complete takeover of our traditions and connection to nature, re-placed with religious traditions. Hence, the light of the world, Jesus' birthday, was placed here so they would accept it, even though we now know that his birthday wasn't even on that date! This merging continued with Easter, the death and resurrection, which replaced the celebration of life in spring, representing the earth rebirthing life, everything coming back to life from the dead of winter. Can you see the parallel? It was a time for us to reawaken to the energy inside us.

The recovery of the Gnostic gospels, especially the Gospel of Mary Magdalene, has led to a rediscovery and remembering of collective wisdom that has been lost to us. This knowledge has the power to rewrite our history and how we see, feel, and act with our bodies as women. Learning more about the true origins of Christianity can challenge your belief system and be very uncomfortable. We have taken a lot for granted over the years and have followed ways, rules, ideas, and beliefs that we thought were there to pro-tect us but, perhaps, in truth, were meant to control us. It's time to look at your beliefs and decide what you want to keep and what you want to live your life by. Living on autopilot in a system designed by the patriarchy, not questioning your mind, heart, and soul, is going to subconsciously affect your life and health.

Knowledge is power; it's time to take your power back.

I was brought up as a Christian, went to church school, Sunday school, church on Sundays, sang in the church choir, and sat through countless sermons telling me how I was a sinner and how I should be living my life. I heard so many stories about all these men who seemed to have all the answers and rules. One day in my late teens, I sat there listening to the sermon preaching, and I remember thinking, 'Where are all the women's voices? Why is it all about men?'

I started to question things; I wanted answers, but no one had them. My parents thought I was going through a phase, and everyone thought I was just trying to cause trouble. I understand now they just didn't know, and not knowing made them defensive because their whole life was built around this belief system.

The church school I attended had separate stairs for the girls because we weren't al-lowed to go down the same stairs as the boys. I used to think it was because the boys had a better position, but now I realise the 'powers that be' feared us showing our pants or getting too close to the opposite sex. Our skirts were measured, our hair yanked up, ties worn—any essence of our female identity stripped away. We were supposed to look like boys. Our periods and our bodies were hidden from others but also from ourselves. This is how shame creeps in. We fear what we don't know.

Studying theology opened my eyes, and I abandoned my faith like I believe it aban-doned me. I didn't find God or love in church; I found sin, blame, persecution, gossip, and lies. The Bible, for me, became another cage, another way to show me how I should behave in this world if I wanted to be loved and accepted. It triggered my core wounds of rejection, perfection, and the need to be loved and belong.

It's Time to Wake Up

My personal belief is that the patriarchy and religion in the past, along with pharmaceutical science today, have wanted and needed us to remain unconscious of the power within. I believe this to be true for many reasons, the most important being control, money, power, and energy. When we are separated from each other, from the source, nature, the power of the body, and universal intelligence, we are very easy to manipulate and control. The truth I want you to hear is that there is no separation of your mind, body, and spirit. You are always connected to God, the universal life force, the universe, or whatever you want to call it. There is only wholism, that feeling of deep inner knowing that keeps us searching, craving, and yearning for an aliveness we can't quite reach but intuitively know exists, even when everything around tells us it doesn't.

Living out of alignment, separated from the whole, leads to dis-ease of the body, mind, and spirit. Your divine human journey is about finding your way back to wholeness. Healing is the journey back home, becoming whole again. As you become more conscious, you will begin to reject the thoughts, opinions, beliefs, and behaviours that stem from the patriarchy, and you will start to see everything, including yourself, through a lens of wholism.

What is in one is in the whole.

Bringing the Sacred Feminine Into Your Life

I often receive questions from clients like, 'How do I bring the sacred feminine into my life?' and 'How does it fit into my religion or belief system about God, the universe, and everything I was brought up to believe was true?' My answer is to feel what resonates as truth in your body and take what works for you.

I invite you to examine how you've been taught to worship something outside yourself. The divine lives in you and in every human on this planet, not somewhere out there in a male version that you can't and were never supposed to relate to.

The sacred is within you.

When we start exploring all the magic and feminine gifts it holds, we wake up to the divine within. As the missing piece, you have been there all along; you just got distracted and were told it was in something or someone outside yourself.

Coming home into your body—your soul's home—can be challenging and confronting. We can use all sorts of avoidance techniques because it requires that we feel everything—the pain, the pleasure, the shadow, and the light. As the layers of fear dissolve and walls start to come down, we find the love that has always been there, patiently waiting.

With this book, I hope you start to wake up to the truth that *you* are who you need to worship—the sacredness in you made in the image of God. Not an off-planet old man god waiting for you to mess up so he can punish you, but a living, breathing universal creative consciousness that lives and breathes in everything. I believe that Christ consciousness, the actual teaching that Jesus came here to teach, is for every human, male and female, to know they are loved and connected to God and the universe within. As above, so below—the sacred masculine and the divine feminine married within. You can have direct contact with your soul, God/Universe, whenever you need and want to. But you won't find it outside yourself and don't need another person to act as an intermediary.

This idea of power and the source of everything that lives within is what I think scares the patriarchy the most. Religion has dictated how we should connect to the outside God, teaching us that there is a guideline, and it's only available for the select chosen few. It gives them power and control over society, allowing men to kill and destroy nations in the name of religion. Religion, to me, is patriarchal, political, and a controlling system of man-made laws and orders that create separation, which eventually leads to conflict. We are all connected to this universal force and are only answerable to universal laws. What is in one is in the whole. You can call it whatever you want, but no one owns the right to God or your energy. As we begin to wake up to this truth, we realise that we are more powerful than we ever could imagine. How we treat each other and our planet, even ourselves, influences every living thing. Start paying attention to your thoughts, beliefs and actions every day. You have the power to raise the vibration of yourself and this planet or lower it. Being powerful and having freedom of choice comes with consequences for ourselves and others, remembering that for every action, there is an equal reaction.

Deep down, we all know there's a voice within our soul, quietly trying to get our attention amidst the busyness of life. We often tell ourselves we're too busy or that we'll deal with it later, as we focus on finding fulfilment in external things—exercise, diets, the perfect body, partner, job, or life we think will make us whole and fill the emptiness inside. But please, take a moment to listen with your heart and your womb. Trust your intuition while still acknowledging your logical mind. You are what you've been searching for all along. Let this truth resonate in your body.

You are a sacred being.

Your purpose is to remember who you truly are. Knowing your body as both human and divine is how you know your soul. Love must exist first between us and ourselves, and then it can exist between you and another. The light of love, God, the great mother, the sacred masculine, and the divine feminine all exist within you, and it is my prayer that you begin to lift the veil and become awake.

We need to remember the past so we can recreate the future.

Practise:

Light a candle, and put on some soft, relaxing music to drown out background noise. I invite you now to go inside your body and look at all the internalised patriarchy and pain that your body is holding on to. Where have you been suppressing, desensitising, and excessively controlling in order to conform? Where do your scars lie?

Take some time, close your eyes, and start to slow down your breathing. Take the breath slowly into your body. Start to be aware of how your body feels. Is there any tightness, numbness, or emotion? Don't judge what you feel—be with it and breathe. Stay like this for 10 minutes, and when you've finished, grab your journal and answer the following questions, allowing your intuition to guide the words that flow:

- What are you scared of?
- What is holding you back? Where do you think it comes from? (Don't go for the obvious, dig deeper.)
- What were you brought up believing that you didn't question?
- What religious views were you taught?
- How were women spoken about and viewed in your childhood?
- How do you feel about your period and sex?
- What does sensuality mean to you?
- Where don't you feel safe to be yourself?
- Where is your worth? Is it based on what you have or how you look?
- Are you striving for perfection in your body and life? Where does this come from?

Research your own lineage so you can learn and recognise how your history and lineage of the feminine have been shaped by the patriarchy. The patriarchy knew if they conditioned women to be fearful, overgiving, sexless, second-class citizens by removing the sacred feminine, we would be controllable. What would happen if this sacred feminine wisdom and magic were reawakened and re-integrated into your body and life?

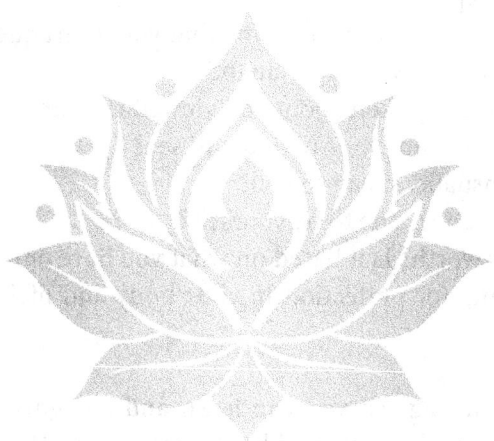

CHAPTER 10
THE MAGIC OF MENSTRUATION

'Nothing in our society, with the exception of violence and fear, has been more effective in keeping women in their place than the degradation of the menstrual cycle.'
—Christine Northrup

Your menstruation is part of what makes you a woman; it's your superpower, yet many women live in dread and hate their periods. Culturally, we've been indoctrinated to believe that menstruation is dirty, unclean, inconvenient, painful, and a curse. I'm here to tell you that it is an archetypal myth made up by the patriarchy that we have all swallowed whole and manifested as our reality.

The ancients referred to menstrual blood as 'heavenly waters.' Menstruation is a healthy purification process. It's a time when our body can eliminate the build-up of excess fats, proteins, and toxins. The body releases these impurities physically and energetically, enabling us to rebalance, restore, and regenerate suppressed emotions and psychological debris. When we allow the flow and invite in this process, we begin to purify, working with our cycle rather than against it. In other words, we move more into ourselves than outside of ourselves. Our health, hormones, and life become more balanced, and we have less pain and PMS.

Throughout history, women's menstrual cycles have been known to be a powerful, mysterious force of nature that should be deeply respected. But today, they are no more than an inconvenient red mark on a calendar—the 'thing' that holds us back, giving us cramps, headaches, pain, heavy clotty bleeds, sugar cravings, and low energy. We're left feeling bloated, resenting our bodies for not being able to fit into our jeans because our stomach is distended with excess water and painful gas. We fear the shame of leaking through our clothes, thinking it's so disgusting and embarrassing. With our rushing, modern, high-paced life, we don't stop to ask the question, 'What is my menstrual cycle trying to tell me?'

When you go to the doctor for a check-up, they take your blood, listen to your heart, monitor your blood pressure, and maybe check your urine, but no one talks about the most important vital sign for women—your period.

Your menstrual cycle tells me so much about you, your lifestyle, choices, beliefs, heart, mind, and body connection. It's also an incredibly useful predictor of health problems, just like the other vital signs mentioned above. It's one of the best ways to identify any underlying imbalances in your hormones and other parts of your body. When our hormones are out of balance, it not only affects our periods but is a precursor for certain hormonal cancers and heart disease.

We are all living in a world that operates on a linear time frame. When you understand your cycle, you begin to understand yourself and life. You start to observe, listen, and intuit special messages from your body that let you know what's happening inside you on a deeper level. The pain and symptoms you experience are the tip of the iceberg. They are on the surface, but to get to the root of the problem, we need to go deeper. These messages become your intuitive feedback system and internal GPS, helping you recognise when something is not quite right in your hormonal ecosystem.

Your body's messages are shown to you via signs and symptoms such as:

- Heavy and clotty periods
- Longer or shorter cycles
- Ovulation pain on either side
- Skipped menstruation
- Skipped ovulation
- Bleeding between periods
- Headaches
- Excessive cramping
- Period pain

We've all bought into the myth that all the above is normal, and when we go to our GP because we feel it's getting worse, we are prescribed the pill, the coil, or antidepressant medication. Something I often say to my patients is, 'The pill is not a band-aid.' It does nothing but hide the symptoms and does not address the real issue. I'm always baffled that women take it thinking it's going to solve all their problems. What we need to start asking is, 'Why is this happening? Where in my body am I out of balance? Which hormones are involved? How can I heal from this rather than treat it as another quick fix?'

Your period is your monthly health check-up. It's when your body says, 'Hello, thanks for listening; this is what's working, and this is what's not.'

When you neglect the underlying issue, it doesn't disappear. I believe it's one of the primary reasons why we see a rise in hormonal cancers and chronic diseases in women. It's just another method to numb the pain, wear the 'good girl' mask, and carry on. The taboo surrounding our female body and its natural functions has always been shrouded in secrecy, not openly discussed, making us feel as if it's an ailment to be remedied. Masking symptoms is another way to silence us and sweep it all under the carpet.

Only a couple of centuries ago, and even in the last century, our menstruation and sexuality were commonly labelled as 'female hysteria.' Medical diagnoses like a 'wandering womb' were employed to assess our female body and its cycles. Symptoms included fluid retention, 'excessive' sexual desire, irritability, anger, and paradoxically, a loss of interest in sex (we just couldn't win), along with a tendency to speak out of turn and cause trouble. This diagnosis reflected how society treated and perceived the female body.

These symptoms have always been normal functions of our body, yet women underwent surgeries, had their wombs removed, were drugged, and placed in mental asylums. To me, this demonstrates another way in which we fear our body and hastily try to contain and hide away our symptoms and our body's voice. We still carry the fear and mistrust of our body—the fear and the patriarchy are still alive in our DNA. Today, though, instead of getting locked up, we take the pill and numb out with depression meds; we live in different times, yet we haven't actually come so far.

Your Cyclic Magic

Let's take a moment to breathe, grab a cup of tea, and delve into the magic of cyclic living. This concept was entirely new to me when I started on this path, and honestly, it all felt overwhelming and a bit 'woo-woo'. My mind resisted it because it was so alien to what I had been taught and had known my whole life. Yet, there was a place deep inside my womb where I recognised this as true. My brain resisted what my heart and soul knew to be true.

We each have both masculine and feminine personalities, archetypes, and essences that make up who we are. The Western world, and increasingly more cultures globally, are designed to operate in the masculine, leading to a more masculine-driven imbalance internally and collectively in both men and women, society, and the world we live in.

Women experience this more profoundly because, as females, we are designed to be cyclic. The sacred feminine within each of us is cyclic; she governs the cycles of life, seen in creation, birth, life, death, and rebirth. This pattern is evident in seasons, nature, the waxing and waning moon, the ebb and flow of tides, and our menstrual cycle. The creation cycle is everywhere and in everything.

Yet, we have forgotten this. We have become so accustomed to the masculine way— the rules, goals, and to-do lists—that we've lost the essence of who we are and all the magic and power our cycle has to teach us. Transformation is a cyclic pattern. When you want to transform your body, health, or life, you must learn to work with this superpower within. When we aren't in flow with our cycle, we are essentially pedalling upstream, which leads to the Modern Disease of the Modern Woman.

On the other hand, when we turn the boat around and go with our inner power and flow, we move endlessly and effortlessly to where we need to be in every given moment, viewing everything as a lesson and insight, always leading us back to who we are. Embodying this wisdom means we can get where we want and need to go because you are always supported. There is a constant flow of wisdom within, guiding you, gently leading the way back to your innate essence. You are not lost. This isn't happening *to* you but *for* you. Trust in your body, your higher self, and the creation process—nature really does know best.

Everything is a cycle:

- A minute has 60 seconds.
- An hour has 60 minutes.
- A day has 24 hours.
- A week has 7 days.
- A month has 28-30 days (mostly).
- A moon cycle has 28-30 days.
- A menstrual cycle is 28-30 days.
- A year has 365 days.

All of the above are cyclic and set on repeat. However, we are getting sick due to our linear way of life. The constant and never-ending lists and calendars lead us into chronic illness and burnout, not to mention an increase in stress hormones that affect our menstrual cycle and mental health. Our bodies are closely connected to the magic and cycle of the moon. Just like the moon, we have four main cycles:

Menstruation: Winter season/dark moon/nighttime

During your period, your body is shedding the lining of your uterus because there is no pregnancy. Your hormones are mostly inactive this week, except for follicle-stimulating hormone (FSH). This hormone helps the follicle around your developing egg grow, preparing it for release during ovulation in the next two weeks.

When we have our period, our bodies urge us to surrender. It's a time to slow down, rest, restore, and recharge. It's an opportunity for deep reflection, to consider the choices we've made over the past month, assess what's working, and identify what needs to be nurtured in the next cycle. We are especially intuitive during this time, making it an ideal moment to journal and connect with our true feelings.

Pay attention to your blood flow. It can provide precious clues about what needs to change or be optimised in the coming month. Your period tells you how you need to eat, sleep, move, and think differently, and perhaps where cyclic honing and supplementation are needed to optimise your health. Keep a diary and fill in the answers to these questions each month:

- What colour is your blood? Is it brown, pink or red?
- Does the colour change throughout your period? If so, how?
- Are there lumpy viscous globs at the start of your period?
- Do you have clots bigger than 2.5 cm?
- Is your period heavy, light and/or spotty? Does it stop and start before it begins to flow?
- How long does your period last?

On a deeper level, when we don't pay attention to our period and the wisdom it offers, we can become stagnant and uninspired in our work and creativity, lacking energy and fresh ideas. Our bodies need this time to surrender, step off the treadmill, reflect, and rest. We must learn to rest fully without feeling guilty or ashamed. Society often conditions us to think that rest means weakness and being unproductive, which affects our sense of worth, especially in the workplace.

Those who take the time to look after themselves are always better able to support others.

Your body needs this rest. In the past, women would come together during their period in a red tent to rest. While this might not be possible today, you can still honour your body and cycle by taking an extra hour to rest, spending time in nature, doing gentle exercise, journaling, taking a long bath, or meditating.

Here's the thing: if you don't give your body the rest it needs, it will eventually take it anyway, often through illness or burnout. Instead of losing time, create time for yourself.

Meditate, journal, daydream, and ask yourself:

- What are my beliefs about this?
- What have I been taught, and what do I truly believe?
- What's stopping me from taking care of myself?
- Creatively, what projects do I want to bring to life?
- What can I draw out from this period of rest?
- What's waiting to emerge?
- What wants to be born in this cycle?

When we take care of ourselves during our period, we naturally have more energy throughout the rest of our cycle. We experience fewer PMS symptoms and generally feel better, so why do we resist it?

We tend to avoid the winter season, both in nature and within our bodies. We're conditioned to love the energy and vibrancy of spring and summer, but winter, like your period and the dark moon, is essential to all other seasons and your cycle. Rest and regeneration are vital for health and nature. Trees may appear lifeless in winter, but underneath, they are preparing for the spring. This mirrors your body. You need to rest and regenerate to fully enjoy the next phase of your cycle, which always comes; you never stay in winter. Spring is always just around the corner.

A Note from a Menstrual Reflection:

Reflecting on my womb and where she is right now, I'm starting to see, or I should say feel, a pattern of how my womb ebbs and flows each month and season. I understand this on a cortical level, but I'm beginning to feel and be with this part of myself through the practises. Last week, I had a heavy menstruation, which I have just come to the end of. What I feel is that this part of my cycle takes me down physically, emotionally, and mentally. How I honour or dishonour myself throughout the month is shown to me during my period. I've learned this month that even when I feel amazing, and it's spring energy in every area of my life, I still need to stay grounded and remember that I'm a cyclical being, or the crash back down will be more challenging. I need to align and find my balance again and again.

My period is my greatest teacher; I need her because she brings me deeper into myself. Another layer of the spiral travelled and drawn deeper into my shadow self. Every month, I've started approaching my period with, 'So where are we journeying to this month? What are you going to teach me this time?' I've been trying to see it more as something that is happening for me, for my growth, rather than fighting it and being a victim of it (even though I still feel like this sometimes). The more I repress during the month, the deeper I go when I bleed, the harder the lesson because the shadow is deeper and more dense.

I imagine the goddess, who is the wise old woman for me right now, sitting in my womb on her rocking chair, knitting, cooking, and being. Every month, she awaits me and asks why I haven't been down to see her more often when I promised I would. She always has a lesson for me. Sometimes bad things come up in life, and I run down there crying and wailing back to her because I know I will always find comfort and guidance, even the type I don't want to hear. When I go there more regularly, my lessons are less severe because I'm learning gradually, resisting less and less. The more resistance and more fear I have, the harder the lesson.

This is my reflection on what the goddess in my womb is teaching me. She will always get me to listen one way or another; I'm either working with her (myself) or against her (myself).

We never fail; we always learn.

Follicular Phase/Spring/Waxing Moon/Morning Energy

My favourite time of year is spring. Growing up in Wales, I loved how nature came to life in the beautiful countryside around me. The sight of daffodils, leeks, and lambs always filled me with excitement, reminding me of rebirth, fresh energy, and the promise of summer.

Spring, with its new beginnings and inspiring energy, is mirrored in the natural world, where everything starts to wake up and come back to life. The birds sing, the flowers bloom, and we begin to plant seeds for new growth. These tender new shoots are like our ideas, planted during the dark moon, now emerging into the light, waiting to be nurtured into reality. We start to bring our attention, dreams, desires, and work into the daylight.

The moon is waxing, bringing more light at night—this is the spring energy of the moon cycle and corresponds to the follicular phase of our cycle.

During the follicular phase, oestrogen levels begin to rise, preparing our bodies for ovulation. Oestrogen plays a crucial role in our hormonal health, supporting reproductive, breast, and pelvic health, as well as contributing to bone and cardiovascular health, among other essential functions. It also boosts our sex drive, as Mother Nature encourages us to conceive. We feel more energetic, and our libido peaks, leading to the most satisfying orgasms during this phase, particularly as ovulation approaches. With an egg ready to be released, sexual desire intensifies, and any sperm present has a chance to fertilise the egg. Remember, sperm can survive in your body for up to six days, so the window for conception is larger than many women realise.

But let's take a step back and focus on your follicular phase, which is laying down the uterine lining needed to support an egg once it's released. This is the time for setting intentions and pursuing new ideas. Everything feels easier; we naturally have more energy, making it a perfect time to get things done.

Ideas flow effortlessly; this is the time for brainstorming, starting new projects, planning, and exploring new adventures.

However, if we haven't fully embraced the winter phase of our cycle, we may miss out on the benefits this season offers, affecting our energy and oestrogen levels. Oestrogen is our friend, but stress and lack of rest can disrupt our cycle and lead to problems like fertility issues, PMS, pain, and illness.

Some women, stuck in cycles of pain and hurt, may fear this season and try to avoid it. Be honest and kind with yourself: what are you afraid to be or do? What are you running from? What's the fear within, and where does it come from? Sometimes, we just need to know when it's time to repot a plant or start something completely new. Remember, your choices and actions affect your body's chemistry; it's all connected. You are a holistic being, and your hormones reflect your beliefs, emotions, and spirit.

We get stuck in one part of the cycle when we resist change. As women, we often fear losing control and not having everything perfectly planned. This fear can keep us trapped—fear of change, the unknown, the what-ifs, the struggle to hold onto everything while trying to grow. We need to learn to embrace our cycles; they are our greatest teachers. Birth, life, death, and rebirth are all part of life. Our cells do it every day, and every month, our womb sheds its lining. Our breath goes in and out, and summer comes and goes. Be honest with yourself. What season are you stuck in? And why? Are you holding onto the inhale, afraid to let go and surrender into the exhale? Understanding this reveals so much about what's happening in your mind, body, and spirit, and this knowledge is key to unlocking the pain you may be experiencing.

Ovulation/ Summer/Full Moon/ Midday Energy

We all love the energy of summer: the sun on your face, long days and nights, fun, travel, parties, high energy, being outdoors, feeling free, magnetic, and abundant. For me, summer means the sea breeze, summer dresses, and ice cream.

I love how summer feels in my body, especially during the ovulation phase. It's when we feel more attractive, we glow, everything fits perfectly, and we feel fantastic. We want to be out socialising, with the energy to dance all night and still wake up feeling refreshed (well, maybe not if you're over 40 with four kids, but you get the idea).

Summer is all about fullness, connection, love, visibility, and magnetism. We are at our peak, making it the perfect time to conceive. Our hormones are in full swing, attracting everything and everyone.

But remember, summer isn't the only season; it's just 25% of the whole cycle. We need the other energies and gifts from the other seasons to fully enjoy and be present in summer. This is also when we feel most alive and turned on, in life and in bed. Our juices are flowing, and if you pay attention, you'll notice your discharge changes during this phase. You crave more intimacy and feel more magnetic.

During this time, our bodies release high levels of luteinising hormone, and the wonderful hormone progesterone is about to rise. Its job is to maintain the uterine lining that oestrogen built the week before and hold the egg in place. This phase is crucial for women trying to conceive and is vital for the rest of our cycle. Issues can arise when women become fatigued or burnt out and may even miss the ovulation phase, which is more common than we think these days.

Stress is the main culprit, as it directly affects our hormones, causing disruptions throughout our cycle. When we don't ovulate, we don't produce enough progesterone, leading to low levels. Progesterone is an amazing hormone that helps balance mood swings, eases heavy periods, and reduces most PMS symptoms. When we aren't producing enough progesterone—and many women aren't—we suffer from PMS. Progesterone is also affected when oestrogen levels are too high. Chronic stress leads to excess oestrogen, throwing progesterone out of balance since they work in harmony. When oestrogen dominates, progesterone can't function properly. By understanding our hormones and how stress, beliefs, choices, and actions impact them, we begin to see how all of this affects our health and sex life.

During this time, the moon is full, and it's time to embrace the wild energy within. It's the fruition of what you planted in spring, now coming into full bloom. It's a time to reflect and release what no longer serves you, considering how you express your energy in the world and how it relates to others.

The full moon is a special time for me. It's a time to write and reflect on what isn't working and what needs to be released from my life. I love using this season and moon phase to let go of any energies that no longer serve me or align with who I am.

When I was diagnosed with skin cancer back in 2009, I developed a beautiful relationship with the moon. After my operation, I developed a fear of the sun and became scared of it because I believed it had given me skin cancer. I started walking more at night, staring up at the moon. I learned to feel her energy, the feminine presence. I followed her cycles, and slowly, my cycle started to mirror hers. I learned a lot about myself and my emotions during this time. Since then, the moon has become my friend, teacher, and a presence that I honour, respect, and commune with. Doing this has helped me develop a more personal relationship with my body and her cycles, and I am always left feeling in awe at the synchronicity and magic we share. I am no longer afraid of the sun, and I respect its power and gifts, but it has also taught me that staying in summer energy and the sun for too long can literally burn us up and cause physical harm, stress, and disease.

Most modern women think we must always be in summer energy. It's the mask we wear, the smile we slap on, the 'yes' we say when our bodies want to say 'no.' Summer is high energy, yet we aren't designed to always be in high energy. The sun is a masculine energy, vital for our health, but it's not how we are meant to function all the time. When we bring in the moon's gentle, deep, feminine wisdom and follow her cycles, our lives will reflect the same. As a result, we feel happier, healthier, and more connected to the magic within.

Luteal Phase/Autumn/Waning Moon/Evening Energy

For me, autumn has always felt like the new year. I love this season… the colours, the feel of the trees, the energy… Everything about Autumn lights me up and makes me feel warm from the inside out. This time is all about regathering, rebalancing, and grounding back down to earth after the high of summer. It's a time in our lives to reap the fruits of our labours in the natural world. Think about the squirrel getting ready to hibernate, tying up all the loose ends. It's a time for letting everything that doesn't serve you fall away—shedding your skin. It's when the leaves turn golden and brown, and the tree lets them fall away as it prepares to go within for winter.

The luteal phase of our cycle is where our progesterone should be at its highest. It's also the time when our second batch is made by the corpus luteal gland, which is produced after we ovulate in the hopes of sustaining a wanted pregnancy. As I talked about earlier, if we aren't making enough progesterone, which most women aren't, we don't get the needed buffer for all the PMS symptoms that begin to bombard us the week before our period. Our happy hormone is empty, making us tired, bloated, and angry, especially as we enter the second phase of the luteal cycle.

This second phase is when we often feel most explosive, setting off a massive cascade of emotions from tears to anger, usually because we haven't been addressing our underlying problems. It's when we feel most out of control and try to suppress our feelings. This is the time to set clear boundaries; this is what the rage is for. You're angry, and the barriers are down. Where do you need to draw the line in your life? Where are you still saying 'yes' when your body screams 'no'? Your body knows and is trying to tell you, 'We're not in alignment here; something needs to change.' In this phase, we need to start getting clear about what we want and don't want instead of doing and being everything everybody else thinks we should be.

Just breathe in and out. You're not broken or crazy, and your kids and husband will forgive you! This gift is your body's way of telling you what needs to change so you can be healthy, happy, and balanced. The problems begin when we don't listen to our intuition. This month's PMS reflects the choices and actions you've made throughout its duration. Your level of relaxation, the amount of stress you've experienced, your dietary habits, and your attentiveness to your body will all be evident in the manifestation of your PMS. The extent of your discomfort directly results from how well you've attuned yourself to your body's signals and followed its wisdom. Avoiding or suppressing these signals doesn't eliminate stress or resolve issues; instead, it compounds into new challenges.

I enjoy taking this time to contemplate what I need to let go of as I bleed every month. Is it a relationship or friendship that no longer contributes positively to my life? It could be a job, a role, or a persona.

Try writing an honest, brutal letter expressing everything, then burn it, releasing the burden into the universe. Ask yourself:

- What does my body signal for me to release to promote its well-being?
- What am I choosing not to carry into the next month?
- What's depleting my energy and life force? Am I willing to let it go for my greater good and health?
- What am I clinging to?

The belief that there's never enough, that we must cling to things, is a learned mindset. It's crucial to acknowledge that there's plenty of money, love, and everything else. However, holding onto excess only prevents us from receiving more.

Releasing hurt, grievances, anger, or frustration is essential. Forgiveness and acceptance are gifts to the soul. When we withhold these from others, we also deny ourselves. Setting others free liberates us. Emotional baggage takes a toll on the heart and soul, sapping precious energy. It's time to let go, allowing those walls to crumble and feeling the relief surge through the body. While forgetting may be unnecessary, forgiving on a soul level is vital.

The dynamic of giving and receiving is an infinite loop of continuous flow. When we cease to give and let go, we hinder our ability to receive. For our lives and health to be in optimal balance, we must be able to receive and give fully. So, release what must go, create space to enter the metaphorical winter—the fertile void—and be open to receiving what's needed for the next cycle of life.

Chemically, by the end of our luteal phase, week three of our cycle, we are either pregnant or preparing to shed our endometrial lining. Progesterone, which hopefully has peaked around day 21, eases us into the winter phase of our cycle.

Other chemical changes happening this week are:

- A substantial drop in serotonin levels, our happy hormone.
- Our plasma levels of glutathione, which acts as an antioxidant and protects us from free radicals, decrease.
- B vitamin levels are lower.
- D3 levels are lower.
- Plasma levels of magnesium are lower.
- Decrease in amino acid levels.

Changes in fatty acid and lipid steroid production, with cholesterol now being used for progesterone and oestrogen synthesis, lead to a decrease in HDL during the luteal phase. This could contribute to increased inflammation due to incomplete or reduced processing of fatty acids in our mitochondria. When the mitochondria aren't metabolising fats, we make acylcarnitines, which produce inflammation in the body, leading to chronic inflammation and metabolic disease. Pay attention to headaches, cravings, brain fog, and aches and pains in your body during this phase of your cycle, as you may need help here.

Halfway through this week, around day 25, progesterone levels fall, decreasing blood and oxygen to the endometrial lining, causing it to wither and die. The endometrium lining is shed, most commonly known as your period.

Summary

Every woman must ask herself, 'Am I authentically aligned with who I am?' When we live incongruently, diverging from the life we're meant to lead, stress creeps in as the truth strives to be heard. It's crucial to examine our daily, weekly, and monthly routines, examining our beliefs, choices, and actions. This mix forms the recipe influencing our hormones and menstruation symptoms each month. Our thoughts and emotions profoundly impact our biology, and aligning with our authentic selves can prompt positive changes in hormonal responses when working with our menstrual cycle.

The menstrual cycle is a valuable gift, allowing us to pause and reflect on our true desires. Even the act of asking oneself this question is nourishing. Our inner voice often signals that we may not be living the life we truly desire, caught in the grip of societal expectations, or chasing an idea of success for validation. We tend to over-commit in various areas of our lives without genuine desire.

Can you slow down enough to heed that inner voice within you? Are you open to listening? When we relinquish control and allow our inner voice to guide us, it illuminates the right path.

Begin by exploring how 'no', integrity, and truth feel in your body. Trust and embrace this intuition—it belongs to you and is genuinely invested in your well-being. Stop worrying about the opinions, thoughts, and actions of others, as it only adds unnecessary stress, impacting your hormones. You don't require external approval; your own validation is enough. Let go of tasks from your to-do list. Loosen your grip, release control, ease the constant striving, and return to your centre. Acknowledge that you are more than enough as you are.

Many women believe it's possible to have it all, saying it might take time but can be achieved. I used to think this too, but I've realised the cost is too high. I no longer want everything; instead, I focus on what truly fulfils me, ignites my passion, and brings love and vitality into my life. I prioritise what really matters and avoid wasting time on things that don't. Chasing it all can harm your health, sanity, and family. Now, I set clear desires that can change with the cycles of my life. By trusting my instincts, I know what to embrace and what to let go of.

Your body has its own wisdom, often signalling when something is wrong before your conscious mind realises it. Many women who suddenly develop physical issues have often missed earlier warning signs because they were too busy with daily life and juggling various roles. The same goes for hormonal imbalances—learning to recognise these signs is crucial.

We need to change how we see our bodies, not just as machines to be fixed with supplements and strict routines. While nutrition, exercise, and supplements are important, true healing comes from connecting the body, mind, and spirit and addressing unmet emotional needs. Instead of constantly looking for external solutions, tap into your inner wisdom as an intuitive woman, and focus on what you really need for deep healing.

Some of my clients feel trapped in their jobs or marriages, and resolving these issues brings them healing. Another client, who felt lonely and unloved, found relief from her menstrual migraines when she connected the dots in her life.

Tuning into your inner wisdom and your cycles means connecting with the part of you that knows the source of your pain and understands what needs nourishment, healing, and love. These things might not always be measurable or logical, but trust your body's wisdom—it always knows what it needs.

Traits like perfectionism, negativity, a harsh inner critic, excessive control, and self-imposed pressure contribute to stress, hormone imbalances, and menstrual problems. Reflect on how often you say 'I should' throughout the day. Consider if you're blaming your body for challenges instead of appreciating it for the gift of life it gives you. Constant criticism, whether from yourself or others, disrupts the delicate balance of your hormones.

*NOTE: If you are no longer menstruating, you can still benefit from living a cyclic life. I advise following the phases of the moon to rebalance and realign to your sacred feminine flow.

Case Study: Susan

Susan, a mother of two in her late thirties, came to me with migraines, PMS, and a recent diagnosis of PCOS. She felt constantly tired, was overweight, and despite trying various diets, she looked and felt ten years older than her 38 years. Working full-time as an account manager, Susan struggled both with her energy levels and financially. She worked long hours, trying to prove she could handle everything, despite having two children. The pressure to perform and the fear of losing her job were constant sources of stress.

When we started treatment, we focused on her energy cycle, even though her menstrual cycle was almost non-existent. We followed the moon's phases, and after a few months, Susan noticed improvements in her energy. We added supplements, gentle exercise, and nourishing foods to support her journey. Susan began reflecting on her life and realised she hadn't felt comfortable in her own skin since having her children. The things that once excited her now felt meaningless. She understood that all her striving had been to feel worthy of love, particularly from parents who struggled to show pride.

There's a reason why PCOS, ovarian cysts, PMS, and other female-related health issues are so common today. Women often feel oppressed, not just by society, but by their own expectations. Subconscious feelings of unworthiness can trigger stress and hormonal imbalances.

When Susan reconnected with herself, she felt immediate relief. She decided to work less, spend more time with her children, and looked into night school to pursue her passion for writing—something she had always loved but was discouraged from pursuing. Now, Susan is pain-free, her PCOS has resolved, and her migraines are rare. When they do occur, she knows it's a sign to reconnect with herself and her inner guidance.

❧

Case Study: Elizabeth

A few years ago, Elizabeth came to me with a severe vomiting issue that began after her grandmother's funeral. For six months, she could barely eat without being violently sick, leading to significant weight loss. During our sessions, we explored her body and energy system, which brought up memories of the funeral.

At the funeral, Elizabeth was in the car with her brother and father. When she saw the coffin, she started crying, but instead of receiving support, her father laughed at her, and her brother told her to pull herself together, saying it wasn't about her. This revealed a pattern she had learned: not to care, not to show emotion, and to see tears as a sign of weakness. As a child, crying led to mockery, which left her emotionally stifled and unable to feel genuine empathy as an adult.

Seeing her grandmother's coffin triggered emotions she had long suppressed to keep others comfortable and avoid feeling humiliated. After the funeral, the vomiting started, and despite medical tests showing no issues, the problem persisted. Elizabeth came to me as a last resort, and together, we worked to release the blocked energy and emotions from her body.

Over the next few months, we focused on helping Elizabeth reconnect with her energy. We cleared areas affected by old beliefs that weren't really hers. We also worked on healing her family line, addressing the idea that emotions are a weakness, which had been passed down through three generations. Today, Elizabeth is a balanced, emotionally healthy woman. She moves in harmony with the cycles and seasons, expresses her feelings confidently, and knows exactly who she is and what she wants.

❧

Are you working 30-40 hours a week, striving to validate yourself and establish a reputation? Despite your efforts, do you still grapple with feelings of inadequacy? What are you truly searching for, and where do you withhold your authentic voice? Are your deepest desires buried beneath layers that hold you back? Uncover the fears standing guard at the entrance to your body and soul, impeding your journey toward self-discovery. Identifying the barriers that keep you from your authentic self initiates the process of unravelling the emotions, memories, and root causes of your pain and imbalance. The answers lie within, patiently awaiting your exploration. This is the profound wisdom that the cycles and seasons can teach us.

Kronos and Kairos Time

Time, consisting of days, weeks, and months, is known as *Kronos* time and is essentially an artificial construct. This quantifiable measurement is how we gauge our days and lives, viewing time in a strictly linear sense. In ancient civilisations, the passage of time was marked independently based on their surroundings, the changing seasons, and the phases of the moon, sun, and stars. Our ancestors recorded time through cycles, as seen in instruments like the sundial. The key difference is that the ancients flowed with time rather than attempting to mould it; it was cyclic, aligned with nature and universally led, not dictated by man-made time patriarchal constructs.

During my priestess training, I discovered that there are 13 moons in a year, not 12 as I'd been taught. The annual calendar, a human creation, led me to assume, like many others, that there were 12 moon phases aligning monthly with the yearly calendar. This realisation prompted me to recognise how man-made time increasingly diverges from nature, impacting our well-being in various ways.

Kronos time, prevalent in our modern, fast-paced lifestyles, is viewed as a commodity we attempt to control. We worry over having enough time, fear wasting or losing it, and adopt masculine expressions like 'time is money' and 'time is of the essence', perpetuating the notion that more money equates to more time.

In its patriarchal, linear sense, time becomes all-consuming, demanding, and a taskmaster that constrains us, moulding us into personas that are unnatural for the feminine psyche. Many modern women find themselves wishing for more time or racing against the clock in an attempt to control it. Kronos time banishes the present moment, restricting expansion and authentic existence. It confines us to a golden cage, compelling us to be excessively productive in service to an unidentified master deeply embedded in our unconscious psychology.

Feminine energy operates in cycles, urging us to step out of the confines of linear time and reconnect with the rhythm and flow of the universe and nature. I'm not suggesting complete disregard for the tick-tock of the calendar but rather an invitation to sense, feel, perceive and tune into your environment. Instead of rushing through life on a high-speed train, missing precious moments, slowing down and realigning with our cycles allows us to embrace Kairos time.

On the other hand, Kairos time manifests as a gentle unfurling, a loosening of the controlling grip, and an expansion of consciousness. In this state, joy becomes palpable in the present, and life is lived rather than merely endured.

Kairos time is qualitative and vertical, connecting heaven and earth. It represents our deepest connection to source, universal intelligence, miracles, healing, and life itself. It's the realm where seemingly insurmountable problems find solutions and blocked emotions dissipate. Kairos moments are accessible anywhere, anytime, if we permit ourselves to experience them. Allowing intuition to unfold, speak, and guide us back home to the present moment can be achieved through activities like walking in nature, deep breathing, self-care, meditation, reading, art, poetry, dancing, or even cooking.

Kronos feels like being stuck in an inhale, unable to exhale, while Kairos is the deep exhale. Reflect on the Kairos moments you've recently felt and experienced. How can you intentionally create space to encounter these moments more often?

To experience Kairos time, we need to gently let go of the control Kronos has over us.

Let's Get Practical

Every week, take a day off. Leave your phone on silent and be 100% present with your kids or fur babies (if you have them)—avoid scrolling or catching up with emails. Relax on the sofa, read a book, get a massage, join a yoga class, walk with a friend, and talk and laugh with people you love.

Every month, respect your menstruation. Try not to schedule big events or important meetings. Engage in less intense exercise, be kind to yourself, and prioritise rest. Follow the phases of the moon. Join a temple which helps you attune to the magic and wisdom of the moon as it moves through the astrological calendar.

Every year, take a break where you allow yourself to switch off and fully experience the people and life you love. Many women use holidays to catch up with deadlines and work, returning from vacation more tired than when they went. Don't let this be you! You will be amazed at how your energy starts to rise as you rise and take back your body. Life begins to flow with you and for you rather than against you. Embrace every cycle and celebrate the turn of the wheel. Learn, create rituals and attend temples that celebrate Imbolc, spring equinox, Beltane, summer solstice, Lughnasadh, Autumnal Equinox, Samhuinn, and winter solstice.

The idea is to learn from each cycle and phase and grow each time you cycle around. Here's what this could look like in everyday life:

A 24-Hour Schedule:

6 am: Spring Energy (Inspired)
Plan tasks and plant seeds. Do the tasks that require more energy and attention.

12 pm: Summer (Visibility, Magnetic)
Engage in online calls, meetings, peak magnetism, and receptivity. Be seen, put yourself out there, and experience full bloom.

4 pm - 6 pm: Autumn Energy
Wind downtime (PMS time of your day). Crave carbs and coffee. Complete tasks, make space, slow down, relax, and finish that paper. Listen to that podcast or read that book you need to read.

12 am: New Moon Menstrual
Rest. Lead up to getting a good night's sleep. Turn off electronics.

In Chapter 19, I will discuss how to eat to optimise your cycle. How and what we eat needs to change to reflect our biochemistry, hormones, and physiology throughout our cycle.

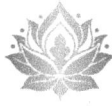

CHAPTER 11
THE LOST ART OF SENSUALITY

You are taught that your body belongs to others... it belongs to you.

As you read this chapter, I invite you to reconnect with your embodied sensual self. A sensual woman is fully alive, with her senses switched on and her body fuelled by her sensuality. She follows her body's intuition and her soul's wisdom, balancing her mind with the natural rhythms of her consciousness.

Your aliveness is your most intimate connection with your feminine essence. Your sexual and sensual energy drives you towards life, love, and connection and away from stagnation. This is a primal need, yet we often suppress it, leaving us disconnected from our life force, which can make us feel sick, tired, and depressed.

There is a widespread issue affecting women today—a disconnection from our bodies. Many women struggle to feel their aliveness, sensuality, and sexual power. They feel numb and often out of touch with their bodies or even unable to feel anything at all. Some may think that what I teach is a myth, like a pot of gold at the end of a rainbow. Sensuality is often seen as a luxury, not a necessity for our health and well-being, and it's marketed to us as something we need to acquire. But the truth is, sensuality lives within us—we are it, and it is us.

Disconnection to our sensuality includes the following symptoms:

- Body shame
- Weight gain
- Bloating
- Low self-worth and lack of self-love
- Hurt, anger, frustration
- Explosive rage
- Tired and low-energy
- Apathy
- Irritable
- Bouts of depression
- PMS
- Disinterest and apathy
- Numbing out

Embodiment is vital for your health and well-being. Connecting with your body and sensuality links you to your life force. When we live in our heads or seek fulfilment outside ourselves, we'll never truly feel whole, content, joyful, and balanced.

The numbness and disconnection from our sensuality can be worsened by things like the pill, antidepressants, and other substances, trapping us in a negative cycle and taking us further away from our bodies and true selves. Society and upbringing have played a big part in this separation from our bodies and the natural cycles of the earth. We've been taught, directly or indirectly, that our sensuality and sexuality are dangerous or shameful. But your power lies in your pelvis—it's where the energy and fire you crave are found. Your vagina, uterus, ovaries, and menstruation are your power sources. So why are so many of us living with our inner flame dimmed and our energy barely flowing?

By exploring your desires, pleasures, and what turns you on, you'll start to discover your true self. Learning to receive energy and love is something society has lost touch with. The habit of overgiving has made it hard for us to embrace this aspect of life. Women have been conditioned to separate their strength, desirability, and femininity from their sexuality, focusing only on the negative aspects. This needs to change. Just as a man's power is often linked to his testicles, your power is connected to your ovaries. When you tap into this energy, you'll realise that your orgasms, touch, and senses are the keys to feeling truly alive. Despite what society suggests, women need sex and orgasms just as much as, if not more than, men.

I know this might be hard to accept, and doubts may arise, but once you understand how your body works and the potential of your sexual organs, you'll see that you've been missing out for too long. I've seen women undergo incredible transformations in this area—shedding stress, losing weight, brightening their appearance, and reducing symptoms of chronic illness. They laugh and love more fully because they've learned to embrace and express all aspects of who they are.

Yet, many women suffer in silence, feeling pressured by society's norms. We either avoid discussing these issues with friends or pretend everything is fine. How often have you faked an orgasm out of disinterest, impatience, or just wanting to get it over with? The pressure to be pleasing and desirable leads to overgiving, and many women struggle with insecurities about their appearance or even their scent, creating tension that disconnects them from their own sexuality.

There are many obstacles for women, both external, like societal pressures, and internal, like the need to conform to certain standards. In relationships, the initial desire to please can turn into resentment when our needs aren't met, leading to misunderstandings with partners. Over time, saying 'yes' when your body says 'no', putting on a smile and going along with things can make you feel bitter and resentful. This pattern extends beyond the bedroom and affects all areas of life. Without a deep understanding of our true desires, we struggle to prioritise ourselves. We've been conditioned to reject our sensuality, creating a gap between who we are and who we think we should be.

Self-pleasure

For some women, self-pleasure has evolved into a means of de-stressing, buzzing out, or even numbing tension with the aid of a vibrator. We often squeeze and contract our bodies, seeking a quick chemical rush, a brief release of endorphins that lasts only a few minutes. While I appreciate the benefits of vibrators and believe every woman should have one, they can contribute to further numbness, especially when many of us are already desensitised in that area. Vibrators can dull nerve endings, making it more challenging to experience pleasure with a partner and hindering the potential benefits of sexual healing through gentle touch and integrated breathwork.

Many of us hold our breath, clench our legs, and push our climax out as if it's confined in a tight box rather than opening up and unfolding like a beautiful flower. This alternative form of orgasm plays a crucial role in balancing hormones, regulating the nervous and immune systems, and transitioning the body into the green zone of rest and digestion. It brings a sense of balance, calmness, and rootedness. The key lies in connection, or more precisely, reconnection—bringing healing and unity to your body, involving the entire body in the orchestration instead of a solo performance by one part. When we lack a sacred connection to our sexuality, we only scratch the surface of what our body truly needs, desires, and is capable of. Vibrators may serve as the power tool for corporate women and busy moms—quick, easy, time-efficient, and effective, but they reduce the experience to a mere checkbox. You are more than that; there are unexplored territories within you that are waiting to be discovered. It's time to unveil the gifts your body holds, recognising that you alone possess the key to unlocking them.

Begin by acknowledging the possibility that there are wild, uncharted, and perhaps perceived dangerous places within yourself that you've been warned not to explore. Identify what barriers prevent you from fully inhabiting your body, become curious about these barriers, and commit to visiting those untouched spaces soon. Let's embrace expansion and breathe into the unexplored rather than remaining confined and stuck in contraction.

Sexual Shame

Sexual shame is widespread in our culture and is a significant barrier to our connection with our sexuality, fuelled by various factors such as past traumas (sexual or related to childbirth), repressive upbringing, core wounds, religious teachings, and the influence of the patriarchy.

Even today, many still struggle to understand what it means to be truly sexy. External influences—from family to media—shape our perceptions, but real sexuality comes from self-love and acceptance. A woman's primary role isn't to sexually please a man; it's to experience the magic within her own body, have orgasms, and embrace her desires. Your sexuality is about how you feel about yourself. Unfortunately, societal pressures often lead us to fake it instead of embracing our true desires.

Personally, my sexual shame revolved around using my sexual power as a form of currency. I sought to make men desire me, love me, and fill the internal void I wasn't consciously aware of at the time. Feeling the need to be seen and desired to validate my sense of self-worth, I adopted the role of a giver and over-giver, neglecting my own desire for sexual pleasure. My focus was on pleasing others, looking pretty, and saying the right things to make my partners feel important. Despite conforming to societal expectations, this self-control and constant pleasing left me feeling unhappy and drained. I struggled to understand why I felt this way despite doing what I thought was expected of me. Questions arose about my unhappiness, resentment, and anger towards my partners, as I expected them to reciprocate my efforts with the love and commitment I was craving.

Fuelled by jealousy, possessiveness, and control, I could become unrecognisable. Trust became a challenge, leading me to question the actions of my partners, ultimately destroying every relationship. In retrospect, I realise that I lacked self-love, self-respect, and self-giving. I had freely given away my life force and energy, becoming vulnerable and weak. My core fear was rejection, and it fuelled and consumed me. This was my shadow to own, reclaim, and love. My sexuality, which I had come to hate and perceive as a curse, became a source of resentment. I refused to feel like a mere object and wanted ownership of my sexuality. My anger was directed towards men, my past, and the world.

Denying my sexuality had resulted in a disconnection from my body, leading me to make choices in my twenties that I might not have made otherwise. Meeting my husband marked a turning point where I began to trust and allow myself to be held through my awakening. Although challenging at first, we stayed together and grew together, and I granted myself the patience and love to grow into my true self. Exploring sacred practises that came online during my priestess training, sacred sexuality, womb work, and tantra further contributed to my transformation. It was a process, an ongoing journey that unveiled the impact of the patriarchy and the sexual narratives ingrained in me and my ancestral line. Healing the sexual wounds in my maternal line allowed me to realise that I wasn't broken; there was nothing to fix. It was about updating and rebooting the beliefs and programming inside me to align with the woman I desired— and was destined—to become.

Many women believe they are broken or need fixing if they don't desire sex or feel sensual. This is a misconception. It's the fearful part within them speaking, the scared part. I acknowledge and hear that part because I've been there. The resistance and rebellion against societal norms come from an intuitive understanding that something isn't right.

You don't just have a body; you are a body!

Let's break free from these mental constraints and rediscover the true power and wisdom of our sacred sexuality. It's time to embrace our bodies, sensuality, and lives, recognising that the beauty within us deserves to be expressed, not hidden away for a distant future.

Some questions to ponder:

- How fully do you allow your sexual body to be present in your life?
- How often do you allow yourself to feel pleasure and sensuality?
- What does your body desire? What makes her feel alive?
- How does your body speak to you?
- What does desire feel like in your body?
- Do you know what aliveness feels like in your body?
- How much aliveness do you feel daily?
- Are you conscious of where you feel shut down or stagnant?
- Have you been living unconsciously in your body?
- Are you wired to feel pain and numbness?
- How does your body interact with the world?
- How do you experience your body?
- What fears does all of this bring up?

Learn to Speak Her Language

Get comfortable with your body! It's astonishing to think that doctors and even partners might be more familiar with our lady parts than we are ourselves. While you may not hold a Ph.D. in female anatomy, nobody should understand your body better than you do. You are her interpreter, her spokesperson, and it's crucial to start speaking in her language because nobody else truly comprehends her unique expressions. She doesn't need an intermediary in the form of a doctor or boyfriend; she needs you.

Deep down, you instinctively know how you feel or want to feel, but at times, the physical or emotional discomfort or inconvenience might make you reluctant to acknowledge it. I'm not suggesting you avoid consulting your doctor; what I'm emphasising is having insights into why you think certain things are happening and what your intuition senses. Learning HER language requires practise. Trust me, I'm no fan of learning languages, and when I moved to the Netherlands, it took me a while to understand and speak Dutch well enough to get by. However, now I understand and grasp the general flow, allowing me to piece myself together and navigate my life here. When I first arrived, deciphering a foreign language was hard, and I often felt isolated and alone—similar to how your yoni might feel—alone, depressed, misunderstood, and outright neglected by you. Learn HER language, and she'll become the best friend you've ever had.

Recently, I had a dream and an intuition that something was wrong with my cervix. I had undergone a pap smear two years ago and wasn't due for another for three years. Upon discussing my concerns with my doctor, they advised waiting, asserting that there was nothing wrong and that the protocol called for a pap smear every five years. Despite having no signs or symptoms, I couldn't shake off the uneasy feelings my body was giving me. After a month, I insisted on another pap smear. I saw the patronising look that seemed to say, 'It's all in your head.' It made me feel small, but my cervix was signalling that something wasn't right, and my close connection with my sacred sexuality and practise compelled me to listen.

The results that came back were not good, and this allowed me to make an informed decision about what steps to take next and uncover some unconscious trauma that was stagnating inside of me, making my cervix sick. If I had ignored my body, three years later my options could have been drastically different. Always remember your body is consistently communicating with you—start listening.

Case Study: Freda

Freda had been struggling with coccyx and Ischial pain on and off for years. When we started working together, I noticed how her muscles and nervous system reacted intuitively when we began exploring her sexuality. She told me that when she was a child, she was sexually abused. She couldn't recall the exact details but had been having therapy on and off for the flashbacks that were coming back to her. Her tailbone was shaped and altered so that it tucked under her, so when she sat, she couldn't help but put pressure directly on it. Her posture mimicked a dog with his tail between her legs to protect. Even though Freda was now 50 years old, her body was still holding on tight to the trauma. It affected how she gave birth, and she ended up having two c-sections because her body refused to open up. It affected her sex life, making sex painful. She was completely disconnected from her body, her aliveness, and her sexual desires. She tried laughing it off, but when we went deeper, she started to cry with relief. 'I thought I was going crazy, I've been living with this fear in my body my whole life. I can't relax, I can't switch it off, and I feel like I'm on guard the whole time,' she shared.

This tension over the years had led to a build-up of stress and pain in her pelvis and nervous system. In addition, Freda had been struggling with chronic fatigue syndrome for the past two years, caused by the exhaustion of trying not to feel and holding back her emotional body. The upkeep of the disconnect was costing her her health. When we started working on awakening her aliveness and freeing up the energy, releasing it and bringing more healing into the body, Freda's body was slowly able to open up and release the pain she had been carrying around for years. What she discovered was that talking about the problem and knowing about it was just one aspect. However, embodying, emoting, and releasing the energy held within was nothing short of life-changing—it was her missing piece.

I worked with Freda using the Sheology protocol, particularly She-Movement practises to re-awaken her body. We also used jade egg practises to reconnect and heal the sexual trauma and shame she had been carrying in her Yoni since she was a young girl. Freda also worked on cleansing her energy body and reconnecting to her feminine body, slowly welcoming her soul back home into her body. It was a return to wholeness.

❧

Sensuality begins with awakening the five senses. In the midst of busyness and stress, we often overlook the richness each sense offers. To become a radiant, sensual being, we must physically engage with the world around us and learn to embody its essence within ourselves. There is a constant dialogue occurring with the things we see, hear, taste, smell, and feel. It's imperative to recognise that we are not separate from this sensory symphony but an integral part of it, with much wisdom awaiting us if we open ourselves to receive.

Awakening the Five Senses—Meditation in Nature

Take a leisurely stroll in nature and find a serene spot to sit. Observe your surroundings, absorbing the myriad of colours and shapes. What do you see? Often, in nature, our minds are preoccupied, whether with thoughts, phones, or step counts. Recall the days of childhood when clouds held shapes and symbols. If you're in a forest, gaze at the trees from a fresh perspective—they are alive and are trying to communicate with you.

Now, tune into what you hear—birds singing, leaves rustling, a passing car, or a distant lawnmower. Once you've identified these sounds, listen with your entire body, feeling for the underlying silence, the sacred pause beneath everything.

Inhale the air around you. What does the scent convey about the current season? If it has rained, the earth may emanate a warm, fresh aroma; perhaps there's a hint of flowers. Engage your olfactory senses, and be attuned to any memories evoked.

Taste the air; let your tongue explore your mouth. What does the saliva feel like, and what flavours linger on your tongue?

Connect with the earth beneath your feet and the trees surrounding you. Rediscover the lost art of grounding—walk barefoot upon the earth, touch trees and bushes, feel the various textures, and sense the awakening of memories and your nervous system. Now, reflect on how much feeling and pleasure you are willing to welcome into your life.

In moments of stress or disconnection from nature and my body, I immerse myself in my environment, utilising my five senses. Whether lying on the ground like a starfish or pressing my forehead against the earth or a tree, I breathe deeply. This instantaneously calms and rebalances my nervous system, serving as a cleansing ritual, particularly after engaging in bodywork with others. Washing your arms and hands with natural salt further grounds, cleanses, and awakens the senses, especially if you work in an environment which requires physical contact with others.

Tips to Activate Your Five Senses

Sight

- Declutter your home. Make the space you live in beautiful.
- Buy yourself flowers and smell them!
- Eat on your best china plates. (Who are you saving them for?)
- Look at yourself in the mirror and see yourself as beautiful in your eyes.
- Take the time to connect and look into your eyes throughout the day, learning to love who you are. See your soul light up behind your eyes.
- Light candles and use soft lights.

- Spend time in natural light and in nature.
- Paint your house and wear colours that make you feel alive.

Sound

- Play music that makes you feel good.
- Put music on when you cook, clean, and drive. Feel the music and sing and dance. Remember, we are vibrational beings, and sound can greatly impact us.
- Listen to how the twigs break as you walk in the forest, how the birds sing, and the river flows.
- Listen to the silence and pause in each moment.

Feel

- Use pillows and blankets that feel good to you.
- Wear underwear that makes you feel sensual.
- Hug your loved ones.
- Get a massage.
- Take time to massage your skin with body lotion. Feel the touch of your hands over your body instead of quickly slapping it on.
- Apply hand cream throughout the day and take time to touch yourself.
- Remember, beautiful textures make you feel sensual because they awaken your senses.
- Feel into what you need, what you desire, and what you want.
- Take warm baths and use beautiful oils.
- Ask your body, 'How do you need to feel or receive love today?' Is it a gym session, a dance, or a walk? Stop putting pressure on yourself to make it be a certain way. Your body knows what it wants.

Taste

Did you know that there are five different tastes, not just sweet and sour? We tend to forget when we are rushing and inhaling our food.

Eating is an intimate act; you are introducing something into your body, and just like sex, food should bring you pleasure. Eating is a sacred ritual of energy exchange, not just a calorie count or intake! Food represents your primary connection to this world—a gift that should be relished, not viewed as a burden, chore, or addiction.

Choose foods that captivate your taste buds. Reduce processed foods and refined sugars that dull your tongue's natural sensitivity. Shift towards a cleaner, plant-based diet that allows you to truly savour the essence and natural flavours of the food you eat. Initially, berries and fruits might not taste that sweet, but as you eliminate excess sugar and carbonated drinks, you'll be astounded by how juicy and flavorful a pear or apple truly is.

Smell

- Wear beautiful oils or perfume without added chemicals.
- Use hair and body products that are as clean and bio-friendly as possible but still smell heavenly.
- Treat yourself like you are beautiful—because you are!
- Treat yourself the way you'd like to be treated rather than waiting for others to do so. When we support ourselves, those around us take notice and see us for who we truly are. They understand how we wish to be treated. How can anyone fully love us if we don't love ourselves? Taking care of oneself and practising self-care is an excellent way to demonstrate to your children or loved ones that looking after oneself is important. We aim for their best, but we must first set an example and embrace self-love. Remember, our children follow our actions, not our words. Be the guiding light they can look up to.
- Use perfumed, non-toxic candles.
- Burn incense.
- Start smelling the air to inhale and smell each season.

My Rules for Eating

- Set the mood with some music while preparing a meal that promises to leave you feeling healthy, vibrant, and satisfied.
- Approach planning, preparing, and cooking as a sacred practise, reshaping your perspective on these daily tasks.
- Chant, in-chant or whisper prayers as you prepare your food.
- Embrace your uniqueness by using your best cutlery. Don't reserve it solely for special guests—you are special!
- Enhance the dining experience by lighting a candle for a pleasant atmosphere.
- Disconnect from distractions; put your phone away. Allow yourself the time to sit and savour your meal without the rush of eating on the run or at your desk.
- Prioritise chewing; it might seem obvious, but many overlook this crucial step, hindering nutrient absorption and leading to bloating and gas.
- Avoid drinking while eating to preserve taste and stomach acid balance, preventing bloating and potential IBS symptoms.
- Take a moment to breathe, release tension from your shoulders, and fully savour every flavour!

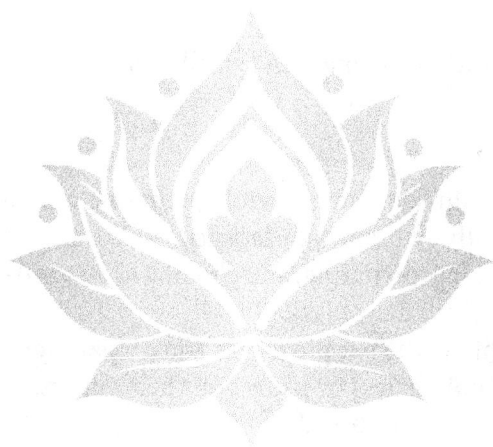

CHAPTER 12
PRIORITISING PLEASURE

'And the day came when the risk to remain tight in a bud was more painful than the risk it took to blossom.'
—Anais Nin

In my late thirties, I had reached a point in my life where I had to get honest with myself. I was dissatisfied, bored, and depressed. The quality of my intimate relationships with friends, husband, and work was a sham. I was tired much of the time, annoyed at my kids, and angry with my husband over small things that, in hindsight, didn't matter. I felt heavy in my body and heart, and every day was an effort.

I was generally dissatisfied with my life and felt extremely guilty about it. At the same time, I didn't let myself feel it deeply and truly allow all the feelings to come into my consciousness. I didn't know how to feel and express all of it, all of me. It felt too much, and I feared it might consume me. I kept myself busy to avoid facing the parts of my life I was unhappy with. I moved quickly, chasing the highs, constantly needing to achieve something—whether it was crossing another task off my to-do list or anything else—to avoid confronting the emptiness and despair that threatened to overwhelm me.

I avoided my own reality by focusing on others—scrolling through social media, playing the rescuer in my friendships—distracting myself from my own life and wasting precious time. I was merely surviving, not truly living. I knew I had to be honest with myself to confront the deep-seated grief I had buried. I had to face the places I feared the most. I was filled with anger and disappointment over the choices that had led me here. My anxiety grew from my inability to be alone with myself, and I felt deep regret for living so disconnected for so long.

I had been lying to myself for far too long, and the truth was surfacing faster than I could suppress it. I faked happiness, orgasms, and joy. I didn't know who I was—I was a patchwork of other people's beliefs and dreams. I knew I was supposed to feel, but I just didn't, and that haunted me. I felt deeply flawed, even though I had spent my whole life trying to do things right. I faked more than I felt, but there was a yearning within me; my body and soul needed more than just survival. I wanted to thrive, to dance naked, to be unapologetically messy! But at the same time, I was scared of expressing myself, fearing I was too much, not enough, that I'd be rejected or not accepted. I wanted sexual pleasure to be the norm, not a chore—I wanted to feel truly alive.

The day I finally saw my life clearly, stripped of all my self-imposed ideas and ideals, I realised how much pleasure I was missing and how deeply unhappy I was. I knew I couldn't continue living this way; something had to change, and that something was me. This realisation led me down a new path, reawakening and initiating me back into my sacred lineage, bringing me here to share this journey with you. The path of pleasure and sacred sexuality isn't just about chasing highs, ignoring lows, or hoping for change through rituals alone. It's not always about pleasure—it's about dancing between pleasure and pain, living a life so full that you can feel and embrace it all because the truth is, we are everything—all of it.

I had spent my whole life denying parts of myself, thinking they were bad, not good enough, or simply too much. Pleasure embodies both light and dark, and it's important for me to acknowledge that here. Your pleasure isn't a one-way ticket to bypassing and suppressing your true self in search of fleeting highs and false security. Embracing my genuine, embodied pleasure and sacred sexuality meant getting honest with myself, and the truth is, it's not always pretty. It's not meant to be!

Wherever you are on your life's journey, you've been brought here for a reason. I've come to believe there are no coincidences, and I honour the part of you that dares to dream a new dream and create a new reality. This journey is about birthing your authentic connection to your unique aliveness, pleasure, and joy. It can be challenging to tune into our pleasure when we have little experience in cultivating true joy and happiness. We're often highly motivated to please and help others, responding like well-trained girls, conditioned to say yes to obligation and responsibility, to be the 'good girl.' For many of us, pleasure feels like an exotic destination or a paradise holiday we dream about. We see the pictures, read a bit about it, and imagine going there, but it remains just a dream—a fantasy reserved for certain women who look a certain way, not a reality meant for us.

Some don't even want to experience such a place, dismissing it as overindulgent and a waste of time. They believe they couldn't or wouldn't be able to relax, feeling the need to stay busy. The constant chatter of the mind, with its endless to-do lists, makes the whole idea seem like too much effort. Women are exhausted from trying, failing, and feeling let down.

Many of us think of pleasure as something we need to seek from the outside, not realising that it actually resides within us. We often subconsciously repress it due to fear and taboo surrounding the idea, or we're simply too exhausted and feel we don't have the time. I understand—as a working mum of four, my life is busy too. But what I didn't realise was that prioritising pleasure actually gave me more energy!

Many of us have our inner 'radio' tuned to pain, stress, and constant doing. We forget that we can change the channel. I know life gets busy, and it's easy to get caught up in the fast pace around us, but your pleasure is inside, waiting to be activated. This habit of living with a 'cup half full,' choosing pain over pleasure, affects how our nervous system communicates with our body. We're neurologically wired to focus on pain and discomfort rather than pleasure. Feeling negative has become normal and comfortable because it's familiar. Many women have never fully experienced pleasure in their bodies because they're unconsciously addicted to self-repressive thought patterns. Often, the enemy is within.

Even though we dislike feeling this way, the predictability of staying in control—even if it's painful—feels safer than breaking free and embracing the unfamiliar. The fear of losing control or not knowing how we'll react comes from this internal conflict.

What if I told you that pain is simply the absence of pleasure? That persistent lower back pain you deal with daily could fade away if you rewire your nervous system to focus on pleasure. Pain and pleasure are processed in the same part of the brain, but we often feel pain more intensely because our thoughts, beliefs, and actions are more attuned to it—like a familiar friend. The voice of pleasure, on the other hand, has often been muted or dimmed. We no longer recognise it; it feels foreign, like something from another world, and can seem alien and unsafe.

Pleasure is the feminine life force that awakens you from years of slumber. No handsome prince will save you and give you the kiss of life for a happily ever after! That was a lie. The true power and kiss of life lie within each of us. How much longer will you live half-awake or with your eyes wide shut? Why aren't we embracing it? Pleasure is the catalyst for change, vibrancy, and new life. It is the fountain of healing, youth, and the balance we crave. Few truly experience it in its full light and potential; it's as if we are afraid of this power and what it might do to us. So, we repress it, follow the rules set by others, and pay the price in our mental, emotional, and physical health.

When I ask women what brings them pleasure or what they do for pleasure, they often look at me blankly as if wondering why I'm asking and what it has to do with how they feel. They might cough, avoid eye contact, fidget, blush, and start talking faster. The unfamiliar topic causes them distress. Once the initial panic subsides, there is noticeable relief because, deep down, we all know we're not as connected to our bodies as we want to be. Most women start talking about their partners, families, children, work, or anything other than themselves. We've been conditioned to find pleasure through others, not from within. This leads women to live through their children or partners, creating control, resentment, and dissatisfaction. It also puts pressure on those we love to fill our emptiness, becoming their burden. This approach always fails because it's not their job to fulfil us; it's ours. This unconscious behaviour results in over-controlling actions, jealousy, and possessiveness. When we believe our pleasure and happiness come from another person, we try to control them and protect that source of joy, making it our purpose and reason for living. Without them, who are we?

We often seek pleasure from food, overeating to get the oxytocin hit or the sense of love that pleasure provides. We eat when we're not hungry because we crave pleasure and have linked it to food and drink. Shopping, buying, and browsing online, even without purchasing, are also ways to get a quick, superficial endorphin hit of pleasure. We're trying to fill up on this feeling, searching for something we can't quite identify. We long for something we cannot describe, but our bodies crave it. How often have you wanted something, bought it, and felt pleasure? How long did that pleasure last before it turned into guilt, leaving you feeling empty again?

Saying 'yes' to your pleasure is what turns you on in life. Pleasure invites you home and back to the feminine of your body. Inside every woman is an innate, unassessed power, packed with sexuality, health, spirituality, self-love, energy, and overflowing confidence—and it starts with you connecting to your pleasure.

The absence of the feminine means the absence of pleasure and life force. When we begin to prioritise pleasure and no longer see it as an indulgence, we open to our emotions, feelings, and soul's wisdom. The feminine helps us surrender and get to know our bodies, our shadows, and how we work.

When we understand how the female body works, we can heal and rewire our beliefs, nervous system, and biology, changing our life story forever. This allows us to move from merely surviving to truly thriving.

Pleasure = Shifting from Surviving to Thriving

There is a new consciousness awakening on this planet, and many women strive to become more spiritual, healthy, and intuitive, but they often do this through the mind. I believe that the way to connect with God/Goddess is through your body. You must go deep into your pain and shadow to emerge into the light. Pleasure awakens the spirit, not just the body. When we ignite the fire within our yonis, wombs, breasts, and hearts, we connect to our soul and Shakti life force, which flows abundantly within. With true self-awareness and an understanding of our feminine landscape, the heart can open, the soul can breathe fully, and we come alive. It's difficult for the heart to open and for our walls to come down until we are warm, know ourselves, and are ready to accept all parts of ourselves—flaws and all.

When I reconnected back to my yoni, I was transported back to when I was a little girl, around the age of four, when I knew that the universe was part of who I was, when I believed in magic, trusted my body, and the invisible world felt more real than the visible one. I could smell the roses from the rose water I used to make. Colours, sounds, and feelings were more vibrant than ever. I tasted the rain, felt the earth under my feet, laughed deep belly laughs, and cried tears of joy. I felt the presence of Mother Nature. I saw how everything is connected and alive through geometry, realising that we are all just vibration and geometry. I understood I was part of something much bigger than I had ever imagined.

My existence and health came from a pearl of profound wisdom, and it now seems absurd that I had tried to control it, tune it out, and fit myself into an acceptable patriarchal box. I come from the whole; I AM whole. The problem was that I couldn't see it and only focused on the safe and palatable parts while others were buried away.

I realised I was connected to everything around me and understood the saying, 'As within, so without; as above, so below.' There was no separation, no compartmentalisation. I saw no boxes or walls, just a divine force maintaining a delicate balance between chaos and order, the duality from which we all come from and exist in. I was part of all of it! I had forgotten and kept myself busy chasing something else. I had no fear; I trusted myself and my body. I was one with nature and the universe, connected to life itself.

Wholism: The ism that fills that hole we are trying to fill.

Pleasure rewires your brain's chemistry by releasing feel-good hormones and endorphins—nature's own antidepressants. It increases oxygen levels, opening us up to love, joy, fun, self-confidence, presence, and self-awareness. With so many of us experiencing pain, health issues, depression, anxiety, being overweight, and feeling overwhelmed, isn't it time to tap into these abundant natural resources within us?

These neurotransmitters naturally dull pain, increase blood flow, lower blood pressure, and prevent heart disease, enabling us to face life differently. Our pain or discomfort no longer has an iron grip on our lives and health.

Orgasms directly affect our hormones and blood chemistry. They teach us to let go and surrender to our bodies instead of fighting them. Pleasure and orgasms flood the nervous system with healing chemicals that spread throughout the body. Activating the pleasure centre between our legs also triggers the pleasure centre in our brain, rewiring our thoughts and feelings and healing us from pain and trauma. It's the ultimate journey of transformation.

The opposite of pleasure hormones is stress hormones, which drain our energy and health, affecting our periods and activating the pain body by wiring us into tension, pain, and constriction. The body always mirrors the nervous system and soul. A woman who is turned on is happy, confident, and experiences pain differently. She is open and understands her body's language. When a woman is disconnected from her body and ruled by stress, she becomes constricted, tight, small, and stuck in a cycle of pain. She feels uptight, often angry, and frustrated. She may feel alone and overwhelmed, quietly suffering from anxiety and depression. Outwardly, she may struggle with lower back pain, headaches, and shoulder pain. Weight is usually an issue because she is weighed down by her over-controlling behaviours and chronic health problems.

Case Study: Hilda

Hilda was always angry. She argued constantly with her partner, finding fault in almost everything. Even when things were good, she found something else to complain about. She was obsessed with keeping her house spotless, constantly cleaning the floors and windows, and chasing after her children with wet cloths to prevent any marks on her pristine white walls. Her temper was quick, and she frequently shouted. She drove like a speed demon, often yelling and overtaking others, always in a rush and running late, blaming everyone else for her tardiness. Hilda complained a lot, had a negative outlook, and felt like everyone was against her or what she believed in. Her energy was seriously depleted, draining herself and those around her.

When Hilda came to see me, she had growths in her vagina and chronic tension on one side of her vaginal wall. It was clear from our conversation that Hilda felt embarrassed about her yoni. She had showered and used wet wipes before our appointment and had sprayed a lot of perfume to mask her natural scent because it disgusted her and made her feel ashamed. She rarely had sex, and when she did, it was more of a task to check off her to-do list than a desire. She felt overweight and was constantly struggling to lose weight.

She craved chocolate every day as it was her only source of pleasure. Hilda felt trapped and was frankly miserable. Her relationship felt more like a convenience and often turned into a battleground. She blamed others and found it difficult to take responsibility for her choices in life and her body.

We focused on reconnecting Hilda with her yoni. I guided her on self-massage and self-pleasure techniques, helping to awaken the energy up to her heart, which had been closed off for as long as she could remember. I introduced her to the jade egg and crystal dildo, and we practised breathwork and movement. Gradually, she started to revive. After three sessions, she walked into my office with a newfound confidence, ditching her baggy mum jeans and oversized t-shirt for a beautiful dress that highlighted her feminine curves. It was like seeing a different woman altogether.

Hilda shared that she had felt genuine desire for the first time in years. She wanted to engage in sex and nearly experienced her first internal orgasm. When I asked about the growths and the pain she had mentioned earlier, she looked at me as if I was speaking a foreign language. She had forgotten about the issues she had come in with. She said her pain had vanished, and she felt more sensation down there than she had ever imagined possible. When she checked her growths three months later, they had nearly disappeared, and a few months later, they were completely gone.

Hilda stopped striving for perfection and stopped pushing herself and her family. She relaxed into life, let go of control, and began to discover pleasure within herself. This is a common story I encounter daily, and it can be your reality, too. When we opt for pleasure instead of pain, we become more attuned to love rather than fear. Fear keeps us small, drains us, and saps our vitality, leading to sickness. We were never meant to live in fear; we were meant to live fully and in love. This is what you've been seeking and what may be missing from your life. Your yoni is the wellspring of your pleasure, and it's time to connect with her more deeply.

ᨆᨆ❧ᨆ

Play

'This little light of mine, I'm gonna let it shine, let it shine, let it shine, let it shine...'
—Harry Dixon Loes

The biggest revelation of my life came when I realised I had been trying to live, create, and achieve everything based on rules and a persona that wasn't truly mine. I was stuck, trying to build my business, connect with the Goddess within, and have healing and mystical experiences, but I felt disillusioned. I lost faith in myself, in healing, and in the universe.

One day, I had a powerful insight after my 'She-Movement' practise. Like many, I had become overly serious. My job, chores, kids, and responsibilities were overwhelming me. When it came to my health and spirituality, I applied the same 'get down to business' mindset, striving to achieve the 'right' outcomes using my mind rather than my body. I realised I was bored and weighed down by constantly overachieving and trying to be everything I thought I should be. It was draining me, and I resented it.

This resentment and boredom were pushing away everything I wanted to create and feel in my life. Like attracts like, and my negative, head-driven approach was suffocating my life force. I was constantly trying to look or be a certain way, say the right things, and have it all together. I was chasing after purpose, the next big thing, and all the social media promises of an amazing life and body. But instead, I felt like a failure, filled with shame and self-judgement. I was frustrated and angry with myself, asking 'Why isn't it working? What's wrong with me? Why does it feel so difficult and heavy?'

The serious voice in my head told me, 'You need to be serious, Michelle. You don't want to look stupid. No one will take you seriously if you don't act the way people expect.' I had been battling my inner critic my whole life. Being serious was my armour, a way to avoid feeling vulnerable, ashamed, or humiliated. Seriousness, dependability, and rigidity were my shields. As a child, I was bullied and constantly teased for being a 'silly little girl,' and the 'dumb blonde' jokes haunted me. I spent my life trying to prove everyone wrong, to show I could be successful, to become a doctor. I pushed myself, overachieved, and tried to escape that feeling of not being good enough, of not feeling accepted or loved. My wounded inner child was running my life, dressed up in a tight, professional persona with a rule book that was bursting at the seams. I was weighed down not only by societal expectations but also by my own inner rigidity and need for control.

I was running from humiliation, believing that by becoming someone important, I could prove I mattered, that I was enough, and ultimately feel safe in this world. But even after becoming a doctor and achieving so much, I still felt like I wasn't enough, like a fraud, constantly fearing it would all be taken away. Inside, I was insecure and empty.

My moment of clarity came when I reconnected with who I truly am—the person I was before I buried her away. I'm a free-spirited, funny, imaginative, and creative woman, but I had silenced that part of me. I had followed a path dictated by the patriarchy, trying to live life in a masculine way while my feminine essence was locked away, both literally and figuratively.

Releasing this playful, feminine energy has transformed my life. When I embrace her, I see possibilities instead of limitations. I feel light, joyful, and connected to a creative flow where ideas come easily and effortlessly. My masculine side is still there to support me, but it no longer constricts me. The love and pleasure I now allow myself to experience are a miracle, and they were within me all along.

When we view life through the lens of the feminine, embracing a light-hearted perspective and flowing with our natural cycles, we connect with our true selves. From this place, we can heal, create, and live authentically. But when we constantly push and force ourselves to fit a mould, we're going against our true nature, and nothing feels or flows naturally.

We need to align with who we are and create from that place. It's a journey, and we'll face resistance because we fear looking silly, feeling humiliated, or not having everything together. But that fear and need for control are draining your life force and making you unwell. You were designed with a unique blueprint—God made no mistakes. So why try to follow someone else's rules? You are perfection, inside and out. You just got caught up in the belief that you needed to be fixed, tamed, or shaped to be successful, safe, and loved. It's easy to get stuck in the 'I'm not good enough' narrative, but what if you asked yourself these questions:

- What am I good at?
- What do I enjoy?
- What brings me joy?

Spending time just being for beings' sake isn't a luxury but is essential for your health and spiritual growth. When you get uncomfortable with doing nothing, congratulate yourself because the answers are close and are going to give you some of the biggest clues to your blocks.

- Why can't I do anything?
- Who told me not to play and that doing nothing is wrong?
- Who am I still trying to prove something to?
- When did I feel stupid or humiliated, and how does that still affect me?
- How much pleasure do I experience or allow myself to experience every day?
- What is it I'm avoiding inside?
- What am I trying not to feel?

> 'You can't solve problems with the same thinking you use to create them.'
> —*Albert Einstein*

Today, I invite you to spend 5 minutes doing nothing—perhaps walk in nature or simply sit and enjoy your tea without any electronics. Gradually build this up to 20 minutes a day. After all, spending 20 minutes on your health and spirituality isn't much to ask, is it? Think about how much valuable mental and emotional space gets lost to scrolling through social media every day. How do you feel after wasting half an hour to an hour looking at everyone else's perfect lives and trying to find ways to improve or fix your own? This habit drains our energy and traps us in the cycle of feeling inadequate, constantly comparing ourselves to others. It leaves us feeling worse, and then we waste even more time and energy trying to fix problems we wouldn't have if we just tuned into ourselves. Start spending time with yourself. I promise you everything you need is within you.

Self-care

Sometimes, self-care can feel superficial, but if you're not taking care of yourself, who will? Let's be honest; we all feel better after a long bath, a haircut, or a massage. So what story are you telling yourself that says you don't need it or don't have the time or money?

- I have kids…
- I have too much to do…
- I have to work…

A belief system within you is probably keeping you stuck in these negative patterns. Whether it's an issue of self-worth, self-love, or feeling like you have to be superwoman, it's crucial to address it because it's holding you back from becoming whole. Here's the truth: women often struggle with receiving. We're just not comfortable with it. From a young age, we were taught not to be too much, too greedy, or too selfish and to always put others first. This inability to fully receive affects every aspect of our lives, even our sex lives and relationships. It's so ingrained that we can't even accept a simple compliment without downplaying it. How many times has someone complimented you on your clothes, hair, or something you did, and you brushed it off? We water ourselves down to be more likeable, more acceptable, and not too much. We fear that receiving comes with a cost, creating an obligation.

I challenge you: the next time you get a compliment, simply say, 'Thank you, I receive that.' Start doing this with everything and everyone. You'll be amazed at how it builds your confidence and energy when you stop tearing yourself down. Now, let's take it further. True self-care is about listening to those negative voices in your head and turning them into more loving, respectful, and supportive thoughts.

These are the voices that say:

- I'm ugly, fat, overweight
- Useless
- I'm a bad person
- I shouldn't eat or drink that
- I feel worthless
- I'm not good enough
- Who do I think I am
- No one likes me

You get the idea… start catching those thoughts and get curious. Ask yourself, 'Whose voice is that? If it's not mine, then whose is it? When did it show up? If I'm observing these thoughts, they aren't the real me—so who is this imposter with all the negativity, and where did it come from?' We all have memories rooted deep within us that form the basis of these limiting beliefs. Often, these beliefs are tied to the very essence of our femininity. Reconnecting with that part of yourself is key to freeing up this energy—it's part of your self-care, specifically for your feminine core.

First, remember who you are beneath all the masks you've been wearing—take them off and tune into your body. I do this by taking deep breaths into my lower belly, connecting with my womb. I imagine opening the curtains and windows, letting in fresh air and light into all the hidden corners. I remind myself that I'm a daughter of the Great Mother, with an incredible energy and creative life force inside me, just waiting to be used for my health and daily life. It's likely been stagnating from disuse.

I thank my womb for birthing my four babies and for the scars around my labia that ensured their safe arrival. I express gratitude to my clitoris, g-spot, and cervix for the pleasure they bring me and for opening portals to my higher self. I breathe into all of these sacred spaces, imagining light flowing in and filling them, clearing away the dark, dense negativity and shame I've carried throughout my life and perhaps even longer.

I massage her and bring renewed blood flow to her. I read poetry that speaks to my heart and womb. I forgive myself and others and surrender to the sacred wisdom within. I let go of self-control. I ask her how she feels, how she wants to feel, and what she wants and needs today. When I'm tuned into this place inside, I can show up whole as myself in the world. Life no longer feels like a struggle, and I can show up as my fully embodied, divine human self.

There's a saying in the Bible taught to all children in Sunday school: 'Love others as you love yourself.' But looking at the world today, it's clear we're not loving each other as we should. It's difficult to love, accept, and appreciate others when we're not doing that for ourselves. The term 'self-love' is often used, but how many of us truly feel and experience love for ourselves? Can we honestly say, 'I love myself completely, with all my flaws and strengths, warts and all?' Or are we only loving parts of ourselves, just as we often love others conditionally? We tend to project blame and judgement onto others because facing those feelings within ourselves is painful and uncomfortable. It's easier to see faults in others than to acknowledge and own them in ourselves.

A key spiritual truth is this: 'If we can see it in another, it exists within us.' Everything is a mirror. We have the choice to look into that mirror, face our shadow, and grow, or we can live on autopilot, ignoring our intuition, burying our heads in the sand, and continuing to play the martyr or victim. The choice is always ours—this is your body, your life, your power. What will you do with it?

Self-care and understanding how we're wired is about learning to love all parts of ourselves so we can fully embrace who we are and become the person we're meant to be. It's not about just accepting the parts we like and pretending our shadow doesn't exist. That's like having a smoke detector that alerts you to a fire, but instead of putting out the fire, you turn off the alarm. This analogy applies to our health, our minds, and everything in between. Many of us function this way unconsciously, treating our inner guidance and intuition as inconveniences we don't want to hear or feel. We walk around with fires burning and our smoke detectors turned off, ignoring the warning signs, and then we're shocked when our life, health, or body isn't working as it should. Developing a relationship that is open, loving, compassionate, creative, and kind—first with ourselves and then with others—is essential.

We cannot give to others what we aren't able to give to ourselves.

Embrace the Pause

In all great musical masterpieces, there is a pause before the best part of the music. It's like riding high on a rollercoaster, and just before you fall and your stomach does belly flops, there's a sacred pause. It tells you to take note and pay attention; something important is about to happen.

Your sacred pause is the time in the day when you make time to tune into that voice inside. You can call it mindfulness, meditation, or quiet time, but it involves taking yourself into yourself to empty, listen, and receive. This is ultimate self-care—listening to what we want and need rather than going into overdrive and pushing through because we're too busy.

Taking a break helps us stay connected and energised while also rebalancing and resetting us. Many women I work with come to me after neglecting these necessary pauses and now find their bodies demanding it without asking. This can manifest as back pain, burnout, or other health issues, with the body effectively saying, 'STOP, enough; we need to reconnect. We can't keep going like this, or we'll face serious consequences that we can't recover from.' Remember, your body's natural wisdom is always looking out for you, and often, these breaks are crucial turning points, signalling the need for change. Embracing this pause can be thrilling because making decisions about your health and life based on wisdom, intuition, femininity, and the 'She' force can transform your life in unimaginable ways. So, if you're experiencing a 'sacred pause,' congratulations—great things await as you welcome rest, play, and reconnection.

In the darkness, we find our light.

The 'good girl' in us has been conditioned to do the 'right thing' and behave in a way that's socially accepted and liked, often at the cost of our own well-being. Our brains are wired to avoid anything uncomfortable or unsafe, so we tend to push down or ignore what we truly feel. This often leaves us feeling quietly ashamed and humiliated by the feelings we try to hide.

But what if we started to change our belief systems and the stories we've been told? What if we created new values that are aligned with our intuition and soul rather than just reacting to fit in and be liked? Many women I work with struggle with health problems because they've ignored their inner guidance for years. Disconnected from their bodies, they're often tired, and their physical, mental, and emotional health suffers as a result.

Reconnecting with your body and living from that place is where real change happens. This is where your whole world begins to shift, and miracles happen. This is what I wish for you.

The body always knows.

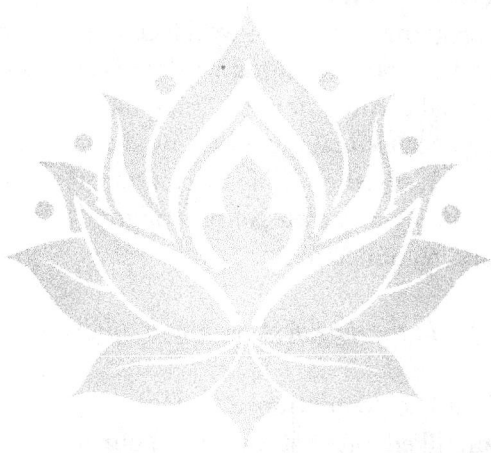

CHAPTER 13
YOUR UNCONSCIOUS SHADOW

'The only thing we have to fear is fear itself.'
—Franklin D. Roosevelt

Thoughts and fears influence our bodies by holding us down, trapped by the weight they hold over us or in us. Every thought carries a frequency and vibration that affects our biology. Thoughts and beliefs are like weights that hold you tight so you can't be free, light, and float up like the hot air balloon I discussed in the last chapter. When we become stuck and weighted with thoughts and beliefs that we can't let go of, they control and possess us.

Phrases such as the following can lead to resentment, procrastination, self-sabotage, and self-hate that we project onto our bodies and others:

- It's not fair.
- I'm entitled to this.
- Why her?
- It shouldn't have happened.
- I need to be better, thinner, prettier, younger.

When we blame everything on our stomach, thighs, or bottom, we have a target and don't have to take responsibility for how we feel. Our primary belief is that when this one thing changes, I will be perfect; therefore, my life will be perfect, too. This anger, frustration, and body shame are a breeding ground for pain and disease. Sometimes, the shame and anger we feel about ourselves becomes too much to bear, so we project this unconscious shadow onto a partner, our parents, the past, a teacher, or a boss.

Present Time

We only ever have the present; the past has passed. We can repeatedly find ourselves stuck in the past, but that's a choice. You hold the power to decide to stay present in the moment. The future hasn't happened yet, and there are no certainties, so start focusing your energy and attention on the here and now because everything else is an illusion—one that's costing you your health. Remember, miracles occur, and healing takes place, but all of this happens in the present, not when we're clinging to old issues from the past or obsessed with how we think our lives should be. Healing can occur instantly, in a moment! If it seems to be taking too long, it's time to get present and examine your thoughts and fears—the burdens you're carrying that freeze time, trapping you in your current reality.

Being present isn't always comfortable; it's direct, honest, and challenging. It's akin to taking away a child's dummy/pacifier, signalling it's time to grow up and take responsibility. My three-year-old daughter still uses one. She wants to stop because she feels embarrassed and hides it with her hand. But she finds comfort in it because it makes her feel safe, and it's familiar to her. She's also worried she won't be able to sleep without it, and honestly, so am I. This situation is similar to when we stick to negative thoughts or habits that don't help us simply because they're familiar and emotionally comforting. We make excuses for these habits, telling ourselves we'll change them… someday. When it comes to your health and happiness, it's about getting honest with yourself. It's time to face the truth and your emotions bravely. A quick, decisive action is often less painful than a prolonged, hesitant one.

Often, when a patient comes in experiencing significant pain, they will exhibit reluctance to the suggested protocol. The fear of life changing too rapidly and the energy required for it to happen becomes a reason for hesitation. But when it comes to healing, it's not always about getting healthy or removing the pain; it's about redefining your relationship with time. I often say to a patient, 'You have a time problem, not a physical one. Your body will heal and change if you do XYZ, yet you don't do it because you're scared to heal that fast. Therefore, you have a time problem built into your thoughts and beliefs about what your body can and should do to heal.' When someone says 'yes,' busts through their resistance and makes the changes, they feel lighter and more empowered, and the universe synchronises to support them. Miracles occur, and they heal extremely quickly.

Other patients who are living in the past, unable to forgive or move on, are dragging the past around with them like a bulging, overfilled suitcase that weighs them down physically and emotionally. How heavy your body feels—how dense and stuck you are mentally, emotionally, and physically—is a good indicator of how much baggage you're carrying and if you're living in the present time or not.

Embracing love, including self-love, is critical to healing. Yet, we often hide behind excuses, avoiding the truth and the wisdom we hold within. We've gotten used to valuing power, status, and material possessions, fearful of empowering ourselves and acknowledging our inner knowledge. We avoid facing our vulnerabilities, ignoring our true feelings and insights. Instead of connecting with ourselves, we prioritise feeling important and separate from others, which ultimately harms us. Our default focus on power and control must shift to embracing love, self-trust, and respect, which requires bravery and self-empowerment. When we connect with this inner love, we open ourselves to grace, healing, and transformation. Choosing love over fear is crucial in every situation. Being honest with ourselves is freeing, allowing us to understand and confront our obstacles, often realising we are our own biggest hurdle. Energy is flexible; recognising your truth is the first step to embracing your identity.

Do you have a hard time making decisions? If so, is it because you understand the power of your choices? Deciding means actively shaping your reality and committing to yourself. Not following through can erode your self-trust and energy. Failure can lead to anger and frustration, setting off a chain of negative events. However, returning to the present allows us to reset and make new choices in every moment. Breaking free from our automatic patterns requires time, love, dedication and ongoing self-forgiveness. Recognising and changing these habits is part of personal growth. Every setback is a chance to start over and continue our journey toward health, whereas dwelling on failures only leads to more pain.

Every decision sets a pattern in motion. As energetic beings, our choices affect us and the world around us. Healing ourselves and choosing love benefits everyone and contributes to global healing. It all begins with choosing love over fear.

I am a body of light. I share that light with myself and the world I love.

Beliefs

'Change your perception and history, and your present life will change.'
—Patti Conklin

Your beliefs shape how you see the world; they act like a lens through which you view everything. These beliefs, influenced by your past experiences and teachings, guide how you live your life and affect your health.

You don't get what you ask for; you get what you believe.
You are either growing or fading.

Our thoughts, actions, and reactions are driven by deep-seated beliefs. How we love, heal, and experience the world depends on these beliefs, which often operate automatically, subconsciously guiding our lives and health. Our words carry significant power, each having a positive or negative impact. Negative thoughts and words build up in our bodies, leading to blockages that can eventually cause pain and illness.

Your words constantly create your reality.
You are the author of your own life and health.

What you believe and how you see things matter. Your body reacts to your thoughts and beliefs, which are shaped by your perceptions, often without you even realising it! Unconscious beliefs can limit your thinking, affect how you experience life, and make you feel disconnected from others. Choosing your beliefs reflects your true self and causes less conflict than simply adopting those around you. Personal beliefs are freeing and bring peace, balance, and a connection to your soul.

In contrast, beliefs ingrained since childhood can feel burdensome, fearful, and unsettling. For example, if you believe you're destined for knee and back surgery because it runs in your family, you might unconsciously make choices that lead to that outcome, proving the belief true. Your biology begins to mirror your biography.

It's interesting how quickly we tend to believe in negative possibilities, often struggling to trust positive outcomes. Beliefs that encourage us to think negatively and fearfully can lead to negative results because we attract what we focus on.

For women, it's crucial to understand our beliefs about our bodies and where they come from. Keep the beliefs that serve you well, but let go of the ones that hold you back. Consider your family's views on healing and pain and how you might have unconsciously adopted them. Looking at how your mother and grandmother saw their bodies can reveal what you believe about your femininity and your role as a woman. We must dig deep to remove the negative beliefs that prevent us from reaching our full potential, like weeds in a garden that block the sunlight and our true brilliance.

Some questions to consider:

- What needs to be cleared away or refreshed physically, mentally, or emotionally in your life to allow you to blossom fully?
- What were you told about menstruation growing up? How does that affect how you see your period? If you see it as painful and inconvenient, can you see it differently?
- What cultural beliefs about women's roles and sexuality, such as being labelled as promiscuous or pure, and norms around premarital sex or the number of sexual partners, have you taken to be true?
- Are you aware of society's views on needing to control, clean, and medicate the female body?
- How have you internalised these beliefs and made them real in your life and body?
- What are your beliefs on healing? Do you believe your body can heal, or do you run to the doctor for medicines or scans when you have a problem?
- What is your belief system around pain and illness?'

Some women avoid their period by continuing to take the pill from month to month; some women have never looked 'down there' as they think it's disgusting, smelly, and sinful. How does this show up in your body as mistrust and denial of the feminine within?

Growing up, I learned to instantly use medication for any discomfort or illness, thinking pain was something bad. However, I've realised that pain signals something deeper needing attention. Even fevers, part of the body's natural defence mechanism, are often hastily treated with medication that can interrupt the healing process. The body can heal itself without compromising the immune system or affecting the microbiome. While I have taken medicines, I now try to support my body's natural intelligence first.

Some people become so identified with their pain and health issues that it becomes a part of their identity, fearing who they would be without it. This attachment can prevent healing because, deep down, they may not want to let go. Consider a goldfish in a bowl;

it's content but confined. If moved to a pond, the goldfish grows, exploring a new environment that fosters a different belief system and reality. Similarly, changing our beliefs allows us to grow beyond our limitations. Sticking to old beliefs or living unconsciously restricts our growth, keeping us in repetitive patterns and leading to fatigue and illness. It's time to aim for more expansive experiences.

Long-held thoughts turn into beliefs that affect our biology. Beliefs influence our health energetically, contributing to the rise in autoimmune diseases. These conditions, where the body attacks itself, may be the immune system's response to negative beliefs and emotions within us. Autoimmune diseases, often accompanied by depression and stress, signify a deeper issue where the body reacts to self-neglect and harmful environments created by negative thoughts, unhealthy foods, and neglectful behaviours.

Can we trust our feelings?

'To thy own self be true.'
—Shakespeare

Can we trust our feelings? It's a paradox. Trusting our feminine intuition is crucial for healing and tapping into divine guidance. However, we must also question the foundation of our feelings. What belief system or conditioning shapes the lens through which we filter our emotions? Are these feelings driven by our ego or guided by the soul?

Clarity is essential for understanding the origin of our feelings because these often-unconscious emotions form the basis of decisions that impact our health and life. Distinguishing between a feeling rooted in deep intuition and one influenced by conditioned beliefs or filters is crucial for well-being.

Start by approaching your feelings with curiosity. Observe them, accept them, and refrain from hastily dismissing them. Feelings frequently stem from fear or a distorted interpretation of facts. Our conditioned mind, entangled in beliefs or past experiences, often perceives situations through a narrow lens that may not align with the truth.

For instance, we might say, 'Look at how she looked at me... she must have been thinking _____; it's true—I felt it.' Often, misinterpretations arise because we're feeling through our conditioned mind, which acts as a filter influencing our perception.

Conditioning encompasses thoughts, memories, traumas, beliefs, past experiences, or what we were taught to think and believe during childhood and through media influence. Developing awareness of these influences is vital for fostering genuine intuitive understanding.

Ask yourself:

- Where do these feelings come from?
- Where do I feel them in my body?
- What are these thoughts and beliefs based on?

- What memories come to mind?
- Is there an emotion attached to it?
- What's the trigger?

Neuro-reactivity is when we unconsciously react to a situation through unconscious feelings. Life gets complicated when we live on autopilot, acting like ticking time bombs ready to explode, often hurting ourselves or others. By taking time to understand our feelings without becoming overwhelmed, life becomes simpler. This way, we save energy and protect our health.

How can we tell the difference between true intuition and ego-driven feelings? Intuition doesn't come from anger, jealousy, fear, or defensiveness. It feels like a calm, clear inner voice that gives us confidence without anxiety. Unlike the uneasy feelings that follow actions based on negative emotions, intuition brings peace, even when we can't logically explain why or how we know something.

Living by the ego adds stress and burdens, pulling us away from our true selves. The ego thrives on drama, connecting with parts of us like the inner victim or child, keeping us trapped in fear and defensiveness. When we react from the ego, we tend to blame others, feeding the ego's need to feel right and leading us to dwell on past hurts as excuses for our actions. We create stories that inflate the ego, seeking validation from others.

However, in quiet moments, we might notice a disconnect between our actions and our deeper truth, which can lead to guilt and a desire for introspection. The ego also tries to control and validate our existence through material things and status, which can mask our true emotions and insights. We must move beyond our conditioned responses and perceptions to see reality clearly, seeking the truth in every situation.

The truth will always set you free.

Reacting from our ego can lead to defensiveness and unnecessary conflict, causing stress and harm to our bodies. When we feel judged or shamed, it can lead to anger, frustration, and resentment. It's important to be honest and recognise how our words impact ourselves and others. Before reacting, it's helpful to pause, consider the situation calmly, and ask how we can contribute positively. How can we see things differently? Reacting defensively often harms ourselves as much as it does others.

Getting caught in a cycle of blaming others or feeling like a victim can prevent us from making healthy choices and healing. We might feel trapped in negative patterns, blaming others without taking responsibility for our projections. Feeling the need to be correct or superior with false feelings of pride can lead to misunderstanding and conflict. It's a common human trait to want to feel powerful, but it often leads to more harm than good.

Reflecting on my own life, I've recognised times when I was quick to blame others instead of accepting my part in situations. Believing I was always right was a way of coping and striving for success. However, real growth and understanding have come from facing challenges and questioning my beliefs.

We always have a choice in how we respond to others and situations. It's not about seeking revenge or labelling others as wrong but about finding truth and justice in a balanced way. Moving away from gossip and judgement has been a journey for me—one that has led to a deeper understanding of myself and improved my relationships. It has also meant letting go of people and behaviours that no longer align with who I am. This can be uncomfortable, especially for someone who has spent much of their life as a people-pleaser and a 'good girl.'

Learning to trust and express my true feelings has been life-changing. For a long time, I focused on pleasing others and seeking external validation, which left me feeling disconnected and unfulfilled. Perimenopause became a turning point, pushing me to embrace my feelings and live more authentically. This journey has taught me the value of freedom and the importance of trusting my emotions and instincts.

Perfection

'A woman who is starved for her real soul-life may look "cleaned up and combed" on the outside, but on the inside, she is filled with dozens of pleading hands and empty mouths.'
—Clarissa Pinkola Estes

Striving for perfection can stress us out and make us ill. It creates a barrier between us and others as we try to feel good enough, loved, and accepted. Perfectionism makes us overly focused, inflexible, and controlling, all to appear flawless and feel worthy. This pursuit keeps us stuck, always chasing an impossible standard and forgetting our inherent value. Media, materialism, and pretending to be someone we're not add to this unrealistic pressure. We hide our true selves, fearing judgement, which feeds our insecurities.

Constantly hiding who we really are drains our energy and leaves us feeling empty and unhappy. Any satisfaction from being 'perfect' is short-lived, and soon, we're chasing another goal, hoping it will make us feel better. But it never does because we're seeking false validation from outside ourselves.

Perfection is an unattainable goal that actually separates us from our true selves, making us ignore our body's signals, intuition, and inner wisdom. It's a harmful cycle that drains our life energy. The mask of perfection often cracks when we face serious challenges like illness or deep unhappiness when we no longer have the energy to keep up the charade. It's in these moments that the light can start to shine through.

Perfection and the Female Wound

Stop shrinking to fit into an idea or ideal you have outgrown.

Striving for perfection traps us in our minds, making us overly focused on logic and external things like achievements. This mindset leads us to compare ourselves to others, causing jealousy, resentment, and stress, which affects our emotional and physical health. We may start seeing other women as competition, damaging our relationships and well-being—what's often called the 'sister wound.' Gossip and hostile behaviour towards others usually reflect our own perceived shortcomings, harming our health and disconnecting us from a sense of unity. Fairy tales like Snow White highlight these patterns, where jealousy and negativity towards others mirror our insecurities. While we don't act out these stories literally, negative talk and thoughts about others can hurt our health and happiness. Speaking badly about others ultimately harms us, making us feel restricted and leading to both physical and spiritual discomfort. Our negative words impact us the most, keeping us from feeling connected and well.

In the darkness, we find our light.

Our 'perfection shadow' is both a friend and a teacher. It's not about eliminating or ignoring this shadow but acknowledging it, listening to what it reveals, and understanding our true feelings and identity. What we project onto others and what we envy in them often highlights our unconscious desires—everything is a mirror. Ignoring our darker aspects and focusing only on our positive traits can lead to unhappiness and poor health. For genuine growth—physically, spiritually, and emotionally—we need to unconditionally love every part of ourselves. Denying parts of ourselves only makes them demand attention more strongly.

The dark side is a part of us, and the best way to handle it is to accept and work with it rather than deny its existence. Allow it to express itself so you can better understand your feelings and find compassionate ways to grow, acknowledging and accepting the fears, beliefs, and emotions driving your pursuit of perfection.

Accepting vs. Resisting

You can't heal what you can't feel.

Feeling easily upset or 'triggered' is common, especially when we're busy, stressed, and tired. Being triggered can start a series of reactions in our bodies and minds that impact our health. If you can't identify and manage your triggers, they can begin to negatively affect you, causing high-stress levels and feelings of being out of control. Continuous triggers can affect your breathing, blood pressure, and hormones, leading to anxiety or panic. It's essential to recognise that only you can break this cycle.

When you're triggered, take a moment to feel what's happening. Move your focus away from your thoughts and into your body. Notice where you feel the trigger physically in the body, and pay attention to sensations such as tightness, pain, fast breathing, or a rapid heartbeat. Let these sensations exist without judging them. Try to understand what emotion the trigger is bringing up and sense where this lives in your body. Imagining this emotion as having a shape, colour, or sound can help you see and feel it as something existing in your body rather than seeing your body as the problem. This approach can also be helpful for those dealing with pain or illness.

Ask the pain:

- Why are you here?
- Where did you come from?
- What are you trying to tell me?

Triggers often come from coping mechanisms we developed as children or during stressful times to protect ourselves. When I practise this exercise, I gently place my hands on the affected part of my body and breathe in white light and love. As I breathe out, I imagine the discomfort becoming smaller and lighter. I also use 'She-Movement' with breathing and sound to change, improve, and move the energy in my body. The sensation usually feels stuck, dense, and heavy and needs to alchemise by expressing itself, becoming lighter and more fluid. When I finish and open my eyes, I feel better and am no longer caught up in what was upsetting me. This way, I don't let the issue weigh me down or control me for the rest of the day. My nervous system calms down, and I feel peaceful.

Emotion vs. Feeling

I want to clarify the difference between emotions and feelings. Emotions and feelings are not the same, though many women have confused them their whole lives, leading to an uncontrollable emotional rollercoaster. Emotions come first—they are the body's response to a trigger, releasing chemicals based on how we perceive and interpret a situation. Feelings, on the other hand, come after emotions. They are more specific and relate to how we think about and interpret those emotions.

Understanding this distinction is important because feelings are the gateway to releasing physical pain and trauma stored in the body. When we ask someone where they feel an emotion, and they describe its colour, texture, smell, or shape, it helps to root into the feeling and release it from the body.

Many of us get caught up in our emotions because they're not just reactions to present triggers but also carry the weight of past, unhealed emotions stored in our bodies. This is why certain triggers feel so overwhelming—the body is holding onto all those unresolved emotions, making the response feel bigger than the situation itself.

Go Hunting

Our minds often keep us from feeling emotions because it seems too overwhelming or unsafe. We might think it's easier to block out these feelings because we're scared of feeling too much, worried we might fall apart or everything around us might collapse. Instead of facing these feelings, we might start thinking negatively about others or ourselves, blaming someone else because it's easier than dealing with what we're feeling inside. I used to criticise myself harshly, thinking I wasn't good enough or that bad things would happen, just to avoid facing my emotions.

Now, when I notice I'm getting triggered, I try not to get caught up in these thoughts. Instead, I focus on what I'm feeling in my body. I call this process 'hunting' for the cause and feeling. I pay attention to where I feel tight, uncomfortable, or numb and try to identify the emotion, whether anger, sadness, or frustration. It is important not to judge or push these feelings away but to sit with them and be compassionate towards myself.

She-Movement practises, breath, and sound can help move these feelings through and out of my body. For some people, simply sitting still and focusing on breathing are enough. It's all about listening to your body and letting it show you what it needs to heal.

Negative Thinking

'A pessimist sees the difficulty in every opportunity.
An optimist sees the opportunity in every difficulty.'
—Winston Churchill.

When we're in a lot of pain or stuck in a negative cycle, it's tough to imagine things being different. We often think bad things always happen to us and say things like, 'I can't imagine that,' which limits our healing. We get used to expecting the worst, partly because of the distressing news and events we hear, making us feel overwhelmed and insignificant. This negative outlook becomes a habit and something we wish to escape, yet we often find ourselves stuck in it.

The idea that 'like attracts like' means that if we focus on negativity, we'll likely experience more of it. This concept has been a challenge in my healing journey and for many women I work with. When you're in pain, it can take over your life, making your world revolve around it and feel smaller.

Our habit of expecting more bad things to happen keeps us in fear, feeling weak and unworthy. Searching for our symptoms online can lead us to fear the worst, creating a cycle of stress and pain.

Instead of focusing on what hurts or isn't working, focus on where you feel good in your body and life. For example, I may have a headache, but my legs and feet are strong and relaxed, and my heart is full and open. When I focus on the positive, I allow that energy to spread through my body and consciousness. This is a powerful way to rewire our biography and biology from pain to pleasure.

The cycle of fear can keep us stuck, drain our energy, and affect our sleep, leading us to worry endlessly about what others think or might say. To break this cycle, keep a diary of your daily experiences and feelings. After a week, look for patterns to understand what's bothering you and differentiate between fear-driven projections and the truth.

Having open conversations with people who trigger us can also be insightful. It can act as a mirror, showing us what we need to work on to preserve our energy instead of losing it. You only ever have power over your reaction to others, not over the actions of others. Your perception is your power; ultimately, it's all that matters.

Change your perceptions, change your life.

The Glass Ceiling—Your Default Negative Programming

We all have limits on how happy, healthy, and full of life we allow ourselves to be, like a personal threshold or glass ceiling. These limits often stem from our childhood experiences and beliefs, including real and imagined events, adopted belief systems, and unexpressed emotions. This threshold represents our comfort zone, where we feel safe, even if it's not the best for us. We all want to grow and achieve more—whether it's finding love, getting promoted, or starting a business. Yet, we often fall short without understanding why. What we desire lies just beyond our comfort zone, in the unknown, where risks are involved and outcomes are unpredictable.

Joy, balance, health, and ease are all beyond this glass ceiling, but reaching them can feel impossible—we hold ourselves back without realising it. Our bodies cling to familiar negativity for safety, even if we long for change. Feeling genuinely good and happy can seem strange for many stuck in negative patterns because positive feelings are unfamiliar. We might stick to old habits, even if we don't like them, because they feel safer than trying something new and challenging. To truly change and increase our capacity for happiness, it takes courage to push beyond this self-imposed ceiling.

When things started going well for me, I would always hit my glass ceiling. I'd start to work more, stress over things that weren't important—anything to feel the familiar negativity I knew. I could not feel, let go or enjoy any small success I had. I would pick a fight with a loved one, start obsessing about my body or my age, look at something that needed to change in my house—anything to make me feel the safety blanket of my negativity. The glass was half empty and not full. I complained about it constantly but could not change it for a long time.

The classic scenario was when I was doing well with my health, feeling fit, looking good, confident, and sexy. This was a huge glass ceiling for me. I would sabotage it all by overeating, binging, or drinking too much alcohol and would wake up hating myself, feeling down, depressed, and angry. I had created the self-sabotage; I was feeling too good, and it was unfamiliar. It was safer to feel terrible; it's what I knew. Smashing my glass ceilings has changed my life and negative patterns. There is always another glass ceiling awaiting us because we are continually growing and evolving, but now I understand what my triggers are. It's easier to push through and up my happiness thermostat. I get to decide how good I want to feel, and I choose to feel amazing.

You never fail—you learn.

If I encourage you to aim higher, dream bigger, and push beyond your limits, it's because growth, the thrill you're looking for, doesn't happen if you always stay in your comfort zone. Here's the reality: there's a gap between where you are now and your fullest potential. This gap is where your growth happens. It's where you'll face challenges, make mistakes, learn, and expand. Through these experiences, you refine yourself and become the best version of yourself, ultimately becoming the person you're meant to be.

So, where do you find yourself at the moment? What's holding you back? And who do you want to become? To heal your body, you must first go in and feel everything you have spent your whole life trying to avoid.

Get Into Your Body

Handling my triggers and realigning myself has been transformative. For most of my life, I grappled with numerous triggers—frustration, anger, and worry. Looking back, I realise I was disconnected from my body, driven by a desire to control everything due to fear of losing security or loved ones. These triggers gained substantial power, running and disrupting my life without my awareness. I thought it was normal amidst the busyness of raising four kids and managing a business.

It wasn't until I delved into working with my sexual energy, my shakti, that I discovered my numbness and the fact that I was leading a half-life. I wasn't fully alive; I was merely surviving. This realisation was a wake-up call. Despite having so much, I felt empty. Awakening and reconnecting with my sexual energy made me understand that we can't truly be alive without feeling and inhabiting our bodies. My body serves as the vessel through which I experience life, and there I was—burnt out, depressed, in a hormonal crisis, and frankly, unhappy. Despite my efforts to get everything right, I wasn't living a full experience because I wasn't present in my body; I was living in my head and to-do lists.

Your body is the vehicle for transformation.

Reflecting on my past, I chuckle at how I was living a half-life, thinking I was doing remarkably well. Successfully managing everything, from chasing after my kids to dealing with work, I realised I was neglecting my own needs in the rush. Amidst my chaotic thoughts about parenting, work, and daily tasks, I was alarmingly numb to my body's signals.

In the midst of busyness, I had learned to override my body's needs, unintentionally blocking its signals. I now understand that this pattern was a dysfunctional coping mechanism rooted in self-protection and survival, typical for those with childhood trauma or a sense of insecurity. Ignoring the body's signals leads to a disconnection that often results in health issues.

Through healing and reconnecting with my body, I've awakened my neural pathways and sensitivity. I've come to appreciate the importance of tuning into my body's wisdom, realising that being present in my body is crucial for living a fulfilling life. Integrating and rewiring my nervous system has allowed me to experience pleasure and joy that was once blocked.

Now, taking care of and listening to my body has become a sacred practise. I find love, safety, and security within myself rather than seeking them from external sources. Even in busy times, I maintain awareness and consciously try to recover and reconnect. This shift has bridged the gap between who I am and who I aspire to be.

Many women live incongruently with their true essence, causing stress and unhappiness. When women reconnect with their bodies and align with their true selves, they experience a transformation—reduced overwhelm, increased patience, increased body awareness, self-love, and improved relationships. I've learned that being the source of my health and happiness positively impacts all aspects of life, making choices that align with my values and embodying the best version of myself.

Integration

Uncovering the underlying reasons for your stress and examining your beliefs is crucial. It's time to let the weary part of yourself rest and rouse the sleeping tiger within. Initiating changes and prioritising your health empowers you to tap into every facet of your being. Break free from the perspective of the past and begin envisioning yourself in a fresh light.

'Believe, behave, become.' This is the language of transformation. Shift your mindset from 'I can't' to 'I can, I have, and I will.' Break free from habitual thoughts that hold you back, such as 'It will never happen' or 'That will never work.' Remember, your words shape your reality. Building new realities and fostering health involves rewiring neural and energetic pathways—physically, mentally, and emotionally. Change occurs when we embody our beliefs.

Here are some practises:

1. Value your precious time; express your true feelings and thoughts without sugarcoating. Be straightforward to save time and energy, minimising frustration in your interactions. Avoid the pressure to be the 'good girl' and embrace your authenticity without needing to prove anything—you are enough as you are. Establish healthy boundaries, making your 'no' clear and your 'yes' definitive.
2. Clarify expectations and urgency; be honest about promptly responding to emails and texts. Prioritise self-care, guarding against the creeping fear of urgency and expectation. Delegate tasks whenever possible; while you may do things quicker and better, consider the cost to your well-being. Delegating fosters satisfaction, team building, and community.
3. Slow down, breathe, and resist the urge to multitask. Connect with your heart, seeking guidance and support from your higher self. Shift your perspective on the to-do list; instead of feeling obligated, view it as an opportunity to accomplish tasks. Ground yourself, take a moment to assess what you realistically want to achieve today, and be content with that.
4. Align your activities with your menstrual cycle and the moon's phases, adapting your approach to reflect your current stage.
5. Be the woman now that you long to be NOW, not in the future. Embody her and watch as the universe aligns to your new frequency and vibration.

Journal Prompts:

- What humiliation, fear, or shame has happened in the past?
- Whose love and acceptance are you still desperately wanting to feel?
- What are you trying to prove, and to whom?
- What will achieving the perfect body or life give you? What's the emotion you are seeking?

Now, think back to when you did something that you perceived as 'perfect.'

- Did it make you feel how you thought it would?
- Did it heal the pain or fill the void?
- When in your life have you not felt loved, good enough, or accepted?
- How are you trying to heal that wound now in your life by being perfect?

Dance

If you feel tight in your body and mind, put on some lively music with a beat and start to dance like a free-spirited woman. Move your body in ways you wouldn't normally. Imagine you are breaking free of the tight contractions you have been holding yourself in. The aim is to be as imperfect and free as possible. Let your mind go, breathe, and surrender to how your body wants to move intuitively, not how you want it to. Remember, the body knows what it needs; it's super intelligent, so get out of its way and dance!

Aim for 5 minutes a day or one song you love every day. I like to do it in the kitchen with my kids when making dinner. It has become like brushing my teeth; it is one way to undo all the conditioning that tightens around me, all the responsibility and pressure that builds up throughout the day. SHAKE IT OFF!

CHAPTER 14
REPRESSED EMOTIONS

What is repressed will be expressed—you get to decide how...

What we repress needs to be expressed, and when it isn't, it gets stored in our bodies, leading to physical, spiritual, and emotional sickness. Emotions can be stored in our cells and passed down through generations. Real healing begins when we become aware of these emotions, face them, and start the journey back to our true selves. This is the true heroine's journey.

As women, we've often been told that we're too emotional and that our emotions make us weak or out of control. Many of us feel wrong or guilty for having them. From a young age, we're taught that happiness and joy are acceptable, but anger, jealousy, and rage make us 'bad.' We hear messages like, 'No one will invite you to their parties or want to be your friend if you act that way.' We learn to hide our true feelings to appear perfect.

Growing up, we weren't always allowed to talk about our emotions or what happened at home because society values a picture-perfect image. I remember after my parents had arguments, my mum would make me promise not to tell anyone. She worried about what others would think; the humiliation was unbearable. We were taught that our worth was based on appearing perfect. Over time, this turned into a deep fear of humiliation and shame within me. I carried this burden for years, trying to seem like I had everything together until it became too heavy to bear.

When a woman shows anger or raises her voice, she's often labelled irrational, hormonal, or crazy. Yet when a man does the same, it's seen as asserting authority and power. This double standard exists because we've been conditioned to believe that women's emotions are bad and need to be hidden. We smile, swallow our anger, and pretend everything is fine, pushing our true feelings deep down and denying them.

Emotions themselves are neither good nor bad—they're neutral. Our thoughts and perceptions about them give them positive or negative energy. When you feel anger or frustration, instead of bottling it up, ask yourself: Why do I think this is bad? Where does this belief come from, and why am I letting it shape my decisions? What am I afraid of? I want you to embrace your emotions, learn to connect with them, and see them as guides leading you back to your true self. But first, let's understand what emotions are.

For years, we were told that emotions were stored in our brains and that we could control them by changing our thoughts. Some self-help methods promote the idea that we can fix everything with positive thinking, saying, 'Stay positive, avoid the pain.' But emotions need to be felt in the body; we need to be present with them and know where they're hiding or being repressed. They are our inner GPS, guiding us when something is out of balance in our body or life. Ironically, we often spend so much time trying to suppress them.

Emotions are made up of feelings that originate in your body—they're visceral. As mentioned earlier, we feel emotions in our body, not our mind, so connecting with the body, feeling, moving, and expressing our emotions is crucial for healing. Your brain constantly communicates with your body, and you perceive events and experiences as feelings that affect all your senses. Think about your gut feeling when you meet someone and instantly like or dislike them—do you listen to that feeling or ignore it?

How often have you realised afterwards, 'I had a feeling something wasn't right,' but dismissed it at the time, thinking you were just being silly? As young girls, we often had instincts about people, places, or situations but were told it was our imagination or that we were mistaken. This led us to doubt ourselves, making us feel embarrassed or ashamed, so we stopped listening to that inner voice because being wrong felt unsafe as a child, which silenced our intuition.

Your body knows—it's that simple. Your body is innately intelligent and intuitive, and when you start waking up and living by this mantra, you will be amazed at how your life plays out.

When you feel an emotion, your body reacts instantly. Your heart might race, your stomach tighten, or you might start sweating. These emotions are felt as sensations in the body, triggering nerves that send signals to the brain, which decides how to respond.

We've learned about the autonomic nervous system and the vagus nerve, which affect our organs. Stress and this system, as well as other parts of the brain, like the hypothalamus and limbic system, influence emotions. However, the chemical changes that emotions cause in the body and their impact on our health are often overlooked.

Many of us have been to therapy, talked about our issues, and felt better but still found ourselves stuck in the same old patterns. This happens because emotions are stored in the body, and just talking about them doesn't fully release them. The body acts as the unconscious mind, holding onto repressed emotions until they become too intense to ignore.

Emotions from past traumas and experiences can be stored anywhere in the body, leading to pain, limitations, or even chronic diseases. These trapped emotions must be acknowledged and released through physical, mental, and emotional expression.

Neuropeptides are key in how our bodies and minds process and express emotions and memories. They are part of a network that extends beyond the brain, affecting cells throughout the body. These cells respond based on their conditioning to various situations, whether or not we're aware of it. This can lead to repetitive behaviours and emotional patterns that keep us stuck. To truly change, we need to address these deeper issues through willpower, understanding, and working with our body's stored emotions.

All of your memories are stored within your cells and receptor sights.

Think back to when a smell triggered a memory or a taste reminded you of something. Or perhaps when you thought you recognised someone while out shopping, only to realise it was someone who looked like someone from your past. These moments trigger memories and emotions.

It's often tricky for our emotional self to distinguish between what's real and what's not. Our perceptions and experiences can be skewed by emotions and learned behaviours stored within us, meaning we don't always see things clearly. For example, if you've grown up believing that pain is bad, you might feel more fearful and sensitive to pain due to past experiences. It's important to remember that we don't control what we remember or how we've learned to react, but we can take responsibility for dealing with this. Our goal is to bring these unconscious emotions to the surface and let go of the feelings that trap us in unhealthy patterns.

The Body-Mind Connection

Your mind and body are deeply connected; they work as one unit. This concept is central in Eastern and holistic medicine, which teaches that the mind, body, and spirit must be balanced for true healing. Ignoring any part can prevent full recovery. Your body reflects your emotions through chemicals, which can lead to illness. Understanding your emotions helps you understand your pain and health issues.

Your body is constantly renewing itself, from blood cells to skin cells. However, emotions and memories can be stored in your cells, affecting new cells as they regenerate. This can keep old, repressed emotions alive inside you. Addressing these stored emotions can stop them from affecting new cells, helping you heal from within.

Emotions that we avoid or fear can become physically trapped in our bodies, causing barriers or pain as signals that something is wrong. This can lead to conditions like tumours, where the body tries to protect itself by holding onto these emotions. Ironically, healing often involves letting go of these physical manifestations, even though they were initially meant to protect us.

Many people develop postures or physical symptoms as a way to cope with emotional pain. We can heal physically and emotionally by reconnecting with and releasing these emotions. In my practise, I see many women whose blocked emotions affect their nervous system, stress levels, and posture, leading to chronic pain and anxiety. This shows how closely our physical health is linked to our emotional state.

Your body communicates with you through pain and illness, often as a sign of blocked emotions. For example, physical discomfort after a stressful experience is your body recording that emotion. Ignoring these emotions can lead to serious health issues like heart disease or fibromyalgia. Your body is your soul's way of speaking to you, highlighting the need to address and heal emotional blocks for overall well-being.

Fascia and Trapped Emotions

Fascia is connective tissue that wraps around every organ in your body, including blood vessels, nerves, bones, and muscles. It's a living system that protects and supports your body's structure and constantly reacts to your emotions, whether you're aware of them or not. It's filled with nerve endings that respond to stress by tightening, which is why stress often leads to muscle tightness, back pain, headaches, or shoulder tension. When fascia tightens, you experience stiffness and pain.

Think of fascia as your body's memory bank, storing all your emotions. It acts like a protective barrier to keep you from feeling pain. However, over time, if we don't process our emotions, there is a build-up, causing the fascia to become even tighter. This can lead to more pain and physical restrictions in the body.

The body is a mirror of the mind.

After working with thousands of people, I've found this to be true. The body doesn't lie; it reveals a lot about a person's emotions through posture, movements, and the way they carry themselves. Even if you're telling me something, I'm closely observing your body language, which often shows what you're unaware of or not saying. This helps me understand how to truly help you heal.

Some might call what I do medical intuition, but I'm not fond of labels. I see the whole person, not just what you think you know or what you tell me. I aim to help you address the root cause of your issues, often found within your energy, frequency, and cells—the things you're not conscious of or have been avoiding because they seem too overwhelming or painful to face. Deep down, you know what the issue is, but your body might be showing it differently to protect you from the pain.

The issue is in your tissues.

Where are you storing your emotions?

Women often store a lot of their emotions in their hips and pelvis. When we're stressed, we might sit with crossed legs or suck in our stomachs, keeping those emotions tightly packed inside. This stress can cause us to breathe shallowly, only into our upper lungs, forgetting to breathe deeply into our lower pelvis. Breathing deeply into the fascia around our pelvis can help us become more aware of the emotions and unconscious wounds we carry.

Have you ever felt emotional when stretching your hips in yoga or doing deep exercises like squats? That's because when we truly relax, emotions we've been holding back can surface. Many women avoid slower activities like yoga because they're afraid of facing these feelings, even if they think they're too busy or prefer other types of exercise.

The psoas muscle, which tightens with stress and is involved in the fight or flight response, can hold onto blocked emotions in the hips. This muscle connects the upper and lower body and is crucial for movement, but it can become tight from too much sitting or constant stress, leading to back pain and pelvic issues.

Allowing emotions to flow without trying to analyse them can be liberating. Movement and therapy can help release these emotions, sometimes dramatically, as if freeing something within that has been protected for a long time.

It's also important to note that emotional pain can be stored around the heart, leading to physical symptoms like poor posture and neck and shoulder pain. Addressing these emotions is crucial not only for emotional health but also for preventing serious conditions like heart attacks and breast cancer. This highlights the importance of a healthy diet, lifestyle, and emotional well-being.

Common Negative Emotional Patterns in Women

The truth is that negative emotions carry weight. They weigh you down physically and energetically. This heaviness takes up space in your body—your cells, heart, and energy field. You start vibrating at a lower frequency because you are weighed down by all of the felt and unfelt unexpressed emotions. Metaphysics teaches us that 'like attracts like.' When negative thoughts and emotions weigh us down, we get stuck in a negative loop of attracting more of what we don't want into our lives and bodies. This builds up until we will eventually have pain or become sick.

The emotional patterns that we, as women, adopt are one of the keys to why we stay on the stressed-out emotional rollercoaster. As children, emotional patterns would have helped us and made us feel safe. Now that we are older, they become more detrimental to our health and often our personal growth. Here are some of the most common negative emotional patterns I see in women, myself included.

Can't Say No

It's very common to say 'Yes' when, deep down, we want to say 'No.' This often happens when we feel pressured by requests, even when we don't have the time, energy, or desire to do something. We might feel our body tensing up and emotions stirring, but instead of listening to these signals and expressing our true feelings, we suppress them and agree anyway. This usually comes from a deep need to be liked and accepted.

The difficulty in saying 'No' often stems from a fear of being seen as unkind or upsetting others, leading us to ignore our feelings. This makes us feel guilty for having those feelings and builds up resentment, which can spill over onto those closest to us.

Women, in particular, often struggle with setting boundaries and may find themselves giving too much, trying to prove their worth through actions rather than valuing themselves for who they are. This constant over-giving can be draining, increase stress, and harm our health. The habit of always saying 'Yes' can come from childhood fears of disappointment or abandonment or feelings of not being good enough.

It is important to recognise when we agree to things we don't want to do. Reflecting on why we feel compelled to say 'Yes' when we want to say 'No' can help us understand and change this pattern.

Pause momentarily and write down all the instances where you say 'Yes' despite wanting to say 'No.' Then, explore the reasons behind these choices.

Needing Acceptance, Approval, and Love

How many of us wished to fit in and be popular as children? How many of us felt the sting of rejection? This desire for approval drives us to seek worthiness and love as adults. Women have learned that their value hinges on how much and efficiently they accomplish tasks. Striving to be 'good girls,' we attempt to prove our worth, often disconnecting from our true selves. The ongoing journey to demonstrate our worthiness leads us to strive to become someone we believe is better, as we don't feel enough just being ourselves.

Many of us have been on this never-ending quest to prove our worth. While we may think we're proving it to others, it's a projection—we are just trying to prove it to ourselves; it begins and ends with us.

When we become aware of our behaviours and gain a bird's-eye view of how they shape our lives, we can change our behaviour and confront the avoided emotions. Understanding the drivers behind our actions is crucial, or we may forget and lose ourselves while trying to be everything to everyone. Recognising why we do what we do and the emotions propelling us is powerful and can help alleviate stress. Taking a moment to pause and breathe, we make our feelings conscious, enabling us to make different choices and craft a new story from this place.

Guilt

Guilt is the emotion I find most challenging; it's the feeling I turn to most often. As a mum of four, I frequently feel like someone is missing out or that I haven't done or said enough, even though I try my hardest. I believe that, as women, we carry guilt in our bodies like a heavy necklace weighing us down. We feel guilty for wanting more or less, not being a good enough mum or partner, overeating, or not exercising enough. It can feel like we're constantly under scrutiny, shaped by our beliefs and conditioning. We've allowed this inner critic—a dominating, patriarchal voice—into our lives, continually correcting everything we say and do.

Guilt is a futile emotion, often arising from assumptions or a lack of self-acceptance. Women often fear letting others down because of guilt, driving us to try to be everything to everyone, which leads to stress and illness.

It's important to remember that guilt is just a perception—a story you're telling yourself. In reality, we are only responsible for ourselves, not for the happiness of others. Our actions and words are ours; others choose how they perceive and respond to us. Their response is based on their beliefs, perspectives, and emotions, which will always differ from yours. If someone feels disappointed or happy, that's their choice and not something you control.

Over-controlling behaviour is a common side effect of guilt and is a widespread issue among modern women. We need to manage everything smoothly, so we analyse and plan every detail. The fear of losing control stresses us out. We even control how we speak to people, altering our words to suit different individuals and using 'damage control' to manage their reactions.

Control and guilt come from the idea that we're not good enough as friends, mothers, partners, or daughters. It's exhausting, and it breaks my heart when I hear women describe how they run their lives under these stressful patterns, often unaware of where it all comes from.

- What makes you feel guilty?
- What stories are you telling yourself?
- What are you trying to control, and what are you really afraid of?

Unable to Put Yourself First

What do we hear on an aeroplane during the safety demonstration? In an emergency, put your facemask on first—not your husband's, not your kids', but yours. When we neglect ourselves, we can't truly help or be there for others as we want to be. If our energy is low and we're stressed, arguments, resentment, and frustration start to surface, and we end up behaving in ways that don't align with who we are. We might lie in bed at night, replaying conversations and outbursts, feeling guilty about what we said or didn't say. We see ourselves becoming someone we never wanted to be, adopting patterns and behaviours that are out of alignment because we're exhausted and stuck in survival mode.

When it comes to our children or loved ones, we often think we must give them everything. But what they really need from us is love, honesty, and the freedom to choose and learn from their own mistakes. I remind myself and my kids every day that mistakes help us learn and grow—they're not failures. I try to show my kids that making mistakes is valuable to their growth.

Life is a learning journey—we're spiritual beings having a human experience. Saying sorry and correcting our mistakes helps us move on without guilt. If we're holding back because we feel guilty toward our family, it's essential to reflect on why. Sometimes, people use their children or partners as an excuse for not pursuing their desires out of fear, which can become toxic over time.

If we always play the martyr, putting others first and never choosing ourselves, we end up placing unfair expectations and guilt on our loved ones, making them feel they owe us. By caring for ourselves, even a little, we teach our children and partners that it's okay to prioritise ourselves. This helps us recharge and have more to offer, creating a positive flow of energy and happiness that benefits everyone.

Taking time for yourself is crucial. Self-care isn't a luxury; it's essential, like an oxygen mask. For me, yoga, sacred rituals, 'She-Practises,' and reading a book in a café rejuvenate my soul. Writing in a journal helps me understand my feelings, needs, and desires. Often, women don't prioritise their own wants, thinking it's selfish. However, allowing ourselves to enjoy life and embrace pleasure can significantly reduce stress and improve our well-being.

She-Movement

What does prioritising yourself look like?

I've developed a method called 'She-Movement' to help women release trapped emotions in their bodies. This can be done in person or online and is a powerful healing tool. In our society, we're often discouraged from fully experiencing our emotions, especially difficult ones like grief or anger. We're expected to show only positive emotions and hide the rest.

However, avoiding our feelings keeps us from fully embracing essential life changes, like becoming a mother or going through menopause. These stages are full of challenges and opportunities for growth, and facing our darker emotions can teach us a lot.

For a long time, I struggled to embrace all aspects of my womanhood and to trust my feelings. I felt disconnected from my true self and avoided my emotions, fearing that facing them would make me weak or overwhelm me. However, real growth and empowerment come from acknowledging and feeling all our emotions, even the uncomfortable ones.

Allowing myself to feel my emotions helped me realise that everything I needed was already inside me. Embracing the fullness and intensity of my feelings was essential for my growth and discovering my inner strength and power.

Just like winter prepares the ground for spring, facing our inner darkness is essential for personal rebirth. I learned to dive deep into my feelings, allowing myself to truly experience them, and, in doing so, found the light within me.

She-Movement is now part of my daily routine. It encourages deep emotional expression and is especially helpful for dealing with PMS, anxiety, or when you're feeling stuck. It can be as simple as dancing to your favourite music, letting your body express whatever it needs to. Movement connects our souls and bodies, serving as a gateway to our inner selves.

She-Movement—Moving Blocked Emotions

Before you start, let everyone in your house know that you're going to let loose for a bit. You'll be making some noise, so they don't need to call the police or send in a rescue team!

Start by writing down how you feel, or just jot down what's going on in your life and how your day has been. Clear a space in the middle of the room, away from anything you might bump into. Keep a big, soft cushion or two nearby.

You can put on any music that feels right to you—it might change every time, so trust your intuition.

Begin with a simple breathwork practise: breathe in through your mouth and out through your mouth. Avoid using your nose—this might be the hardest part. As the emotion builds, you'll feel physical resistance in your body. Start with 20 breaths, then work up to 50, and eventually 100 or more.

Let your body move, shake, and rock. Stamp your feet, pulse your hips, or shake your head from side to side. Make sounds and noises as you exhale. Some women feel like screaming, but for others, opening the throat chakra is tough. Try sounding the letters 'Eee,' 'Ohhh,' and 'Ahhh' as you exhale to help get started. The key is to keep breathing through your mouth and moving your body however it wants.

After about 10 minutes, you might want to get on all fours, grab a pillow, and start thumping it hard. Raise your arms high as you inhale, then bring them down forcefully on the pillow as you exhale with a scream or shout. This really helps release emotions.

Another tip is to imagine you're a small child having a tantrum. Kids are great at expressing their emotions fully. Roll on the floor, kick, scream, let it be messy. Allow yourself to feel and express everything inside—you naturally know what to do if you let yourself.

After about 10 minutes, you might start to feel sad and cry. Hold yourself like you would a child, soothing yourself by stroking your hair and skin, surrendering to the feelings.

When you're complete, thank your body for opening up and expressing, and go about your day feeling lighter and more in tune with yourself.

Some days, I skip straight to the pillow punching and tantrum-throwing. Listen to your body and let it show you how it wants to express itself—your body is your greatest teacher.

*Visit **www.drmichelleboycedc.com/resources** for She-Movement practises.*

Fibrocystic Breast Disease

My journey with fibrocystic breast disease has deeply influenced my career in health and wellness. Despite being a professional in the field, facing the disease for the third time made me question my expertise and integrity, which affected every part of my life. This wasn't my first encounter with the condition—I had surgeries at 17 and 19 due to similar growths. Driven by my family's health history and my childhood experiences of being bullied for my weight, I was determined not to let my genetic predisposition define my health.

This determination led me to a career in health, fitness, chiropractic, and holistic medicine. But despite all my efforts, I often felt like I was missing a key piece, especially when dealing with clients whose issues seemed more than just physical.

The discovery of another lump and the need for surgery became a turning point. I turned to meditation, journaling, and ancient practises to reconnect with a part of myself I had forgotten. I began to see the tumour not just as a problem to be removed but as a sign of deeper emotional issues. By connecting with this part of my body, I uncovered old pains and traumas from my childhood, like being bullied and feeling unsafe and unlovable.

Acknowledging and releasing these trapped emotions and memories allowed me to complete cycles of trauma I had unknowingly carried all my life. This realisation brought a profound change in my health and outlook. I understood that my physical ailments weren't just happening to me; they were manifestations of unresolved emotional pain.

This journey taught me the power of self-awareness and the importance of healing my emotional body. It also allowed my body and breast to heal without needing another invasive surgery. Healing isn't just about addressing physical symptoms but also about recognising and releasing the underlying emotions and beliefs that affect our health. True healing comes from within by acknowledging and letting go of what we've held onto for too long.

Learn To Feel It All

Embrace pain, for within it lies a transformative magic;
avoiding it only deepens the sense of being lost.

All your feelings and emotions are meant to be felt. The idea that some emotions are 'bad' needs to end. Feeling everything won't make you fall apart. Pain signals that something needs to change—physically, emotionally, or spiritually. It's part of our journey, turning challenges into opportunities for growth instead of getting stuck in the fear of 'what ifs.' Your emotions are valuable gifts, guiding you to listen and make changes.

Avoiding pain means missing out on life. We're often tempted to seek quick fixes—through purchases or medications—to mask our hurt. But this keeps us numb, trapped in negativity, and feeling broken. Avoiding pain leads to more suffering, making us lose trust in ourselves and our bodies. We end up feeling lost, afraid to embrace who we truly are. Your pain doesn't define you; it's not an excuse to opt out of life. You're meant to be vibrant and full of adventure.

It's time to stop waiting for someone to rescue us and face our challenges head-on. Like a Phoenix rising from the ashes, we can break free from what holds us back. Welcome your emotions like an old friend, and allow yourself to experience them fully.

Healing is more than treating symptoms; it's about becoming whole, embracing self-discovery, and trusting your inner strength. Your body has an incredible ability to heal itself when treated with love and respect. Trust in this inner wisdom that keeps you alive rather than relying solely on external solutions. It's time to take your power back.

CHAPTER 15
WHAT IS ENERGY?

Change your energy, change your life.

The body is a mirror of consciousness, where the invisible becomes physical. The physical is always the final manifestation of all your beliefs, thoughts, emotions, and feelings. It's much easier and energy efficient to go to the root, to the invisible energy, before it manifests into the physical.

The Energy System

Cleansing, balancing, and awakening our energy is essential to our health and vitality. Through years of working with patients, I've developed an understanding of energy, enabling me to consistently diagnose patients by reading and sensing their energy anatomy.

Observing specific postures, for instance, provides insights into how individuals perceive themselves and life. It reveals the activity levels of certain centres and indicates potential imbalances in chakra points, which contribute to discomfort and pain.

It's essential to recognise that your spine, energy, and nervous system are an integrated system. Addressing one area affects the whole. This holds true when attempting to change a pain pattern or resolve a health issue—all energy centres must be addressed to restore balance to your body, health, and overall life.

Within you is an intelligent energy system that connects you to your true self, the world around you, and the entire universe. This system consists of 12 chakras, or energy centres, also known as lifeforce—or Shakti. When these centres are balanced and functioning well, so are you.

This book focuses on the first seven chakras:

Chakra 1 — Root Centre
Chakra 2 — Sacral Centre
Chakra 3 — Solar Plexus Centre
Chakra 4 — Heart Centre
Chakra 5 — Throat Centre
Chakra 6 — Third Eye Centre
Chakra 7 — Crown Centre

Each chakra governs different aspects of your life, from physical and emotional health to spiritual well-being. All your chakras contain a blueprint of your internal and external environment. Your body and energy system continually read and communicate unconsciously with the world around you.

Organised and coherent energy forms intricate geometric patterns, storing light codes of DNA and the fractal blueprint that defines who you are. This information plays a crucial role in organising your cells. These remarkable energy centres collectively constitute your 'energy system,' similar to how various parts of your body form your physical being.

All of your chakras hold a blueprint of your internal and external environment. Your body and energy system are constantly reading and communicating with the world around you without your knowledge or cortical input. Cleansing and balancing your energy is essential for optimal health and life.

How the Autonomic Nervous System Influences Our Chakras and Can Cause Pain

Your autonomic nervous system, responsible for regulating your heartbeat and growing your hair, nails, and even babies, unconsciously influences and controls all your chakras.

Imagine each chakra having its own personality and brain, with distinct intentions and consciousness. These chakras constantly communicate information to the brain. Each chakra point also affects our cells, tissues, and organs, possessing its own glands, hormones, and chemicals for internal communication.

Like our nervous system, our chakra system seeks to maintain balance and homeostasis within our life and body, and it will strive to do so at any cost. Stress is a major contributor to the autonomic nervous system most of the time.

In our fast-paced, perfectionist world, stress is seldom turned off. It leaves us in sympathetic dominance and impacts our health in ways we may not even be aware of. Many of us only become aware of how stress affects our energy body and Shakti life force when we experience burnout, chronic health issues, or live with pain or illness.

Now, let's relate this to you. If you're dealing with chronic pain and health problems, you might be caught in a negative pain cycle, consuming vital life energy needed for healing to cope with increasing stress. Imagine the potential energy you could free up by using your energy differently.

Most women find themselves drained of health and vitality due to the constant demands of modern-day life and external expectations, creating a vicious pain cycle. An imbalance or incoherence in a cortical centre and its corresponding hormonal centre leads to cascading effects affecting cells, tissues, and associated organs, resulting in pain, stiffness and disease.

When our brain perceives stress, triggered by limiting beliefs or repressed emotions, the nervous system fires non-coherently, impacting the spine and creating incoherence within the body. Thoughts and perceptions trigger belief systems, producing emotions and feelings with different frequencies, leading to a cascade of neurotransmitters and hormones affecting cells, tissues, organs, and energy centres.

This negative feedback loop, where the brain and hormone sites exchange information, perpetuates chronic pain. Movement becomes affected, fear sets in, and stiffness increases, leading to more pain and disease. This cycle can continue for months or even years until the body becomes numb and unresponsive, eventually manifesting as more significant health issues.

Depression, burnout, and chronic pain often coexist, as pain affects not only the body and energy but also thoughts, feelings, and emotions, shaping future limiting beliefs.

Each energy point or chakra has its own brain and assignment, using the frequency of information it receives. If our thoughts, beliefs, and emotions don't align with who we want to be, this misalignment is reflected in our physical world, particularly in our health and life.

Chakras 1-3 are the centres where most women lose their energy, which correlates with pelvic and lower back pain and other hormonal diseases. It's crucial to emphasise that issues like neck problems, shoulder problems, breast cancer, and heart disease can be traced back to a blockage in one of the first three chakras. This highlights the importance of looking at a person holistically to address the root cause of disease and pain.

The Energy Flow of the Chakras

It's time to acquaint yourself with your chakra system and understand how healing these energy centres can positively impact your body and life. Your chakras are constantly receiving energy from the universe. While this might sound a bit woohoo, trust me, it's measurable.

From the root chakra (Chakra 1), we draw up earth energy and also pull down and rejuvenate energy from above through our higher chakras. I believe the root chakra is linked to Mother Earth, serving as the channel for Shakti life force, also known as kundalini energy, which rises up the spine. The energy from above tends to carry a more masculine quality, while the feminine energy is deeper and resides within the lower chakras. This feminine energy ascends from the earth through our feet, rising into our legs, pelvis, and lower abdomen. These energies continuously spiral up from the Earth and down from the heavens in a torus geometry, creating our energy field that spills out from the top and bottom of the body.

Furthermore, all energy consists of different vibrations, with lower chakras carrying lower vibrations and higher ones exhibiting higher vibrations. A low vibration doesn't always equate to negativity; it's a matter of high or low vibrations, depending on how the energy point is spinning and its openness and can vary based on the location in the body. For instance, Chakra 1 naturally has a lower frequency than Chakra 6 due to its location and function, yet both are equally important.

While meditation and mindfulness are often emphasised, what's frequently overlooked is 'embodiment.' We must be present in the entire body, not just the mind. The lower chakras ground us on earth, focusing on physical survival, while the higher chakras are more connected to our spiritual essence. Women need to be grounded and embodied before achieving the magic and gifts of the higher chakras.

Blockages in your chakras can disrupt the proper functioning of your energy flow and life force, hindering your ability to receive essential information. To illustrate, envision these blockages as boulders obstructing the flow of water in a rushing stream; the water can't flow as easily as it hits the rocks, which creates currents and ripples and slows down the flow of water and, in our case, energy.

Why do we have these blockages?

Blockages in our chakra system can be attributed to our belief systems and perceptions of life. These factors are closely followed by trauma, inherited beliefs from childhood, and past lives, forming patterns that affect us.

- You may feel anger due to a lack of support from a loved one.
- Experiencing pain and frustration with your health may also contribute to feelings of anger.
- Negative self-talk about your body image or self-criticism can also lead to negativity and anger.

These perceptions release neurotransmitters, affecting thoughts and emotions that impact specific chakras. For instance, Chakra 3 is linked to anger and resentment, which affect our breathing and posture. When this centre is not functioning properly, we may experience various physical issues like kyphosis, shoulder tension, headaches, liver problems, and stress.

Over time, these emotional patterns activate survival archetypes. Guilt may bring up childhood perceptions and fears, leading to relationship sabotage and distractions. This activates the victim archetype, creating a defensive mindset, escalating stress and anxiety within cells, affecting hormones and chakras, resulting in energy depletion.

Negative thinking and behaviours often become ingrained, and we may not be fully aware of them and the damage they cause. This lack of awareness contributes to physical changes like upper and lower cross syndromes, functional scoliosis, and kyphosis. Pain or disease doesn't always lead us to connect the dots, so addressing deeper belief patterns is essential.

Our beliefs, influenced by parents, media, education, and lineage, significantly shape our choices and actions. Factors like birth charts, rising signs, moon phases, sun signs, and ancestral influences also contribute to our energy system, affecting our body and life. Knowing your astrological makeup can help you lead a more aligned life. Astrology, the moon, and the sun affect your energy body, which can change cyclically.

The importance of your chakra and energy system is part of how you heal from disease and chronic pain. Evaluating belief patterns, discarding and working through those that no longer serve, and adopting soul-enlivening thoughts and behaviours are crucial for optimal health. It's like an energetic detox for the mind, body, and soul.

While positive affirmations are beneficial, true healing requires changing underlying beliefs, patterns and energy. Cleaning up your energy leads to transformative shifts, bringing about miracles and positive energy flow in your life.

Chakra 1—Root Centre

Physical Manifestation:

- Pain in spine, legs, knees, feet and ankles
- Collapsed foot arches
- Sciatica, hernia, and pain radiating down the leg
- Trapped nerves in lower spine
- Stiff and painful hips and Sacroiliac problems
- Lower cross syndrome
- Loss of lumbar curve
- Varicose veins, broken veins
- IBS, constipation and problems going to the toilet
- No connection to nature
- Lack of exercise, low energy
- Overweight, unable to lose weight easily
- Poor diet and self-care
- Iron deficiency
- Low immunity, gets sick easily and frequently
- Fibromyalgia or other autoimmune disease
- Unable to manifest desires
- Feel ungrounded, unbalanced, and disconnected from your body and others
- Fall easily
- Cross legs when sitting
- Stand on one leg, shifting hips to one side

Manages:

- Spinal column and nervous system
- Legs
- Feet
- Hips
- The body
- Energy levels
- Rectum and descending colon
- Our grounding in human form
- Survival, safety, and security

- Self-trust
- Community, sisterhood, friendships, and belonging

Energy Problems:

- Chronically tired, burnt out, stressed
- Depression and anxiety
- Laziness, general fatigue, malaise
- Forgetful, unorganised
- Attract drama in life
- Unable to own faults
- Stuck in survival pattern
- Hoarding; focused on material possessions and wealth
- Struggle to make ends meet
- Make love and friendship decisions from a place of lack and need for security
- Low sex drive
- Disconnected from the womb, femininity, and sexuality
- Not in touch with nature or the feminine cycle
- Numb, often on the pill or antidepressants, cut off from intuition and body
- Struggle with lack of time and energy
- Neglect friendships and loved ones in the struggle to survive

Nourish:

- Chakra 1 loves the colour red: eat red food, wear red colours.
- Dancing, Tantra, movement with breath and sound.
- Be in nature, walk barefoot on the earth.
- Paint, write, draw, decorate.
- Declutter, make space, purge what you don't need.
- Spend time with people you love.
- Nurture friendships and relationships.
- Practise Yoga, especially postures that help you balance and ground.
- Walk with a goal of 5,000 -10,000 steps a day.
- Hug a tree.
- Create a safe, sacred space in your house and spend time there every morning.

Beginning the Journey...

Chakra 1 is our connection to the earth, linking us to our roots and culture. In the world of the esoteric, where the mind often dominates, this chakra is often overlooked. Many people I encounter lack a strong mind-body connection to this chakra, and this contributes to much of the physical, mental, and emotional suffering we see today.

This chakra is the densest and keeps our spirit grounded during our human experience. It has the lowest vibration and accumulates heavy baggage over the years—things we've suppressed, like unspoken emotions, unresolved issues, unrealised dreams, fears, shame, and guilt. These suppressed emotions build up, creating a kind of emotional 'storage' that we try to keep locked away. When this chakra shuts down, we disconnect from this part of ourselves, losing sensation and sexual desire, often feeling ungrounded and numb. Our energy gets trapped, trying to contain these buried emotions and desires.

This stagnant energy drains our life force, causing stiffness and pain. It's like a blocked drain that prevents emotions from fully releasing, leading to a backflow that saps our energy. This is why we experience pain, fatigue, hormonal imbalances, depression, and burnout.

This energy centre is deeply connected to the earth, grounding us like the roots of a tree. Our energy meridians run deep into the Earth, while our higher chakras act like the sun, nourishing and replenishing our vital energy. This interconnected system links us to all life and the Shakti life force of the Earth, providing grounding, nourishment, and balance for a healthy, fulfilled life.

When we think about gravity and our physical connection to the Earth, we should also consider what we give weight to in our spiritual and emotional lives. This means examining the beliefs, narratives, grudges, and negative emotions that hold us down. These attachments keep us stuck in the past, creating patterns like victimhood, self-righteousness, blame, and resentment. These patterns stop us from being present and prevent healing. They shape our identity and influence our decisions based on past experiences, causing us to repeat the same stories in our lives, often in ways we don't even realise but that our body feels.

What you think and feel shapes who you are.

Letting go of this emotional weight and choosing what we give gravity to is essential for healing. Healing requires letting go because holding on to outdated beliefs and behaviours has long-term consequences—like a boat that can't sail when it's overloaded. The empowering truth is that you have a choice; you're always in control. This is your life, and you can shape it through your perceptions and choices.

Forgiveness is the key to inner freedom. Take note of where you're holding on to patterns, beliefs, and judgements—both of yourself and others—that drain your energy. Love has an expansive, healing quality, while fear tends to contract and diminish us. An unbalanced Root Chakra often signals a state of fear, which controls our actions and thoughts.

Love expands, fear contracts.

Think of your energy body like a tree. Just as a tree is nourished by its roots, we are sustained by our own 'roots,' even though we only see the visible parts—our bodies, like the tree's branches and leaves. Ignoring the importance of the Root Chakra, especially in a world that often focuses on the mind, is a common mistake. Many people lack a strong connection to this chakra, contributing to widespread physical, mental, and emotional suffering.

This chakra invites us to examine where we are pushing too hard or over-attached to our agendas and to-do lists. Where are you trying to over-control or overcompensate in order to be who you think you should be? What fear are you running from? This base chakra asks you to find the empty space within and surrender to life's natural rhythm. The energy of Mother Earth encourages you to stop pushing and striving against the flow of life. Peace comes when we surrender and work with the energy in this chakra; we start to have more energy, feel more supported in our body and life, and can let go of what no longer serves us.

Building new, firm, grounded foundations in our body and emotional life based on what we believe and who we want to be is part of how we begin to heal this chakra. But first, we must face what is there and look into the dark. By letting down some walls, we begin to let the light shine through.

Chakra 2—Sacral Centre

Physical Manifestation:

- Lower back pain
- Reproductive issues
- Sexual problems
- Bladder, colon, pelvic issues
- Digestive issues, IBS IBD, leaky gut

Manages:

- Individualism
- Survival—fight or flight
- Pleasure
- Creativity
- Intuition, gut feeling
- Money Mindset

Energy Problems:

- Becoming or being an individual
- Creative blocks
- Fertility issues
- Intuitive blocks
- Money
- Sex
- Power
- Mood swings
- PMS
- Envy

Nourish:

- Chakra 2 loves the colour orange: eat orange food and wear orange colours.
- Sunsets.
- Pleasure.
- Self-pleasure.
- Massage, hugs, romance, joy.
- Be in the present moment.

This chakra, found below your navel, is like a magnet that attracts what you desire, from people to opportunities. It's the centre of your power and creativity—where you bring new things into the world. However, chronic stress and hormonal imbalance can drain this chakra, affecting your energy, creativity, and relationships. When stressed, we might put on weight around our abdomen as a protective response.

This chakra deals with our relationships and their power dynamics, including our need to control or be controlled, which can lead to giving away our power to others. Recognising that we only have control over ourselves is a crucial life lesson.

Many of us use our energy to please others, losing our sense of self-worth in the process, paradoxically trying to prove our worth at the same time. These behaviours can manifest as health issues, especially in a woman's reproductive organs. When we give away our control and drive to prove our self-worth, we can become lost and disconnected, struggle with decisions, and feel out of balance.

Growing up, we may push against authority to define our independence, but societal or familial expectations can lead us to make choices that are not aligned with our true selves. Finding a balance in this chakra means making decisions that reflect our authentic desires, not just trying to unconsciously seek approval.

Relationship changes can make us insecure, but self-discipline helps us stay true to ourselves. Neglecting our strength leads to dependency on others and drains our energy. Reclaiming our power can transform our lives, even if it challenges those around us.

Many women I work with struggle with an imbalance in this chakra due to internalised shame and a conflict between seeking fulfilment and fearing it. Societal expectations often exacerbate this, making it hard to enjoy life's pleasures without guilt. A balanced second chakra allows us to pursue and enjoy life freely.

I spend a lot of time with women focusing on Chakra 2, the energy centre where we connect with emotional fluidity. This chakra is key to feeling, accepting, and releasing our emotions, allowing our Shakti—our life force energy—to awaken and flow. However, this healing process is often avoided. Many women are unaware of how they think, believe, and act, usually feeling numb because they've spent most of their adult lives suppressing their emotions. The energy it takes to bury these feelings can eventually manifest as physical issues. Many women unconsciously yearn for the life force and vitality that resides within them, but it feels out of reach. When this chakra is blocked, you may experience low energy, a diminished sex drive, and a sense of dullness and lifelessness. This blockage is often found in women with severe PMS, burnout, depression, and lower back pain.

Chakra 2 is closely tied to the cycles of birth, life, death, and rebirth, both physically and metaphorically, within our wombs. Our natural response to these cycles often involves fear, leading to a blocked and stagnant Chakra 2. We fear change, loss of control, and endings because we've lost touch with our intuition, which resides in this centre. Instead of trusting our inner wisdom, we rely on logic and evidence, getting stuck in the 'how' rather than following our unpredictable, mystical intuition. When we learn to embrace our cycles, listen to our intuition, and face the challenges they present, we start to trust ourselves, our bodies, and our connection to the universal intelligence of all life.

Your navel connects you to your mother in the womb and, energetically, links you to the universal womb of Mother Earth. Many women aren't aware of this life force energy they can tap into for nourishment and support.

When this energy centre is not functioning properly, it can lead to repressed desires, especially sexual ones. Reawakening our sexual desires, clearing our sexual shadows, and connecting to our pleasure and womb wisdom is a powerful process available to every woman—it's your birthright. When women are unaware of their sexual shadows, they may behave in ways that are draining and often toxic, leading to difficult situations, behaviours, and relationships that don't align with their true selves. Guilt, shame, and negative feelings can build up and become part of a 'pain body' that weighs us down.

Understanding what you want and need sexually is a source of strength and joy for a conscious woman. Knowing and living from your desires and sexual fulfilment are often overlooked but are essential aspects of inner transformation and healing.

Restoring balance to this energy centre creates emotional fluidity, which is the gateway to sexuality and orgasmic fulfilment. For women, sexual pleasure and emotional fluidity are deeply connected, yet we often compartmentalise our sexuality, unaware of the natural integration between the two. If we're not in touch with our emotions, we won't have a deeply satisfying sex life. Fully integrating our emotions, spirituality, and sexuality is vital for health and happiness. Your body is an instrument of pleasure and joy; Chakra 2 is the doorway to this. Every woman has the divine right to explore and discover the powerful, life-changing potential hidden in her yoni, breasts, womb, and voice. Weaving together our sexuality and emotions creates a sacred connection that brings peace, joy, deep healing, and intimacy into every area of your life.

Chakra 3—Solar Plexus Centre

Physical Manifestation:

- Stomach issues, stomach ulcers
- Reflux and GERD
- Liver issues
- Oestrogen dominance
- Gallbladder problems, gallstones
- Digestive issues, IBS, and small intestine issues
- SIBO, diarrhoea, bloating, and constipation

- Pancreas issues, diabetes, or hypoglycemia
- Eating disorders
- Eating fast
- Spleen issues—immunity, blood cell production, anemia
- Adrenal, chronic fatigue syndrome, and burnout

Manages:

- Personal power—self-esteem and self-empowerment
- Personal choice
- Your honour and your word
- Boundaries
- Inner strength and personality

Energy Problems:

- Giving energy away or relying on others for energy; energy vampire issues
- Lacking boundaries and saying 'yes' when you want to say 'no'
- Misalignment between what you feel and what you say
- Victim mentality, disempowerment
- Over-controlling, bullying, and stubborn—either the victim or the bully
- Can't keep your word
- Can't be honest with others and yourself
- Scared of conflict
- Self-absorbed and lacking motivation and discipline
- Lack morals
- Unhealthy competition.
- Difficulty standing up for yourself or what you believe in
- Rescuer or saviour complex
- Dealing with secretive anger, resentment, and frustration

Nourish:

- Chakra 3 loves the colour yellow: eat yellow food, wear yellow clothes, and visualise the colour yellow filling up your third chakra.
- Create healthy boundaries.
- Practise holding your centre.
- Strengthen your core stability.
- Work on your posture.
- Start saying 'no.'
- Align with who you are physically, mentally, and emotionally.
- Delegate.
- Ask yourself what you want and who you are, and take small daily steps to embody it.

I struggled with my third chakra, which showed up as an overwhelming sense of responsibility for my actions and words, a crippling fear of rejection that held me back in many areas of my life, and an inability to handle criticism that turned me into a perfectionist. My relationships were built on the need to feel safe. I chose people I could help and rescue because it made me feel validated and secure, thinking it would keep them from leaving me. However, my inner child remained undeveloped, and I soon realised, especially through challenging experiences in friendships, that this way of living was unsustainable and left me unhappy.

Speaking your truth from this chakra is vital. When we speak from a place of love, it's not our concern how others react to our boundaries or responses. Our responsibility is to be truthful and honour our sovereignty, allowing others to do the same. When we agree with others just to keep the peace or to be liked, we dishonour our intuition, drain our power, and leak energy from this centre.

Building self-esteem is crucial for how we approach and navigate life. In the second chakra, we learn to listen to our intuition; in the third chakra, we learn to act on it. When we can't express our feelings or pursue our needs and desires, our body and mind become out of sync, leading to illness.

Focusing on the third chakra helps us prioritise our soul over our ego, choosing truth over illusion. We become aware of the power of our will and choices, understanding how they affect us and those around us. Taking responsibility for ourselves is the start of building our inner strength and establishing our presence in the world in a balanced way. In the past, we might have blamed others and seen ourselves as victims, but accepting our role in our lives shows us that we have more power than we realised. Blaming others only gives away our power; we must acknowledge our role in shaping our lives and circumstances. We are the co-creators of our reality. People often say that rejection is protection. I also believe that projection is a form of self-protection because it's easier to blame others than to face our own part in things, whether we're aware of it or not.

As we balance the third chakra, we stop drifting through life, influenced by others, and begin making deliberate choices and actions, understanding that they have consequences—our vitality depends on it. Every personal decision we make and every step we take in life reduces the physical world's control over our body and mind because we have always been the creators of our lives. We take charge and steer our lives rather than being passive passengers. Each choice that aligns with our true self strengthens our energy body and chakras, becoming healthier, happier, and more vibrant. We start to let go of negative influences, and the universe brings situations that help us remove people and things that no longer fit who we are. Naturally, this process can be complex and may cause anxiety, as it can feel like life is falling apart. But as women, we are natural weavers and begin to create a new life that is in tune with our soul.

Each new phase of life brings fresh beginnings, reminding us to trust in the death and rebirth process within and around us. When everything seems to collapse, and a thread comes loose, we realise that these threads were always there but were too tightly woven for us to see before. By following these loose threads, we start to weave a new pattern, a new life that we couldn't have imagined if what we thought was perfect hadn't fallen apart. Sometimes, we need to feel as though everything is lost in order to be found and that everything has died to be reborn into the life and energy we were always meant to embody.

As we open to our unique life force, life becomes a blessing rather than a burden. We become aware of the mystery, the feminine path of spirituality, and the 'She' power within us. You were born to embody your unique soul essence, which begins to awaken and bloom as your third chakra comes to life.

Chakra 4—Heart Centre

Physical Manifestation:

- Heart problems—Cardiovascular disease
- High or low blood pressure
- Circulation problems
- Breast cysts and cancer
- Kyphosis of the thoracic spine
- Breathing problems, anxiety, feeling tight in the chest
- Upper respiratory illness yearly, pneumonia, asthma, allergies
- Chronic pain in neck, shoulders, and upper back
- Tingling, pain, and numbness in arms and hands

Manages:

- Heart
- Lungs
- Upper chest, neck, and back
- Arms and hands
- Circulatory system
- Emotions
- Receiving and giving love
- Compassion and forgiveness
- Present moment connection

Energy Problems:

- Bitterness and resentment
- Jealousy and regret
- Depression
- Anxiety
- Feel cold, distant, and detached
- Fear

- Can't trust or love
- 'Good girl' complex
- Searching for love to feel fulfilled
- Inability to attract love and finances
- Being controlling, critical, and judgemental
- Conditional love
- High expectations of friends, partners, and children
- Feel victimised, hurt, and betrayed
- Lack joy

Nourish:

- Chakra 4 loves the colour green: eat green food, wear green colours, and spend time in nature.
- Practise heart-opening exercises using yoga.
- Posture! Sit and stand with an open heart. Imagine a light beaming out of your chest area rather than hiding away as you hunch over.
- Practise forgiveness; let go of old wounds.
- Start a gratitude journal.
- Tell yourself and others how much you love them.
- Meditate on opening up the heart.
- Offer yourself and others compassion, kindness, and prayer.
- Smile.
- Practise being able to receive compliments and kindness—stop deflecting.

Your fourth chakra is the gateway and power source of your being. It's where your mind and emotions meet and where your body and soul come into balance, determining your energy and health. For most of us, the fourth chakra is underactive and closed off due to past wounds and unresolved trauma. As women, these wounds run deep. From a young age, we were all taught to be 'good girls,' whether at home, school, church, or by well-meaning carers. Women are raised to be good, kind, patient, obedient, and ignore their feelings, while men are often brought up with different rules.

For many women, unconditional love means serving others, staying quiet, putting up with things, following orders, and being what others want or need. We were taught to do as we're told, not to question, and to keep smiling. This stems from the fundamental message we received as little girls: our worth is based on how good we are, how much we do, and how well we do it. This manifests in adulthood as overgiving, running a tight ship at home and work, perfectionism, over-controlling behaviours, and prioritising everyone else's needs while keeping our emotions in check.

This pattern of overgiving and putting your needs last creates a weak and underactive fourth chakra. A healthy and balanced fourth chakra requires both giving and receiving without attachment. Yet, many women are stuck in overgiving, unable to receive fully, and often resentful when they don't receive recognition for their efforts.

A healthy fourth chakra also depends on a balanced third chakra and maintaining healthy boundaries. As mentioned earlier, many women have an imbalance in the third chakra, which causes problems in the heart area. Energetic and physical boundaries are essential for heart health. When the third chakra is underactive, it can lead to misplaced love in unhealthy relationships or withholding love altogether, leaving you feeling drained, burnt out, and unhappy.

We've been conditioned not to listen to our intuition and instincts, which leads to energy leaks and the overgiving syndrome. Our third chakra receives information from the second chakra; we need to listen to our lower chakras, but because we've been taught that our wants and needs don't matter, we ignore these messages and gut instincts until we can no longer hear them. This creates passive, victim behaviour, which eventually leads to aggression, suppression, bitterness, and a shut-down heart chakra.

Think about how resentful you can feel when you are overgiving and not receiving. If you're doing something you don't want to do, you have two choices:

1. Accept it, or…
2. Stop doing it.

It's that simple. We waste so much of our vital energy complaining and resenting, and this is making us sick.

I often see women who say they want love but are closed off to it. There's a mismatch in their energy, with a defensiveness and an unrealistically high standard. No one seems good enough, or they pick apart the smallest flaws and blow them out of proportion. Beneath this lies a fear of opening their heart and getting hurt. These women often blame others for everything that happens in their lives and struggle to take responsibility for their actions. They play the role of the good girl, the victim, or the martyr, believing they have no power, while everyone else is cast as the villain. This mindset is disempowering, and many women aren't aware of how their passive-aggressive behaviour is affecting their lives and bodies. It leads to bitterness and fragility, both physically and emotionally. Physically, it can manifest as conditions like osteoarthritis, osteoporosis, Alzheimer's, high blood pressure, and atherosclerosis. Their blocked emotions turn into physical inflammation and plaque buildup in their arteries.

Keeping a healthy and balanced fourth chakra is essential; we must stop polluting our minds, bodies, and the planet with unconscious thoughts, fears, negativity, and behaviours. All of these contribute to disease in the body, mind, and soul.

The fourth chakra is also about your dreams and doing what you love. It's essential to have something or someone you love in your life. I see many women trapped in dreams of future happiness, unable to appreciate what they have in the present moment. They often say, 'If and when I have this, then my life will be better.' But having dreams and love in your life is as important as breathing—and I'm not just talking about romantic love.

-   Cuddle your kids or a pet
-   Walk in nature

- Stroke an animal
- Get a pet and care for it
- Bake something
- Grow a garden or tend to a plant
- Make wholesome, nourishing food
- Take time to enjoy your cup of coffee or tea
- Take full, deep breaths
- Feel the sunlight on your face, or use a SAD lamp in winter

Romantic love can be tricky because we often look to another person to fulfil us or make our dreams come true. We need to enter relationships as whole, independent individuals, not needing someone else to complete us.

On the other hand, some people struggle to have a relationship because they haven't fully processed or let go of their Father wound. Maybe you had a difficult relationship with your father growing up, or perhaps there's some unhealed trauma in this energy centre. Until you can fully let go and forgive, you may find it hard to love and be loved by another. This can also apply to the Mother wound, but in my experience, the heart chakra is often more closely linked to the paternal line.

Do you feel like you've missed the boat?

Reflect on any broken or unfulfilled childhood dreams. Where has your heart lost faith or been wounded? Life rarely unfolds as we imagine. Our inner child, along with her lost dreams, needs to be recognised and embraced. The resentment in our hearts—the thoughts of 'I wish that were me... I want to be that... I should have that life by now...'—must be confronted but without judgement.

- Listen to what you want.
- Develop an honesty policy with yourself; stop lying to yourself.
- Don't discard your feelings; they matter and are there for a reason.
- Release judgement.
- Listen and journal about what's in your heart.
- Manage your expectations and get real with yourself.
- Do you want a dream for you, or do you think it will fill the hole you have from childhood wounding? Many dreams can come from wanting love and recognition from our parents.
- Decide which dreams to pursue and which you need to let go of.

Forgiveness

Take a look at how you're carrying upset, resentment, anger, and bitterness towards others and, most importantly, yourself. We all need to let some things go. Because we respond to others and the world around us based on our beliefs and conditioning, we develop perceptions that aren't necessarily true but become our truth, which we then live our lives by. We are quick to judge and validate our perceptions because our ego needs to feel right.

Learn to be neutral in your expectations of others.

Most of us expect people to behave in a certain way, and this can cause us much unhappiness, especially in our relationships. Often, we wait, expecting the worst of others, and we miss the best in them and ourselves and feel hurt because of our unrealistic expectations.

Nothing outside of you can make you whole or happy; happiness comes from within. You are the one generating love; love comes from within. When we peel back the layers around the heart one by one, we let things go, and what is left is just you and love. You come into this world alone; you will leave it alone. People and things will come and go; it has and will always be you dealing with yourself; your feelings and emotions are transient—it's painful but true. It's all about generating love for yourself first, which can then ripple out to others and the world. When we stop judging others, we stop judging ourselves, and this sets us free.

Female spirituality begins in the heart, not the mind, rooted in love, trust, and surrender. When you strip everything back, the most important thing you can do is relax into your feminine essence and love yourself completely, embracing every part of you, flaws and all. Female spirituality awakens the heart to the language of universal love, a language we all understand unconsciously. Learning to transform the fear and pain in our hearts back to their original state is deeply healing. Through the heart chakra, we remember that we are the love we've been searching for—the missing piece we've been longing to find.

I am the one generating love. It's all coming from within me.

The Power of 'I Love You'

Spend a few minutes each day looking yourself in the eye through a mirror and saying, 'I love you, I love you, I simply love you.' Repeat this ten times daily, and you'll be amazed at how your heart begins to open. The eyes are the window to the soul, and truly looking at and connecting with yourself is incredibly healing. When I first started this practise, I found it difficult to fully meet my own gaze. I wanted to avoid the emotions that surfaced. But as I continued, layers of self-rejection and fear began to peel away, revealing a deeper sense of self-acceptance.

I also have 'I am Love' written in lipstick on my bathroom mirror. Every day, as I brush my teeth, it reminds me that I am the love I seek, right here and now, in every moment, and that everything I need comes from within me.

Chakra 5—Throat Centre

Physical Manifestation:

- Stiff neck and reduced range of movement
- Tight jaw; may grind teeth at night
- Headaches referred from the neck due to poor posture
- Thyroid problems and hormone imbalances
- Weak voice
- Mouth ulcers and dry lips
- Problems swallowing or eating certain foods
- Swollen lymph nodes around the neck
- Hunched-over shoulders with a forward head position
- Chronic coughs and sore throats

Manages:

- Self-expression
- Authenticity
- Communication
- Truth
- Getting needs and desires met
- Surrendering your personal will to a divine will

Energy Problems:

- Can't communicate well, leading to miscommunication and frustrations
- Creatively blocked
- Gets out of breath quickly
- Talks about others behind their backs
- Tells tales about others and exaggerates stories
- Envious and judgemental of others
- Feels alienated and misunderstood
- Can't speak about how they feel
- Unable to express themselves fully and confidently
- Tends to become more introverted than they are, coming across as shy and nervous
- Thinks one thing and says another
- Feels floaty, lacks the determination to see things through
- Can't make decisions and speak up

Personal Power Challenges:

- Anger outbursts
- Uses food and alcohol to numb feelings.
- Bites fingernails; habitually puts things in their mouth.
- Food issues and cravings.
- Usually has a weak second chakra with low sexual energy.
- Feels they have no voice and their opinion doesn't matter.
- Adopts a 'grin and bear it' motto.
- Change what they say depending on who they are with because their words lack weight.
- Has a shadowy or ghost-like presence in a group

Nourish:

- Chakra 5 loves the colour blue; wear it and surround yourself with this colour.
- Singing—try it in the shower or while driving to work.
- Make noise when you exhale.
- Engage in somatic movement and dance with sound.
- Speak what's true.
- Speak from the heart.
- Engage in conversations that light you up and inspire you.
- Eat nourishing food.
- Drink warm herbal tea.
- Receive neck and face massages.
- Focus on lymphatic drainage.
- Move the neck in all directions/doing neck rolls.

Chakra 5, also known as the throat chakra, is key to authentically and confidently expressing ourselves. It's about feeling our intuition and being able to communicate who we are and what we feel in every moment. Many women struggle to speak their truth, often finding that what they feel and say doesn't match up. This disconnect can lead to illness.

Earlier in this book, I mentioned the connection between the throat chakra and the cervix. This link is vital in addressing modern women's health issues, so it's crucial to recognise this connection within yourself.

Women often say 'yes' to sex when they really want to say 'no'. This starts when we're young, as we might have sex to feel liked and loved, even if it doesn't align with our true selves. As we get older and enter long-term relationships, sex can feel like a chore if we're not connected to our sexuality and yoni. We do it because we think we should, because there's pressure, or because we don't want to lose the person we love. This disconnect between what we want and what we do with our bodies can trigger various health problems.

Our voices are how we communicate love and bring it into the world.

We recognise truth because it resonates within us, like a bell. When someone lies, we feel it in our bodies; something doesn't sit right, and we don't fully trust them. We feel guilty when we don't speak our truth, and it weighs on us. That's the power of your words and expression—they can turn thoughts into action, creation into reality... they are spells. When we're unhappy with a situation, we must be honest with ourselves: *Where am I not speaking truthfully? Where did I ignore my truth? Where did I suppress it for the sake of convenience?* When we betray others, we betray ourselves. We break a vow to our soul, further distancing ourselves from who we are.

Every woman carries the wound in the throat chakra. We've been silenced, shamed, mocked, ostracised, and feared for speaking our truth. We were taught to keep our truth hidden, much like the great mother, and her essence has been forgotten. Now, more than ever, the feminine voice must be heard to heal ourselves and the planet after being long ignored and ridiculed.

Our words have power. Truth spoken from the Yoni can heal and change the world, cutting through personal and collective illusions. When we awaken the energy of our lower chakras and let it speak through us, we tap into deep wisdom that needs to be heard. Speaking from this deep place is like performing magic, freeing ourselves from the constraints of patriarchy and repression. By letting go of the past, we stand strong in the present, rooted in our truth and strength.

When we don't use our voice or disconnect from our lower chakras, we get stuck in our heads, which can lead to headaches and neck pain. Suppressing our truth creates tension in the neck and shoulders, leading to chronic pain. The physical strain of trying to contain ourselves and appear as perfect superwomen is overwhelming, and our bodies respond accordingly.

Releasing this energy, connecting to your womb and yoni, and speaking from deep wisdom is liberating. Your upper and lower mouths are connected; the larynx and vulva mirror each other physically and energetically. Many of us who feel disconnected from our bodies also silence the inner voice and intuition that come from our womb. This leads to holding patterns within our bodies, often experienced as tightness and constriction in the head, neck, and shoulders, manifesting in chronic pain. Reconnecting your body's energy pathways can heal this wound.

Breathing doesn't just come from the throat and lungs—it also involves the yoni, but most of us only use a small part of our lungs, neglecting the lower diaphragm. This shallow breathing creates stress and a sense of unworthiness because we're not fully occupying our physical space, which is reflected in our behaviour. Women often make themselves small, careful not to take up too much space or time, trying to be invisible and pleasing, which stifles their power and life force, sometimes with serious consequences.

Your vagina has a voice, a memory, stored deep within your body. The Vagina Monologues by Eve Ensler in the 90s started the process of women reclaiming the power and voice of their yoni, encouraging open conversation. Your yoni has a powerful voice that can break through limitations, helping you to manifest your desires. Manifestation starts with the pleasure generated in the yoni, where energy is created and birthed. But without true feeling and an open third and fourth chakra, affirmations and words are empty, lacking the energy needed for manifestation.

Speaking truthfully, with wisdom, honesty, and compassion, allows us to tap into our deep emotions, clearing away the blocks and reigniting our inner fire. Letting go of masks and superficial interactions reconnects us with our inner wisdom.

Speaking your truth can be daunting, but it's the path to inner freedom. When you stay silent, ask yourself what you fear losing. Hiding behind masks attracts people who love the facade, trapping you in a cycle of people-pleasing and slowly draining your energy and spirit.

Truth energises your spirit; without it, your energy fades. Lying and maintaining facades drain the energy that could be used to improve your health and happiness. Compassionate speech is powerful; it offers clarity and leads to heart-, womb-, and gut-led solutions. Words can be weapons or shields, so connecting with your body's wisdom is essential.

For years, I numbed myself with diets, exercise, and alcohol to avoid feeling pain. I stopped trying to protect myself because expressing my truth was often mocked. This pattern repeated in my relationships leading me to silence myself, become a pleaser and doer, and disconnect from my truth to avoid rejection. I lived defensively.

It took some therapy and blaming others before I realised I wasn't trapped; I had imprisoned myself and handed over the key. Blaming others and playing the victim was easier than owning my shadow and taking responsibility. Speaking my truth, acknowledging my mistakes, and recognising my self-denial was painful but liberating. Embracing my truth transformed my relationships and healed a family pattern of feeling inadequate, staying silent, and striving for perfection. By healing this ancestral wound, I freed my daughters from carrying the same burden.

Can you remember when someone put words in your mouth, finished your sentences, or spoke for you? Or when someone accused you of something you didn't say or do? Do you recall how that felt in your body? I get really angry and frustrated when this happens to me—and rightly so. When someone puts words in your mouth, it weakens your power, especially in this energy centre, affecting how you function as an energetic being. Be mindful of people who do this, always speak up, and reclaim your voice.

Reconnecting with your truth after long periods of numbness requires a gentle, careful awakening. If you're emotionally numb due to unsatisfying work or relationships, facing the truth can be frightening. Commit to breaking the silence, recognising childhood patterns, and cutting ties that silence your voice. Your ancestors' silence doesn't have to be yours. Liberating yourself frees them and prevents the cycle from continuing.

There was a time when speaking our truth was unsafe, but that time has passed. It's time to free your soul, let her sing your truth, and restore your wholeness.

I'm bent over my knees, screaming and vomiting from the depths of my soul. All the suppressed emotions, the feelings of not being enough, the hurt, shame, and anger, I hear myself screaming, 'I'm enough, I'm not stupid, and I matter.' I see my parents and feel my truth. My whole body starts to shake. My head begins to turn rapidly, my neck shaking uncontrollably as emotions fly out of my throat with a sound that seems to come from deep inside my body, transporting me through my life back to the core wound that separated me from my truth. As I arrive there and feel with my heart the child who was always trying to please, say sorry, and rescue everyone and everything, my heart breaks. I sob uncontrollably for the loss, the hurt, the pain that I have held onto throughout my life and probably many more. Snot and tears run down my neck as I shake uncontrollably. I feel free.

All the neck pain and constriction in my throat are freed up and expressed. My neck can turn fully; I can breathe into my chest, the ringing in my ear is gone. There is silence, there is me, and I am connected to my truth. I vow to no longer suppress her, to quiet her down, to make myself more palatable, people-pleasing. I promise to let my 'yes' be a yes and my 'no' be enough, knowing that I've always known my truth, but now I'm no longer afraid to speak it. I feel aligned with my Yoni, her voice, her deep wisdom. I know that when I listen and speak from her, everything will fall into place.

This first practise for cleansing the throat chakra comes from my beloved mentor, Diana Dubrow:

Throat Chakra Exercise

- Find a stone that speaks to you; it may grab your attention. It doesn't have to be anything special; perhaps you come across it on a walk.
- Paint it turquoise, the colour of the throat chakra.
- Find a quiet space, preferably when everyone is out of the house. Light a candle and set your intention to free your truth.
- Hold the stone to your neck, close your eyes, and take three deep, slow inhalations and exhalations through the nose. Bring the breath down deep into your womb space.
- Holding the stone to your neck, speak out your pains, regrets, and how you really feel about people and things that are happening and have happened. What are you not saying? What are you blocking? Speak out your pain, denial, and truth into the stone. You can speak it, shout it out, or sing it.
- The idea is to free up the silent scream and rage that has been locked up inside. Don't judge the words or feelings—just let them come free from your body.

What helps me is inhaling through my nose and making a sound that comes deep from my yoni, rising up through my lower chakras and into my throat chakra. You will be amazed at how long your exhale and sounding can go when you open your jaw and let the sound start to escape. After a minute, primal screams and anger may begin to come up from the depths of your soul that you didn't know were there. Don't control, tame, or shut this process down; keep going until you get to the root cause of the pain. Scream it, cry it, shake it; let your body lead you.

Speaking Truth to Yourself

What does your body want to tell you? What does she need you to know? This is a mental and emotional process that can be confusing when we've been shut down. Your truth grows as you grow; give yourself permission to make mistakes and get it wrong, forgive yourself, and learn from them. This is about growth, trust, and rebuilding our nervous system.

Sit quietly and breathe into your lower belly. Feel into your intuition; invite her in. Give her a seat at the fire. What feelings come up when you ask yourself the truth? Imagine she's sitting on a cushion in front of you; ask her:

- What's going on with me?
- What's not working?
- What are you trying to tell me?

When we arrive at the truth within, you will feel a resonance, a deep knowing throughout your entire body. The urge to start to flow; you may find yourself starting to cry, or your heart may begin to race. Sit with the truth and ask:

- What's the most healing thing I can do right now?
- What's the next step?

Some truths are hard but need to be felt and acknowledged. Honour what comes up and write it down.

Freeing Up Your Voice

- Sit in a quiet space and light a candle.
- Ground yourself and take some full, deep breaths into your yoni. Relax your jaw and pelvis, and allow the breath to flow freely from your mouth and deep into your root chakra.
- Unclench your buttocks, relax your stomach, let go of the pulled-in tummy muscles; let it all hang out.
- On an exhale, connect to your breath and make noise, starting with the sound 'ah' coming from your root, up through your chakras, and out of your mouth.
- Repeat this ten times, playing with different tones and expressions that want to move through you. As you exhale, stick your tongue out as far as you can, extending the physical exhale even longer, deepening the connection to your yoni.

Singing is another wonderful way to liberate your voice. As a little girl, you may have loved to sing, shout, and let it all out. It's only when someone tells us we can't sing well or we must be quiet that we disconnect from the voice within. Sound is your birthright; you don't have to be the next Mariah Carey, but you do need to make noise—and lots of it. Sing in the shower and in the car, and put your favourite playlist on when you cook. Singing along and moving your body frees up all the stagnant energy and teaches you how to show up and express yourself in life.

Learning to listen to yourself speak is also healing. So many of us don't like the sound of our own voice. Recording yourself saying loving, heartfelt affirmations or reciting poetry is truly healing. Knowing and loving your voice helps you open up and express your truth.

This process helps you reclaim everything stuck inside that you didn't realise was even there, held in lumps and swollen glands causing you strep throat, sore throats, gum disease and vocal problems. It's the reason you can't speak up or be seen. If you can't listen to yourself, how are other people supposed to? This process helps us to trust ourselves again. Our word is our power; it's our sacred bond with self. When we clear out all the pain and repression, we can hear and speak our truth to ourselves first, then to everyone around us. Hold yourself with high esteem and sovereignty. Release all the times you quieted yourself or changed your words to please another. Release all the times a person of higher authority has looked down on you and called you stupid or dumb or acted like your voice didn't matter.

- How many times have you left a meeting or situation and wished you had said what you really thought?
- When did you agree to something when your inner voice said no?
- Where are you saying yes because you want to be loved, liked, and accepted?
- How have you denied your truth and compromised your body and soul?

Women are often people-pleasers. We say yes to keep the peace, deny our truth, saying it doesn't matter or we'll get to it later. This makes us sick; we have to feel and speak our truth. The truth sets you free, and it also sets others free. When you keep saying yes, you are as much to blame as the person who is pushing you. Your role is to break the circuit and pattern; you're now changing everything.

I recently had a situation with a friend telling me about her dilemma. As I listened to her, I found myself going along with her story and began to see an old pattern in myself. In truth, I wasn't being honest with her because I was responding from a place of fear rather than love. Afraid of her reaction, of offending or hurting her, but ultimately worried that she might not want to be friends anymore or that it would cause conflict, I fell back into my old habit and went along with her to keep the peace.

Afterwards, I felt out of alignment; my body was unhappy, and my throat felt constricted and tight. I knew I had betrayed myself and her by not saying what I intuitively felt. As a friend, being loving and truthful, regardless of how others can receive it or not, is what love does. This has been a hard lesson for me over the years, as being truthful about what I feel and think can be seen as judgemental and has cost me friendships. It was easier to shut up and say nothing, but is that real friendship? Is that fair to the other person we are in a relationship with? Once you start working with your energy, this is no longer an option; self-betrayal is no longer your default, whatever the cost. As you walk the spiritual path, your soul and integrity ultimately are the only things you are responsible for—the rest is none of your business.

A few years ago, I made the ethical choice to be truthful in my relationships. I believe in treating others honestly, even when the truth is hard to hear. The truth is always welcome as long as it comes from a place of integrity, love, and for the highest good of everyone involved. However, I don't have a large circle of friends because I've learned that not everyone values honesty. Some friends prefer you agree with them and play along with their stories, making their ego feel safer, justified, and more powerful.

When you stay silent and hold back your truth, you weaken your energy and empower their ego, draining yourself in the process. This fear of being honest often stems from a fear of conflict, but living in fear means living only half a life—one where you're too afraid to love and express yourself fully. Your truth is your integrity, and no one should be able to shake or take that away from you. How someone reacts to your truth is their business, not yours—based on their values, beliefs, and past experiences. Don't take it personally. Love them unconditionally, but for the sake of your well-being, speak what's in your heart and soul.

True friends will come to appreciate your honesty. They'll turn to you in times of crisis because they know they can rely on you to speak the truth, even when it's uncomfortable. Those who aren't true friends or whom you may have outgrown will naturally drift away. Although that can be difficult, it's better in the long run, as pretending to be someone you're not just to keep others happy will only make you ill and hold you back.

The truth is like a sword that frees you from everything and everyone who isn't meant for you. Find your sword, and use it to free yourself and your voice.

Chakra 6—Third Eye Centre

Physical Manifestation:

- Headaches
- Migraines
- Blurred vision
- Eye problems
- Sinus problems
- Stroke
- Tinnitus and deafness
- Seizures
- Night terrors and nightmares
- Circadian rhythm imbalance
- Sleep problems

Manages:

- Eyes
- Sinuses

- Pineal gland
- Melatonin and serotonin hormone release
- Cranial bones: sphenoid, orbital
- Sight
- Vision: physical and psychic ability
- Insight and intuition
- Connection to our dreams and their interpretation
- Memory
- The ability to think
- The ability to learn and retain information
- Concentration and focus

Energy Problems:

- Narrow-minded
- Live in a small world
- Black and white thinking
- Can't concentrate or focus
- Often multitasking
- In the head, can't be present with people
- Dizziness
- Ungrounded
- Inflated ego, not based in reality
- Repeat mistakes
- Disconnected from the body
- Poor memory
- Live in the past and future
- Relive past experiences and project the feelings and circumstances into the now
- Inflexible in thought and body
- Learning difficulties: ADD, Autism, ADHD

Personal Power Challenges:

- Unable to connect with and feel self and others
- Lack empathy
- Socially awkward
- Closed-mindedness
- Feel like an outsider
- Lack perspective
- Live in a dream or fantasy world
- Lack of self-awareness; feel less than

Nourish:

- Chakra 6 loves the colour indigo. Wear it and surround yourself with this colour.
- Meditation
- Mindfulness
- Visualisations
- Manifesting
- Harnessing psychic abilities.
- Relaxation techniques to connect mind and heart
- Balancing thinking and feeling
- Facial massage
- Chiropractic adjustments
- Journaling dreams
- Natural sunlight, regulating sleep patterns and circadian rhythm.
- Use an SAD light box, red light therapy, and blue light glasses.
- Breathwork
- Plant medicine

Chakra 6, the third eye, is the psychic centre of our intuition and wisdom. It connects how we perceive and experience the inner and outer worlds, acting as a gateway to the unknown, ancient wisdom beyond time and space.

Many women I work with have blockages in this chakra. This is because we often live in our heads, disconnected from our bodies, and caught up in the stresses of modern life. Our minds are often on autopilot, filled with endless tasks and internal chatter. This leaves little room to relax and truly feel. Women often say they can't relax or don't understand why their bodies are stressed even when they think they feel fine. Their third eye chakra operates like a computer with too many windows open—constantly processing, analysing, and overthinking, which disconnects them from their bodies and lower chakras.

Most of us need help knowing where or how to start addressing this. Our brain's dominance leaves us numb to our emotions, stuck in survival mode rather than truly living. We take pride in ticking off tasks, briefly satisfying our need for approval, but the feeling doesn't last. We normalise feeling jittery, experiencing anger outbursts, headaches, and tight shoulders, often reaching for painkillers instead of recognising these as signs we need a break. We ignore our body's signals, pushing through because we feel there's no time to stop.

These women often pride themselves on managing everything, judging themselves and others harshly for any sign of weakness. They may be in denial about their true feelings, competitive, and goal-oriented. They might unwind with wine or seek endorphin highs through intense exercise, inadvertently increasing their stress. Yoga, mindfulness, or meditation may seem unappealing, yet these are exactly what they need. Deep down, their bodies know that slowing down would mean facing suppressed issues, leading to a disconnect between body and mind. The body keeps score, even when the mind tries to ignore it. High achievers often face the hardest breakdowns when their carefully constructed realities begin to fall apart, leading to not just physical but also psychological and emotional struggles. Their need for control and perfectionism traps them, as they wear their 'capes' to prove their worthiness—something their inner child never received.

Meditation

Everyone tells us to meditate and practise mindfulness, and we all know we should, but many of us struggle with it. Whether it's racing thoughts, lack of time, or discomfort from sitting, let's be honest—most of us have a love-hate relationship with it. There's nothing wrong with you; you've probably just been doing it in a way that doesn't work for you, which is why it feels so hard!

For women, meditation isn't best achieved through the mind or even the third eye (Chakra 6) alone, but through the body. We need to move our bodies and create emotional flow so our energy can rise into our third eye. Tantra teaches us that men and women reach higher consciousness differently. Men can open their third eye by sitting still and meditating, while women need to feel, move, make sounds, and breathe to connect to theirs.

'She-Practises' are ideal for opening and healing the chakras, especially the third eye. They prepare the body for stillness and meditation by releasing, opening, and emptying so we can fully receive and embody our energy and light. It's important to remember that men and women are wired differently—physically, emotionally, and energetically. Women need to understand the power of their bodies and work with them, not against them. There's nothing wrong with us; we've just been following the wrong instructions!

Once we've raised and embodied our energy, meditation becomes a powerful practise from which everyone can benefit. Meditation isn't pseudo-science; plenty of research supports the benefits of a regular practise, with new discoveries being made all the time. When we meditate, we bring our energy and brainwaves into coherence. Brainwaves are electrical signals that create different states of being, with the four main types being Beta, Alpha, Theta, and Delta.

1. **Beta:** Active, awake state, 14-21 cycles per second. People who are stressed and anxious tend to operate at 18-21 cycles per second.
2. **Alpha:** Light meditation, 7-14 cycles per second. This is the level of healing, energising relaxation and mindfulness.
3. **Theta:** Deeper meditation, 4-7 cycles per second. This is where we tap into ideas of inspiration and intuition. It is also known as the pseudo-dream state.
4. **Delta:** Even lower than Theta, 1-3 cycles per second. This is found in the deepest levels of relaxation and restorative sleep states.

Meditation done right brings science and spirituality together.

A good meditation and energy practise involves embodying and moving your body through She-Movement and then taking your mind through 3-4 levels of meditation states using brainwave frequencies.

Chakra 7—Crown Centre

Physical Manifestation:

- Headaches
- Migraines
- Vertigo
- Chronic fatigue
- Burnout
- Depression
- Overstimulated
- Scalp and head issues
- Dizziness, lightheadedness

Manages:

- Head and cranium
- Cortical brain
- Nervous system.
- Skin

Energy Problems:

- Lack of focus
- Lack of purpose
- Can't make decisions
- Confusion
- Blocked creativity
- Stuck in a negative heavy pattern
- Insomnia
- Stiffness in body and mind; the body is always a mirror of the mind.

Personal Power Challenges:

- Connection to the universe
- Lack of trust and faith in themselves and the universe
- Difficulty quieting the mind and thoughts
- Fear-based
- Uses addictive substances, especially food, alcohol, and excessive scrolling, to escape reality

- Lives and projects their life through others, especially famous people or celebrities
- Copies others due to a lack of individuality
- Lacks symbolic and mythic sight

Nourish:

- Chakra 7 loves the colour violet. Wear it, eat it, surround yourself with it.
- Use lavender to help calm the mind.
- Meditation
- Mindfulness
- Exercises to centre oneself
- Believe and have faith in something greater than yourself.
- Prayer
- Nature—immerse yourself in it!
- Inspirational reading, myths, folklore, legends to awaken ancestral psychology
- Get in your body, and do some movement.
- Cranial sacral therapy work
- Chiropractic adjustments

Chakra seven, or the crown chakra, is the final chakra in the body and acts as the gateway between the physical and non-physical realms. When this chakra is weak, it can lead to an overfocus on the physical body, often showing up in our eating, drinking, and exercise habits. Women might become overly concerned with their appearance and ageing, not realising that their energy body, which is essential for their vitality, isn't functioning well. Just like a plant needs water, our energy body and chakras rely on a healthy crown chakra to receive the energy required for us to thrive and grow.

Many women today have an underactive crown chakra, leading to feelings of overwhelm, burnout, chronic fatigue, and depression. This happens because of a disconnection from and underdevelopment of our energy body. It's not your fault—it's difficult to understand something you've never been taught. Owning your energy makes you self-reliant and less likely to conform, which challenges the patriarchal system.

We've been led to believe that spirituality must be mediated through others, often in a church, but our spiritual connection to the universe and God is direct through our energy body. Integrating sacred spirituality into our daily lives is the ultimate goal. Practises like yoga, ecstatic dance, breathwork, tantra, plant medicine, prayer, and meditation help us connect with the divine. The body is always our starting point in this journey. Searching for this connection outside ourselves is exhausting and can be harmful.

The crown chakra is where energy and life force from the universe and God enter, nourishing our physical and energetic bodies. Like a water filter, this energy supports all our bodily systems, calms the nervous system, and keeps our heart beating and blood flowing. Without this energy, we are lifeless. Upon death, you can see the life force leave the body, leaving behind an empty shell.

A healthy crown chakra is vital for our spiritual well-being. While we understand how diet affects our health, the impact of spirituality—or the lack of it—on our health and the planet is often overlooked. From my experience with thousands of women, what we often call burnout, depression, and psychological problems are actually symptoms of a spiritual crisis and a disconnection from our sacred bond with spirit and God. When the crown chakra isn't functioning properly, we fail to recognise this spiritual crisis, focusing only on the physical. While medication has its place, especially for chemical imbalances, we also need to explore our darker feelings and emotions, as they have their own reasons for being. In a world that avoids discomfort, embracing all feelings, even those hidden deep within us, can guide us back to our true selves. To find ourselves, we must first allow ourselves to be lost, to sit in the dark, and to feel everything we've been taught to avoid.

Women who experience a spiritual crisis display specific symptoms:

- Feel something is missing; they should be happy but just aren't.
- Feel that they need something or someone, but nothing quenches their thirst.
- Things that used to make them happy no longer do.
- Loss of self; they don't know who they are anymore.
- Don't know what they want out of life; they have lost their purpose and meaning.
- Struggle with feeling and moving past grief
- Can't let a deep grudge or the past go.
- Fear starts to arise as they feel their old life slipping away, which can make them controlling as their world becomes increasingly more out of their control.

Signs of a spiritual crisis:

- Depression, anxiety
- Severe PMS and perimenopause
- Burnout
- Stress
- Chronic fatigue
- Autoimmune disorders
- Chronic pain
- Brain bleed

This spiritual crisis is a dark night of the soul, and it's a place we all reach in life, some more times than others. Developing a sacred and spiritual practise and balancing the feminine and masculine energies within help us navigate this healing journey. This cyclic journey, this rollercoaster of life with its ups and downs, with its cycles of birth, death, and rebirth, pushes us to shed more layers to become more of who we truly are. The surrender, the release and acceptance and the ability to be with what is without trying to change anything in the present moment, knowing there is a divine plan to all that we are and do whilst also being able to let go of the past and future is how we heal a spiritual crisis.

This is the physical and spiritual medicine; this is how we come home to our soul, letting go of how we want things to look and trusting that we are exactly where we need to be, being comfortable with being uncomfortable without numbing and dulling our feelings. There is no linear endpoint; we are constantly evolving or dying slowly or quickly. Each choice we make in the present moment brings us closer to death or life. Faith, surrender, prayer, and connection to something greater than ourselves bridge the gap and reignite the power and energy of Chakra seven.

'The dark night of the soul is when you have lost the flavour of life but have not yet gained the fullness of divinity, so it is that we must weather that dark time, that period of transformation when what is familiar has been taken away and the new richness is not yet ours.'
—*Ram Dass*

Releasing Stuck Energy

There are many ways to release stuck energy within the body. Here are three ways—you can decide which one works best for you:

1. Chakra Cleansing
2. The Five Tibetans
3. The Microscopic Orbit

1. Chakra Cleansing

Chakra cleansing realigns, strengthens, and cleanses your chakras. I like to think of it as chiropractic for your energy system. I use it when I feel blocked or stuck in one area of my body or when I'm experiencing a specific health challenge or pain.

Sit in a comfortable cross-legged position or lie down on your back. Feel your sit bones or feet on the ground, surrendering the weight of your body to the earth. Start by breathing in deeply and exhaling deeply, relaxing your muscles, and bringing your awareness to your first chakra. Now begin by imagining an anchor going from your belly button all the way through your pelvis, legs, and feet down deep into the earth. In your mind's eye, envision a deep ruby-red crystal. This crystal is pulsating slowly, like a heartbeat, the heartbeat of Mother Earth. Wrap your imaginary anchor around the crystal, rooting yourself firmly into the earth. Pull up on your pelvic floor and imagine the red light from the ruby coming up through the anchor and into your body. See this beautiful ruby-red colour filling up your first chakra. You can place your hands on the area of the body where the chakra resides if this helps focus your attention. Breathe in the colour red and imagine the colour as a ball filling up your pelvic area. Stay here for five breaths or longer if you feel intuitively guided.

Repeat the process through your seven chakras, using the following colours for each energy centre.

Chakra 1—Root Centre—RED
Chakra 2—Sacral Centre—ORANGE
Chakra 3—Solar Plexus Centre—YELLOW
Chakra 4—Heart Centre—GREEN
Chakra 5—Throat Centre—BLUE
Chakra 6—Third Eye Centre—INDIGO
Chakra 7—Crown Centre—VIOLET

When you get to Chakra 7, move your awareness above your head to the higher chakras that reside outside your body. These chakras range from 8 to 12. Keep breathing in and out for five breaths. Then, imagine a ball of white light above your head and breathe in a few more rounds. The ball of white light then enters your crown chakra, lighting, filling, and cleansing each chakra as it descends through the body. Keep breathing in and out, and let the white light go wherever it feels intuitively led to go. If you have any areas of pain or illness, direct the white light there with your inhale while visualising any dark, stuck energy leaving your body on the exhale. Feel this energy fill you up, washing you clean from the inside out. Breathe, and when you are finished, see it moving through your legs and feet and into the earth. Relax and hold an upside-down triangle with your hands over your pelvic area, sealing in this energy.

Sometimes, my body craves a complete cleanse with a specific colour. If I'm experiencing period pain, I ask my body what colour it needs to heal, and I intuitively sense that colour in my mind's eye. Then, I imagine this colour entering my body through my feet and feel it moving through me. I focus on exhaling any negativity or pain as I do this. I breathe the colour into the areas where I intuitively feel it's needed. Sometimes, the colour changes, sometimes it stays the same. Don't overthink it; just go with the flow. When I'm finished, I bring in white light, let it wash through me, and seal the process with an upside-down triangle mudra. This practise is an adaptation of Patti Conklin's Colourworks therapy.

2. The Five Tibetans

*Visit **www.drmichelleboycedc.com/resources** for demonstration videos*

This ancient healing system, developed by Tibetan monks 2,500 years ago, is designed to reconnect us with our life force energy. I see it as a way to clear out stagnant energy and blocks in our cells, rejuvenating and healing us simultaneously. The exercises work by cleansing and improving the function of your chakras, organs, and meridians throughout your body. They are especially helpful for hormone imbalances and low energy because they directly affect your endocrine system.

What I love about these exercises is that they build core strength while clearing energy, creating stability and strength in the body. Practising daily helps balance emotional and mental states, improves spinal and joint flexibility, and aids sleep. I've also found that they help reduce pain, especially in the lower back.

The Five Tibetans are a series of five exercises that should be done daily, ideally first thing in the morning. If you're fit and healthy, start with seven repetitions of each exercise, gradually working up to twenty-one. If you're not as fit, begin with three repetitions, always listening to your body and doing what feels right. Twenty-one is the maximum number of repetitions, so don't go beyond that! It's a powerful routine and a great way to get active and move your body.

Because these exercises detox your energy, you might feel lightheaded, dizzy, or nauseous when you start. Listen to your body, reduce the reps if needed, and adjust according to what feels right.

Tibetan 1

- Spin like a sufi!
- Stand upright with your arms stretched out wide.

In the Northern Hemisphere, you want your right palm facing up, and you will spin clockwise, with the left palm facing down, and vice versa for the Southern Hemisphere.

Tibetan 2

- Lie on your back with your palms facing down on the floor. Lift your legs up straight as you exhale. Lift your torso slightly at the same time. With control, lower your torso and legs back to the ground. A variation on this would be placing your palms face down under your buttocks; this is important if your core is very weak and you have lower back pain. It will get stronger soon.
- When you're finished, place your hands in the shape of an upside-down triangle with your thumbs touching your navel and the fingers beneath, creating the triangle. Inhale and exhale three times to seal in the energy.

Tibetan 3

- Come onto your knees. I like to place a folded blanket under my knees for extra padding, and I advise this if you have knee problems. Place your hands on your lower back with your fingers resting on the upper part of your buttocks.
- To begin, inhale and arch your back and neck into extension, tilting the upper body back and hips forward. Exhale, returning to an upright position while flexing your head forward, stretching into the back of the neck.
- When you're finished, place your hands in the shape of an upside-down triangle with your thumbs touching your navel and the fingers beneath, creating the triangle. Inhale and exhale three times to seal in the energy.

Tibetan 4

For me, this one is the hardest!

- Sit on the mat facing forward with your legs slightly bent in front of you. As you inhale, press yourself up so your hips and stomach are in one straight line. Pause at the top, clenching all the muscles in your buttocks and body. Exhale and return to the ground, keeping your core nice and tight. The idea is that you don't just fall to the ground, which you will want to do, especially when you first do this. The movement should be slow and controlled, but trust me, you will be tempted to drop! *To modify this, bend the legs more.*
- When you're finished, place your hands in the shape of an upside-down triangle with your thumbs touching your navel and the fingers beneath, creating the triangle. Inhale and exhale three times to seal in the energy.

Tibetan 5

You will recognise this one if you've ever done yoga. It's two moves blended into one.

- Begin in a downward-facing dog (sneak in some hip and calf stretch). As you inhale, move the body forward, hips resting away from the mat. Roll over your toes as you come down into an upward-facing dog. Pull your shoulders down and back and look up, stretching the anterior neck and torso. Exhale and return to a downward-facing dog.
- When you're finished, place your hands in the shape of an upside-down triangle with your thumbs touching your navel and the fingers beneath, creating the triangle. Inhale and exhale three times to seal in the energy.

3. Microscopic Orbit

Over the years, I've learned this practise from various teachers in different forms. I'm sharing my version, one that I use and that has helped hundreds of women. The Microcosmic Orbit is a Taoist practise focusing on the body's primary energy pathways. This pathway forms a loop, starting from your perineum, travelling up your spine to the top of your head, and then flowing down the front of your body. These energy pathways exist in everyone, and as you focus on them, you'll begin to awaken them. When I first started, I didn't feel much because I had become desensitised to my body's subtle signals. As you practise, you might feel tingling sensations, numbness in your fingers or toes, or even feelings of pleasure and the urge to giggle.

I also use the Microcosmic Orbit when working with my sexual energy, and I teach this to the women I work with. This loop is a powerful way to move sexual energy and shakti through the body. Your sexual energy does more than just give you pleasure; it energises you! As you move this energy around your body, it cleanses and revitalises all your organs and cells. The energy intuitively knows where to flow, sensing what needs to be flushed out and unblocked. When you start this practise, it may take some time and attention as this energy circuit creates new neural pathways in your body.

By the age of forty, most women have a weak pelvic floor, which can be due to poor nutrition, childbirth, hormonal changes, body composition, or lack of strength. There's no need to feel ashamed, but it's important to understand that a weak pelvic floor can contribute to lower back and neck pain, hormonal issues, and symptoms of perimenopause and menopause. We often overlook how a weak pelvic floor can also cause us to leak vital energy. A strong pelvic floor helps you hold onto the energy you'll create through this work. The pelvic area acts as a reservoir, storing your energy and creativity so you can move it through your body, revitalising your mind, body, and soul. A weak pelvic floor means you're not just leaking urine but also your shakti energy. Strengthening these muscles, perhaps with a jade egg, can help stop this energy from draining away.

Practising the Microscopic Orbit

I prefer to do this lying down, but you can also do it sitting up. Your imagination is important here as we use it to visualise the flow of energy. Imagination, visualisation, and dreams connect us to the liminal world—just because you can't see something with your eyes doesn't mean it's not there. Use your imagination and, while breathing from your perineum, inhale and visualise a ball of energy moving up your spine to the top of your head. As you exhale, guide it down the front of your body. I ask my body what colour the ball of energy needs to be today, or I simply imagine the brightest, purest light possible, seeing it move through the loop you are creating, waking up and cleansing your cells. This loop is a closed circuit; it slightly contracts your pelvic floor, about 20%, to hold the energy in the loop and within your body. The energy you create can be used later throughout your day. Do this practise daily for 3-5 minutes.

Personally, I also visualise the Microcosmic Orbit when I am self-pleasuring, practising with a jade egg, or during sex. I imagine my sexual energy circulating in the loop I've created, knowing I have a beautiful reserve of energy stored up whenever I need it.

CHAPTER 16
RECLAIMING YOUR PERSONAL POWER

'With great power comes great responsibility.'
—Ben Parker (Spiderman)

When it comes to our health, our personal power is critical—it's directly linked to disease and pain and how this shows up in the body. Imagine for a moment that your energy is like a battery. Every battery has a certain amount of power before it needs to be recharged. Different tasks require different amounts of power from a battery, depleting the energy from the source, and your body is the same. You were born with a full battery. However, certain beliefs, thoughts, emotions, and actions will drain your energy and life force throughout the day, leaving you tired, overwhelmed, and running on empty. Taking time to recharge is essential to your health, and each day you've had a good rest, you have recharged your battery to a comfortable set point. It's so important to spend more time recharging.

Your choices determine whether you leak energy and if you get ill. When reading a patient's energy field, I look for disruptions or ruptures due to energy leaks. In a torus field, the energy comes in and down through the crown chakra and up and in from the root chakra. When a person loses energy, their energy field becomes smaller, denser, and less energetic—also known as low vibration. Rips and tears may also be visible when a person is leaking energy. This may be due to consistently negative thought patterns, a person in your life acting as an energy vampire, or behaviour in a certain energy centre.

Other issues that affect your energy field are childhood and family problems, past life karmas, ancestral patterns, trauma, attitudes, habits, cravings, addictions, fear, shame, humiliation, and interpersonal power struggles. The constant need to control people and situations, the desire for the perfect body and life, and negative self-talk are chronic, slow punctures to your precious energy and life force, and when all your energy is invested in holding back these issues, it causes stress and pain in the body. It can feel like you are carrying the weight of the world on your shoulders.

So many women I meet are caught up resisting what is and living in the past. Dwelling on what could have or should have been causes resentment, bitterness, and jealousy. Reliving past trauma, arguments, holding grudges, being unable to forgive, stubborn pride, frustration, and unexpressed anger weighs you down spiritually and can show up as physical issues.

When I see a woman struggling with her personal power, it's often reflected in her posture—her shoulders are slumped, her breathing is shallow, her energy is flat, and she's lost that spark in her eyes. The space around her feels heavy and contracted. Her voice carries this loss of power, and her words mirror the unconscious pain she's experiencing, both inside and out. Physical pain, like shoulder, neck, or back pain, might be what brings her to me, but it's usually just the surface—the real issue runs much deeper. To truly heal, we need to explore her energy field and uncover the underlying causes. We'll also examine universal laws to see how they relate to her power and energy—and where it might be leaking.

When I struggle, I remind myself that I am a divine being with the capacity to experience bliss and joy. I am the universe expressing itself through creativity, sensuality, intuition, and power. I know that sadness, negative emotions, or depression may accompany me at times, but they don't define who I am. I am not sad, fat, depressed, or lonely—these are just feelings that will come and go.

Let's start by changing the language from 'I'm sad' to 'There is a feeling of sadness with me.' You are not the problem or the feeling you identify with. When you say 'I am that,' it becomes an identity that takes your power away.

The Law of Cause and Effect

With every action, there is a positive and equal reaction. Every thought, emotion, and behaviour that you have on repeat in your head has a reaction that you can see and feel in your physical world. For example, physically, if you eat cake every day and binge on sugary food, this action will create a reaction that may result in diabetes and obesity, adversely affecting your health. Alternatively, if you exercise and move your body daily, the response in your body will be equal to this action. This operates not only on the physical aspects that you can see and feel but also on emotional, chemical, and spiritual levels beyond just our five senses.

So, for every negative action, you get a negative reaction, usually in your body and life, which drains your power and energy. If we flip the coin, every positive action creates a positive response, maintaining and preserving your energy and power.

Thought and Consequence

The universe doesn't give you what you want.
The universe gives you who you are.

All our thoughts, actions, and words have power. I want you to reframe your victim thinking from: 'I can't do this,' 'Someone must fix me,' or 'It's in my genes,' to powerful, life-affirming thoughts. You get to decide how you perceive things; you are the filter and are responsible for every emotion, spark, and act created in your life and body. This law of the universe shows us that we are always developing and the universe is always in motion, bringing our thoughts into reality. In addition, these thoughts determine how clean our energy is and whether the thoughts are adding to or draining our energy. Take a moment to reflect on how you talk to yourself daily. Do you engage in negative self-talk, like the following examples?

- I'm so fat.
- I hate my body.
- I wish I looked like her.
- It's not fair.
- I hate this pain.
- I want a new body.

All this sludge acts like a parasite to your energy field and slowly eats away at your life force. Every thought has a consequence, so choose them wisely. Think how you would speak to a friend or someone you love. Treat yourself with the same care, patience, and respect you so easily offer others.

What is in One is in the Whole

Everything is connected; what affects one part impacts the whole. This universal law shows us that our beliefs, thoughts, and actions influence our physical bodies and lives. We are all spiritual beings, and we can't separate our minds from our hearts or our bodies from our souls. Just like adding a drop of dye to water affects every particle, anything we put into our bodies, like painkillers, affects not just the symptom but every cell. The body then has to work to detoxify and eliminate these substances, which uses energy.

I'm not telling you not to take pain medication; there are times when it's necessary. But it's important to understand how your body works and not rely on medication blindly. Be a detective—find the root cause of your pain and address it. Painkillers mask pain; they treat the symptoms, not the cause. Often, they simply dull the message your body is trying to send. Pain is your body's way of getting your attention, signalling that something needs to change in your inner world. Pain is often the first sign that something is off in your energy body. It's like a smoke alarm going off, alerting you to investigate. Would you just turn off the alarm and go back to sleep, or would you get up and see what's wrong?

Realising how powerful you are and the impact you can have on your health is liberating. Many of us were raised to believe that we need a doctor and medicine to heal us and that we can't trust our body's natural ability to heal. While there are times when medicine is necessary, it's crucial to understand when external help is needed and when it's not. We've been conditioned to feel disempowered and to fear our own bodies. Taking responsibility for your health can be daunting. It requires self-awareness, effort, and determination. It can feel overwhelming, and it might seem easier to hand over control to someone else because we don't feel powerful or knowledgeable enough.

I value Western medicine and use it when appropriate. But I view health holistically, and ultimately, I am my own healer, just as you are yours. I want to help you develop this skill so you can be your own physician and heal yourself. Yes, guidance and medicine have their place, but true healing comes from within. I'm done with putting plasters on pain because we don't want to deal with what's going on. Sometimes, even though it hurts, we must rip the band-aid off and let our pain breathe so we can deal with what's really going on.

Energy medicine can have a bad rap. Sometimes, it is ineffective when done by well-meaning people who aren't as competent as they portray themselves to be. When we do just affirmations, or we're trying to heal our energy and focus on the light, we bypass the essential process of the descent before the ascent.

We have to get down, go into the depths of ourselves, into the shadow, and dig deep in the dirt to be able to rise. Diamonds are born from irritation. Every butterfly must first go through the alchemy of putrefaction. The trees need to die and retreat to be born again, and so it is with us. We have been distracted by the light, avoiding the uncomfortable, bypassing the true spiritual journey. I call this 'Neo-spirituality,' and it's another way we lose touch with the depth of who we are because we are distracted—on the shore, never truly entering the ocean within.

Letting it Go

Healing takes longer when we're drained of energy, stuck in the past, and caught in negative cycles. Holding onto things, be it physically, emotionally, or spiritually, literally weighs us down. Like a ship, our body is likely to sink because it costs too much to keep it afloat. When we are utterly unaware of how and why we are blocked, we resemble a boat with holes attempting to navigate the sea. We become engrossed in trying to bail out the water because we are frightened and wish to remain afloat when, in fact, we need to stop and repair the holes and do the hard work instead of focusing all our energy on the superficial. The holes represent power leaks that must be addressed so that we can stay afloat and gradually start to sail forward again. Your inner power is the centrepiece of your health—spiritually, physically, and emotionally.

Healing and miracles occur in the present—the here and now—not in the past or future. If we keep choosing things that act as dead weights, we'll find ourselves stuck and sinking quickly. It's important to remember the principle of cause and effect. I like to imagine letting go of negative thoughts and beliefs as if they're weights pulling down a hot air balloon. As these weights are released, my energy increases, and my body, like the balloon, becomes lighter, more free, and more vibrant.

Letting go of these burdens and feeling our energy lift changes how we view life. From your window, you might see traffic and buildings. In a city, the crowds and movement can feel overwhelming. However, imagine seeing it all from a hot air balloon. Your perspective changes as you begin to rise above the chaos and see life from a different viewpoint or perspective. We can always choose to see things differently.

I experienced this when I went on a hot air balloon ride for my anniversary a few years back. Floating above my home, I was surprised to see the proximity to forests, lakes, and wildlife, contrasting with the usual noise and activity I noticed from my window. This shift in perspective can also apply to our health and to pain, offering a broader, more truthful view of what is really happening. Pain can give us tunnel vision, focusing only on the problem, whereas freeing up our energy and creating a new perspective allows us to see our health holistically, which is liberating and leads to greater awareness, healing, and energy.

So, I invite you to intuit and feel—not think—your way through this process. Become conscious of what's going on around and inside of you. Start looking at where you lose power.

Contemplate or journal the following:

- How is my self-esteem?
- Am I able to self-reflect truthfully?
- Do I get stuck in the past?
- Am I projecting blame onto another?
- Am I able to see my dark as well as my light?
- What am I scared of? What is it that I truly fear?
- How do I rate my inner power on a scale of 1-10?

One of the hardest parts of healing is moving past what has or hasn't happened. I understand it's difficult, especially if you've experienced terrible things, but holding onto anger and resentment harms you more. I encourage you to release it. It's holding you back! Let it go; life is a learning journey, and we all have lessons to learn and share with others that aid our growth. How can we judge others when we're unaware of their own life agreements or karma? It's their journey—not ours to fix or fixate on. Your primary focus should be on your own healing and growth. You need all your energy and attention for yourself. The reality is that we can't change others, only ourselves and how we perceive things. The most loving thing to do in any situation is to work on yourself—that is how we can help others and heal our planet.

Take a moment to journal on the following:

- How can I lighten my load?
- What am I ready to release?
- What's not worth holding onto any longer?
- Who do I need to forgive?

Ritual: Burn It

For releasing, I find a burning ceremony powerful. Start by writing down everything you want to let go of—whether from this lifetime or another. You might want to write a letter to someone who has hurt you. Offer these burdens to a higher power you believe in. They're no longer yours to carry. When you're ready, place the paper in a burning dish or fireplace and watch it burn. As the flames consume the paper, visualise all the negativity burning away. Imagine the smoke carrying it out of your body and soul.

I also like to visualise a bridge between myself and these old beliefs and thoughts. Crossing the bridge into a new perspective is a choice you can make if you're ready. As you walk across, feel the flames and smoke rising behind you, and don't look back. You are closing one chapter and stepping into another.

It is done, it is done, it is done.

PART TWO
SHE-PRACTISES

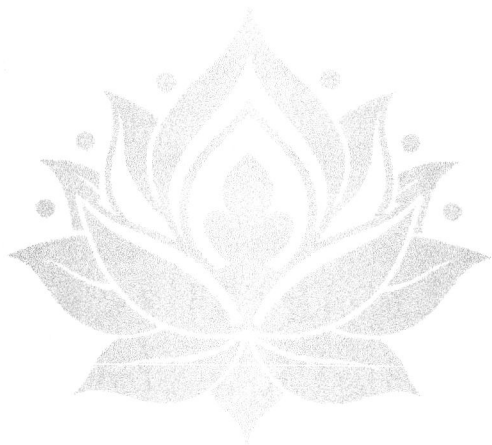

CHAPTER 17
SHE-PRACTISES—AN INTRODUCTION

You don't need to know the path—it will be revealed. Just know that it is You.

My greatest hope for you is to discover the power and magic within yourself. These practises are like a roadmap guiding you back to who you truly are. The magic, your true self, and your hidden treasures are always within you, found in the shadows and the depths of your being. This is the ultimate heroine's journey, one we take many times throughout our lives. Where you are right now is exactly where you'll find your strength and vitality if you choose to walk this path.

Many of us long to be saved, but the truth is, there's no saviour—no doctor or guru who can fix or heal you. There will be great guides and teachers (like the ones in this book!), but the journey is, and always will be, an inward one. It's a solo venture into the depths of yourself to find your hidden treasure. You are the heroine of your own story. In every fairy tale, myth, or legend, the heroine always saves herself. This is especially true in goddess myths. The goddess within us all emerges from her trials with a precious gem, and so will you.

Finding alignment with myself has been crucial in my spiritual journey. When you have a deep connection to yourself, anything is possible. A world of endless possibilities and magic opens up when you truly align. These practises will help you come back into physical, emotional, and spiritual alignment. Welcome home.

The Practises—An Introduction

Both science and spirituality teach us that before we can fully commit to making a change, we need to understand why it's necessary. I also believe we need to feel and embody these changes, as not all understanding comes from the logical brain—much of it comes from the deep wisdom in our emotional, spiritual, and feeling bodies. The solutions offered here form the foundation of the 'She-Method' I've created, which has helped hundreds of women like you reclaim their bodies and power.

This is just the foundation, and there are many layers and depths to this work, as each person is unique in their desires and needs. Simply reading about these practises won't heal or change your life. True healing and transformation happen when we commit to a practise that's devoted to ourselves, our health, and our lives. It's about showing up as the person you were born to be. Devotion means investing time, energy, and sometimes money in yourself. Consistency is key; your body is your instrument, and your life force is the music you create. Just as you can't learn to play the piano with one lesson, these practises require regular effort to truly take effect.

As you begin this journey, these changes will become part of who you are; your chemical, neurological, and physical pathways will be rewired, and you'll become a different version of yourself. What you do, say, and think will reflect who you become. Everything starts and ends with you and your choices—you have that power.

> 'Be the change you want to see in the world.'
> —Mahatma Gandhi

The following chapters are not another to-do list or a simple set of instructions. You can use them as gentle nudges or invitations from your soul. They are here to inspire and ignite her in you, to reconnect you back to your body, nature, and everything you truly are but have forgotten. When you have little time, simply read to remind and motivate you, and when there is more time, explore a topic that resonates with you. I recommend starting with less than you think you can and slowly building up from there.

Start by creating new habits so you develop new patterns. When we begin anything, it feels time-consuming and often overwhelming, and we can feel out of our depth. That's because it's unfamiliar, and we crave the familiar; it's how our brain works.

Remember, this is an integrated approach, combining the mind, emotions, and your physical and spiritual body. These practises are designed to connect you to your body's wisdom, which will change you from the inside out.

Just 5 Minutes...

Little and often is the way to approach this; even eating one healthy meal, lighting a candle at your desk, or dancing to one song will positively affect your body and mind.

Listen

Do what speaks to you. I invite you to see this section as something that nourishes you, something you want to do, not as another chore. Be realistic and kind; perhaps when you show up to practise, you only want to rest, and that's fine. Always listen to your body.

Exploration

Everything in this book is here to awaken something in you and help you find a missing part of yourself. Sometimes, the things we resist the most are the ones that will be the most transformative for us. Explore and question why you feel excited about some practises and not others, and investigate your feelings around this. Many of the practises are designed to give you insight into how you function and why you do things the way you do, which can bring up resistance. Don't be scared of the unknown; welcome it with open arms. What we don't know about ourselves and what we haven't yet experienced will reveal so much about what's going on, who you are, and what you want. By engaging in these practises while allowing emotions to flow and feelings to be felt, you become present to the layers of masks and expectations you hold for yourself and others. When the masks and armour begin to fall away, tears may flow. Let them; they will help you heal. Emotional fluidity releases our physical and mental rigidity. This always leads to breakthroughs if we are willing to flow with it instead of fighting against it. In my experience, it's always better to float downstream rather than struggle and paddle upstream against the flow of what is.

The Importance of Ritual

Before there were churches and organised religion, there were circles where women would gather, share, and be fully seen in their sacredness. They met in caves, forests, and homes. They celebrated the moon, the seasons, and nature in all its forms. There was a deep gnosis and relationship between the land and her body, an invisible red thread that anchored her back to who she really was. Every sacred movement starts with ritual; ritual is the portal to the sacred. I believe the reawakening of the sacred feminine and her rise back into our consciousness at this time is what will save this planet. It starts with us, with you, with ritual.

Sacred ritual is the structure and cauldron our body and soul yearn for. It is the missing link in the mundanity of our daily lives. It connects the liminal space between the seen and unseen world. In our modern-day culture, ritual has been stripped back and removed, rites of passage gone, and sacred worship of the feminine and connection to our ancestral heritage has been virtually wiped out. As women, the path of reawakening and remembrance starts, continues, and ends with ritual. It is profoundly needed in society today. As part of my priestess work, I hold temple space where women can delve deep into who they are. It's a place where we are in the betwixt, the in-between of who we are and who we want to become. Ritual is a space and container that holds a woman's transformation. It's the place where the caterpillar can safely turn into the butterfly, where a woman is held, seen, witnessed, and supported as she transforms out of the old and into the new. Creating such space requires ancient priestess technologies and training, which have profound and life-changing effects on the physical, mental, emotional, and cellular body. Most women I work with are yearning for this space, yet they have no idea what it is or how to find it. As part of my work with women, I offer temple and ritual spaces to help women through their life transitions, and sacred space is something I teach all women who first come to me. Creating sacred space and ritual is something you can do at home. It is one of the most important yet overlooked steps in any transformational journey and change you want to create in your body and life.

Creating Sacred Space

Creating a sacred space at home links you to your physical life and body and to the spaces between time and space, which I call the subliminal space, timeless in essence. This place, which has an altar at its centre, is where you can deeply connect and tap into your true self, your soul, and the essence of who you are. When I'm connected and spend time in this space, I can access my true feelings, my shadow, my light, and my magic. I find answers and truths that my cortical brain can't reach. It's like coming home to my true self, where I discover my inner wisdom and intuition and where I can meet and connect with the wise woman who lives within me.

I recommend making this sacred connection a part of your morning routine. I rise earlier than my children and dedicate at least 15 minutes to it. The way we start our day influences the entire day. Taking time to prioritise yourself with self-care helps build neural pathways, calms your nervous system, and connects you to your soul. Seeking guidance from your intuition and inner wisdom for your day should be as routine as brushing your teeth. Learning to tap into the unseen and your own magic will assist you in every aspect of your life and health. Remember, everything you need and desire originates from within you, not external to you. So, set the intention to start your day in a sacred manner.

Everything you need and want comes from *you, not* to *you.*

Creating Your Altar

This doesn't have to be overly complicated. Your altar can be created from anything, such as an old coffee table, bookshelf, desk, or even a tray you pull out and keep under your bed. Your altar should inspire and energise you, connecting you deeply to your femininity and the sacred parts of yourself.

Things on my altar include:

- A cloth to lay over my altar; I may switch up the colours with different seasons or moon cycles.
- A candle.
- Incense.
- Smudging herbs such as white sage or herbs from my garden.
- Crystals such as clear quartz, amethyst, rose quartz—anything that speaks to you.
- Figures: I have a Sheela na gig and a Mary Magdalene, but you may have a spirit animal, Buddha, or a Christian symbol. Choose what resonates with you.
- Photos of people or yourself when you were full of that fun, divine spark. I have a picture of me as a little girl, full of life and energy, radiating femininity, love, and happiness.
- Paintings and vision boards.
- Oracle cards.

Starting Your Sacred Practise

- If you're doing this in the morning, sit with a cup of tea or coffee, ensuring you're comfortable and warm.
- Light a candle and some incense, and smudge your body.
- Take five deep cleansing breaths, counting to five as you inhale and exhale for five.
- Imagine the breath reaching every area of your body, lighting you up, and waking you from the inside out.
- After breathing, begin by sitting in 'Empty Presence.' This process, as the name suggests, empties you of all thoughts and negative energies. You can achieve this by focusing on a spot, such as a candle, or with your eyes closed if you're new to this. When you feel empty, ask your inner wisdom for guidance. The answer may come in thoughts, images, words, or feelings. If clarity eludes you, ask for it to reveal itself throughout the day.
- If you have any aches, pains, or illnesses, ask your body what colour it needs to heal or release tension or pain. Sit in empty presence, allowing that colour to fill you up and cleanse your body. Conclude by flushing white light through your entire body to wash away anything that needs to go.
- At the end of your process, journal any thoughts, words, or symbols in your consciousness. Free writing is a compelling way to connect to the sacred. I ask my guides, 'What is it that I need to do?' and the answers always come as my pen hits the page. (Some days, I read sacred literature, such as poetry by Rumi or a spiritual book, and I ask my guides to direct me to what I need to hear and read today. I then follow my intuition. I'm always amazed at the page and messages I receive.)
- You can also pull cards from your Oracle deck for clarification on any questions you have. Observe the colours, numbers, symbols, and words—take notes in your journal so you can observe the patterns as they begin to appear in your life. Be aware of how synchronicities start to manifest, making the unseen seen and the invisible visible. You will be amazed at how magical life becomes.

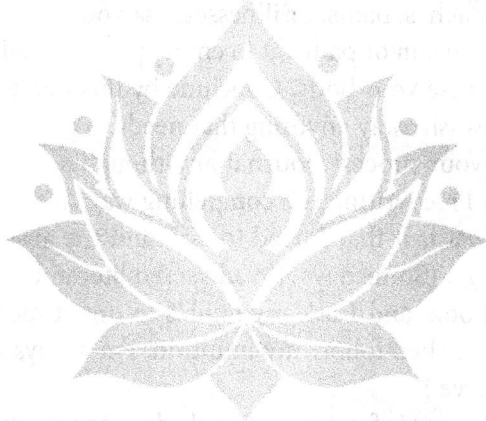

CHAPTER 18
SHE-PRACTISES—POSTURE & STRENGTH

The first phase of the She-Method is to change the top layer of stressful input into the body so we can lower sympathetic dominance and switch out of the red zone into the green parasympathetic zone.

Get Regular Chiropractic Adjustments

Vertebral subluxation, slight misalignment or partial dislocation of the vertebrae in the spine, is very real—most of us are walking around with a spine that is not functioning correctly. Vertebral subluxation affects the health not only of your spine but of your whole body. The spine is not an isolated structure standing alone. Your spine is the house, the lifeline to your whole physical being, and without your spinal cord and nervous system, you wouldn't be here right now reading this! Your heart wouldn't beat, you wouldn't be able to breathe, you wouldn't be you! Did you know that the nervous system and brain are the first things that form in an embryo? Everything else comes after the nervous system is developed. Your nervous system controls and coordinates all organisms and structures within your body; it's a big deal. Your heart would be unable to beat without your nervous system, yet most of us never give it any thought. It is vital to grasp how important a well-functioning nervous system is to your whole being and how vertebral subluxations can make you sick.

Vertebral subluxation not only leads to structural issues in the spine, such as reverse curves, degeneration, and other related problems, but also causes nerve dysfunction. Your brain controls the alignment of your spine and sets the tone for your nervous system. It's not enough to just physically align the spine; we also need to ensure proper motion and alignment in the brain, creating coherent proprioceptive movement both internally and externally. Restoring motion to a joint helps improve overall health and re-establishes communication between the brain and the joint.

According to Hilton's law, any synovial joint, especially in the spine, requires an optimal range of motion. Anything that crosses a joint, such as a nerve, tissue, muscle, or ligament, is mapped in the brain. The brain detects issues not because it sees them but because it senses them—this information comes from the joints and surrounding tissues. Reduced range of motion, nociception, or damage to a joint creates a disconnect between the joint and the brain, leading to degeneration and further injury.

A fixed joint also 'fixes' the part of the brain that controls it. Over time, disrupted synapses in the brain lead to a loss of motor control in that area, resulting in situations like 'I just bent down to pick up my pen, and my back gave out.' Chiropractic care restores motion and coherence between the joints and the brain, leading to better recovery and a reduced risk of future spinal problems.

When joints aren't moving properly, we lose mobility, and postural changes can develop, leading to arthritis. I've yet to meet anyone who moves their spine through its full range of motion daily, which is why getting our joints moving is so important. This is achieved through movement and, most importantly, spinal adjustments. Chiropractors identify restricted joints in the spine, restore movement, and re-establish brain communication, which helps to regulate the nervous system.

Simply doing exercises and stretches is like brushing and flossing your teeth but not going to the dentist to fix a cavity. Many people visit the dentist and discover an asymptomatic cavity. Would they say, 'Leave it, I'll just brush my teeth,' or would they get that cavity fixed? We need to think of our spines in the same way. Most of the time, we're unaware of spinal problems until we feel pain, but these issues have often been building up for years. Pain is never an accurate indicator of spinal health, yet it's usually only when we experience pain that we seek help.

You need to look after your spine just as you do your teeth—if not better! You can get new teeth, but you can't get a new spine or nervous system. Get checked regularly by a chiropractor, and don't rely on the absence of pain as a sign that everything is fine. Learn to prevent problems rather than waiting to fix them. Your health and vitality are closely linked to the health and flexibility of your spine, so start taking care of it as if your life depends on it—because it does.

Develop A Supporting Posture

Posture correction is essential so the nerves can travel without interference between the brain and nervous system. Remember that poor posture sends the wrong messages to the brain and pushes us further into stress, so what better place to start than here with how you sit and stand?

How's your neck?

Check-in and see if you can fully turn your head from side to side without moving your shoulders. Can you easily bring your head to the side and tip your head back?

Upper cross syndrome is a modern-day disease of the spine that sits for hours behind a computer and needs to be addressed.

The best place to begin your posture journey is to retrain and strengthen the muscles that are supposed to extend, rotate, and lengthen the muscles that are stuck in flexion. It doesn't matter how bad your posture is. It can always improve. Remember, your skeleton renews itself every 2-3 years. With the right exercises and movement, you can improve the quality of your spine, prevent osteoporosis, align the curves in your spine, and address the symmetry and balance of the muscles.

Here are a couple of my favourite go-to posture exercises. Create movement breaks, stretch and move when you get up for the toilet, and set an alarm on your phone to move every hour, especially if that hour has been spent bent over a keyboard.

Visit **www.drmichelleboycedc.com/resources for a demonstration of posture and rehabilitation exercises for lower back, neck, and shoulder pain.*

Stargazer Stretch

This stretches the sternocleidomastoid muscles in the neck. These muscles help the neck flex and rotate. These get tight with computer work. This exercise can be done standing or sitting down. Place your left hand on your right collarbone, and put your right hand over your left, stretching out the neck muscles on the right-hand side. Now, turn your head to the left and look up at the sky or ceiling. Try to tilt your head back a little further, feeling the stretch through the front right-hand side of the neck. Hold for 30 seconds, then repeat on the other side.

Ear-To-Shoulder Stretch

This stretch stretches the side of the neck, which can become tight due to poor posture. Tip your right ear to your right shoulder. To increase the stretch, place one hand on the head and one hand on the shoulder. Feel the stretch on the left-hand side of the neck. Hold for 30 seconds, then repeat on the opposite side.

Cat-Cow

I love this exercise, as it stretches all the flexors and extensors on both sides of the body. Get on the floor on all fours. Place your hands shoulder-width apart and your knees hip distance apart directly under the hips. Inhale slowly and deeply, curving your lower spine while bringing your head up and tilting your pelvis up like a cow. Exhale slowly and deeply while bringing your stomach up and in and bringing your head and pelvis down like a cat. Repeat this ten times, moving from cat to cow. Finish with a free movement cat-cow, letting the head and neck move and unwind any areas of tension that may have built up over the day. I love moving my hips from side to side, opening my legs and going deeper into my hip flexors to release and mobilise these often stiff, underloved joints.

Finger Follow

Sitting at your desk, place your arms straight out in front of you with your index finger pointing upwards. Move your arm/finger to the side and into the top corner of the room (right arm goes to the right, left arm goes to the left). Follow the movement of your finger with your neck so you are also rotating and extending the head to look at your finger. Try to keep your upper body stable so you don't cheat, and move your body instead of your neck. Do this ten times in one direction, then ten on the other. This move uses neck extension and rotation and is excellent for increasing the cervical range of movement.

Hold the Grapefruit

This exercise addresses the long and weak muscles in the posterior neck. Most of us have a head that is stuck out in front of us, which leads to headaches and neck pain. This exercise works on restoring cervical lordosis, which is quickly lost as we age. Sit or stand upright and imagine you have a big grapefruit under your chin; hold this position for 15 seconds, repeat a few times, and then release it to the chin into extension. I also encourage my patients to imagine holding a grapefruit while working, on the phone, driving and sitting on the sofa. Learning to get control of your cervical lordosis is important to an optimally functioning spine and nervous system.

Side Dips

Great for adding an increased range of motion to your spine, side dips and twists help keep your spine healthy and flexible; it's like flossing for the spine. Flex and twist the body from side to side. Repeat at least 10 of each. I love to do this to music and add a leg left across the body or out to the side. Get playful and feel where your body feels stuck and how it needs to move; this can change from day to day. Feel into the deep core muscles. Remember, great posture comes from a strong core.

Seated Figure 4

This is my prescription go-to exercise and a must for anyone who has hips and a sitting job, so basically everyone! It stretches out the deep gluteal muscles and increases the range of motion in the hips, helping to alleviate symptoms of lower back pain. Seated, place your right leg bent over your left knee in a figure four position. Lengthen your spine and lean forward through the centre. You will feel a stretch into the right buttock and the side of the leg. If you are super flexible, apply pressure to the upper right thigh. It's common for one side to be more flexible than the other; just be with where you are and breathe. Do this for up to a minute on both sides, at least four times per day if you struggle with lower back pain.

Pec-Stretch, Baby

Our pectoral muscles all need love, and our lifestyle means we are always hunched or bent over some device. Our lovely pec muscles are getting shorter and tighter, causing more wind up, poor posture, and stress in our bodies. Ideally, we want to strengthen the back muscles to pull us back and stretch out the front of the body with regular practise of pec stretching. Stand next to a wall or door, stretch out your right arm and place your hand flat on the wall slightly higher than your shoulder. Twist the upper body and neck to the left and feel the stretch in your right arm and upper chest area. This can be quite challenging to begin with. You may experience tingling in your arm and hand, which is normal as your brachial plexus and nerves from your neck also benefit from this stretch. Be patient, breathe, relax, and feel what is right for you. Begin with this exercise at least three times a day and do it throughout the day. When your coffee or tea is brewing, find a door or a wall and hang, baby! Hold for 30 seconds, then repeat on the opposite side. Feel it in your shoulders, arms, wrists, and fingers.

Maximise Your Multifidus

Sitting all day does nothing for this highly proprioceptive spinal stabilising muscle in our spine. Grab a weight—start at 2 kg—and lift the arm from the hip out to the side. This exercise works on the opposite side of the arm that is moving.

Releasing Lower Back Pain

You can do this at home when you are struggling with acute or chronic back pain. But remember, pain is not an indicator of spinal health. This is my first aid prescription that helps treat the symptoms of lower back pain. I recommend going to a chiropractor who uses spinal adjustments to get to the root cause.

1. Firstly, identify where the pain is.
2. Breathe into the pain; don't avoid it; allow yourself to get angry or frustrated. Release the story about why you have it or what you did. Just be with the pain and observe your thoughts and feelings, but don't become attached to them. You are the witness here to your pain, not the pain itself. Pain is an emotion!
3. Make your breathing slower and longer. Breathe in for 5 and exhale for 5, exaggerate the out-breath, and make a sound or a sigh, letting go of the pain and tension you unconsciously or consciously hold in your body. It can help to visualise white light entering your body on the in-breath and black smoke or a colour releasing from your body on the out-breath. Ask your body what colour it needs to heal, then fill the area of pain up with this colour.
4. Next, create space, stretching away from the pain and lengthening the muscles. Let your body guide you; listen, feel, and become curious.
5. Feel and massage the pain with your hand or a tennis ball, or simply push your lower back into the ground as you stretch. When you have back pain, you need to increase blood flow to the area, as most pain is due to a lack of blood flow, nociception and reduced range of motion (movement), which keeps you stuck in the pain cycle, creating an increased perception of pain in the brain. We don't feel pain in the body; we experience nociception. Pain is an emotion that is experienced in the brain.

6. Strengthen your core and pelvic floor so you stop hanging in your body. The intrinsic muscles in the spine are often under-conditioned and underworked, especially for those who sit at desks.

7. Your hips don't lie! Tight hips always go hand in hand with lower back pain (and emotional and mental rigidity), which reduces the range of motion in the pelvis and lower back. Move your hips in BIG circles and make figure eights with your hips. Put on your favourite tunes that made you run to the dance floor back in the day. Dance like Shakira for 5 minutes every day as you cook or do the dishes. Get your family involved, and make it fun. You will be amazed at how good you start to feel physically and emotionally. If you sit all day, your lower back needs movement in other directions rather than bent over your desk or your car's steering wheel. Tight hip flexors contribute to much lower back pain, so go and shake it, baby.

8. Begin to sit straight and use the curves of your spine as they were intended. Sit on both of your Sit bones rather than your coccyx. Use a pillow behind your bra strap area and stop yourself from slouching forward. This can help to strengthen the small postural muscles in the spine. Make sure you're stretching out your pectoral muscles daily, as when these are tight, they pull you forward into a humped-over posture, leading to spinal degeneration and kyphosis.

9. Ground your legs into the floor as you sit and stand. Use them to support and strengthen yourself. So often, we hang forward over our bodies and sit with our legs tucked under the chair or legs crossed. Maybe you stand on one leg, throwing your posture off balance and creating compensations that are contributing to your back pain. Start to become conscious of how you live in your body.

10. The position of our feet and legs is often overlooked, yet it is the foundation of everything. Think about building a house: if the foundations aren't good, that building will fall or look like a melted lopsided cake over time. Check if your feet are turned out, and be aware of how you stand. A healthy spine is built on a good foundation, and that starts with your feet.

11. Just get into your body and feel! Pain is your body's way of trying to get your attention. Listen, feel, and investigate.

Strength Training

Strength training is incredibly important for inner and outer strength; there's no way around it—you need to lift weights. Resistance training becomes your best friend as you head into perimenopause and beyond. After age forty, we need to start thinking differently about how we move. By 35, we are already losing muscle mass and bone density, so we must build and maintain it. During our pre- and post-menopausal years, we are at a higher risk of metabolic disease and many other illnesses. Stubborn, often difficult-to-shift toxic fat starts to accumulate in our abdomen, underarms, and mid-back area, and it needs to go. Not because you need to look thinner or because you're not good enough, but because it's an indication that you are on a one-way ticket to heart disease, diabetes, and an increased risk of cancer, not to mention other diseases.

My mission is to help women live longer, healthier, happier lives. It matters how strong and flexible your body is. As part of my 'She-Woman' transformation programme, I assist women with this; it is the foundation of the work because your body is how you experience life, so it needs to be in optimal health.

Optimal body and nervous system = Optimal life

What I have learnt is that most diet and exercise regimes are male-focused and don't take into consideration a woman's unique body composition, stress, hormones, and different nutrient and emotional demands that also change during her life phases. A woman in her forties needs to approach health and fitness more holistically. What worked for you in your twenties and thirties isn't going to yield the same results anymore. When women get stuck in the techniques of years gone by, they experience injuries, back pain, feel stiff, and can't burn fat no matter how much they calorie count or how long they run or walk. When it comes to getting strong, burning fat, and feeling fantastic, it's not magic; it's female brain and body biochemistry and physiology. There aren't enough trainers out there looking at women's bodies holistically, meaning we become stuck in an old paradigm of one size and way fits all when it doesn't. Women over forty have different needs and demands than ever before, requiring a different approach than men.

The science of how gender affects exercise, fat burning, reactions to medicines, and susceptibility to certain diseases is still developing. Only in the 1990s were women allowed to participate in clinical trials for disease prevention and medicines. This is significant because, until then, all medicines and disease studies were conducted solely on men, who, as we now know, differ from women in many ways—physically, hormonally, chemically, and mentally. Thankfully, female-focused science and medicine are making strides, although there is still progress to be made in some areas.

A few recent discoveries have uncovered:

- Women are more likely to die each year from heart attacks. In addition, the presentation of a heart attack is different in a man than in a woman, often leading to misdiagnosis and reduced early prevention.
- Women with diabetes have a six times higher risk of heart disease than men with diabetes.
- Women smokers are twice as likely to develop cancer as men.
- Women are more prone to depression, anxiety, and burnout than men.
- Women over forty lose more muscle and bone density than men of the same age.
- Women are at a higher risk of diseases from drinking alcohol than men.
- Women need additional and often different vitamin and mineral support than men.

Extensive research now shows that women who lift weights and stay active in their forties and beyond gain less weight, reduce stress, alleviate perimenopausal and menopausal symptoms, and lower the risk of metabolic diseases. This also helps to reduce toxic stress and prevent chronic degeneration.

Tip:

Perimenopause is a transition that requires a plan. You are going to be in this phase for around a third of your life, and that's a long time to suffer. It's time to drive the body rather than let it pull you along. You get to choose how you look and feel. How do you want to experience the rest of your life? What do you want to do, feel, and create? Whatever the answer, you will need a body that supports you physically; there is no getting around it.

She-Woman exercises are crucial for addressing the modern health challenges women face today. How we move is important. Women can become overly focused on burning calories, losing fat, and counting steps. We go to the gym and lift weights that target the muscles we can see in the mirror, such as our biceps and chest, which can push us further into a state of sympathetic dominance and lead to neck and shoulder pain.

Earlier in the book, I discussed upper and lower cross syndromes, which are common among those with these modern health issues. We should focus on toning the upper back, around the bra strap area, and stretching the front of the upper body. Additionally, we need to tone and strengthen the lower front part of the body, concentrating on building core stability and incorporating stretches that lengthen the back of the lower body. Strengthening the glutes—our bottom muscles—is also essential, as these muscles can weaken and sag with age.

After age 35, we lose muscle mass, especially in the glutes, which is worsened by sitting for long periods. Weak gluteal muscles lead to overcompensation in the lower back and sacroiliac joints, causing lower back pain. When we exercise correctly, we move from a slouched, stressed posture to an upright, optimal one, enhancing neurological function. All of your exercises should support this transition as you journey through perimenopause and beyond.

Focus on lifting weights and moving in ways that strengthen the extensor muscles and stretch the flexor muscles in the upper body while doing the reverse in the lower body—strengthening the front and stretching the back. This approach improves posture and prevents the hunched, bent-over appearance. Remember, poor posture can add years, weight, and health problems, while good posture can take years off and improve overall well-being.

Running, walking, and cycling are beneficial, but be mindful of your head position. Many runners and walkers look down at the ground, leading to tight shoulders, neck pain, and headaches. Instead, try focusing your gaze ahead, keeping your head in a good position and preventing shoulder rounding and the development of a hump in your spine. I often advise my patients to look ahead as if they're searching for rainbows and unicorns!

Tip:

Imagine you have a light between your breasts. When you sit and stand straight, the light shines forward rather than on the floor. When you engage in any sport or class, even a 30-minute walk, take 5 minutes to stretch your calves, hamstrings, and pectoral muscles; you get out what you put in.

Core stability, working your abdominals, is the magic ingredient that holds everything together, and it is the weakest in most women past the age of 40. Years of sitting behind a desk and caring for babies take their toll. This is not about having a flat stomach or body shaming at all! Most women are unhappy with their midline because they think it's too fat or bloated. I'm not focusing on that here; most bloating and excess fat are related to hormone imbalances, stress, and diet. Core stability concerns the muscles underneath; it's those muscles that have been sleeping, just like Sleeping Beauty, waiting to be awakened from their slumber.

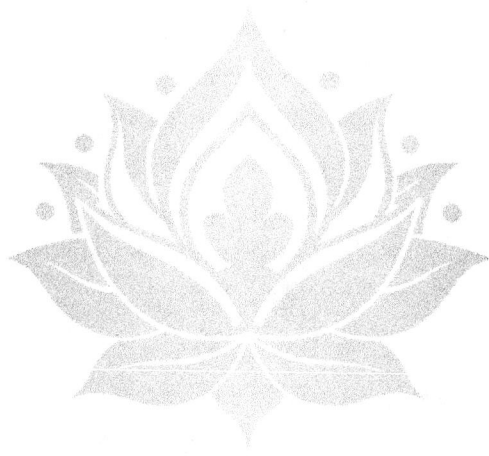

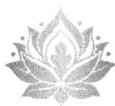

CHAPTER 19
SHE-PRACTISES—RELIEVING STRESS

Insomnia is one of the most frequently reported symptoms of stress, perimenopause, and menopause. Sleeping less than 6 hours per night disrupts your cortisol level, creates insulin resistance, and affects your cognitive function, wreaking havoc on your emotional and energy regulation and leaving you tired, stiff, bloated, and depressed.

Sleep

Sleep is the key to everything. It's the foundation of how we think, move, and eat. We cannot be healthy unless we get enough sleep. Poor sleep can lead to:

- Hormonal imbalances.
- Sympathetic dominance and high cortisol.
- Obesity.
- Type 2 diabetes.
- Poor adaptation to stress.
- Reduced libido.
- Back pain.

Causes of disrupted sleep:

- Stress and cortisol levels are too high.
- Hormone imbalance.
- Temperature regulation.
- Where you are in your menstrual cycle.
- Anxiety.
- Alcohol.
- Too much caffeine.
- Obesity.
- Timing of meals and snacking late at night.
- Working night-shifts.

When the sun goes down at night, and if you live in the northern hemisphere, especially in winter, you tend to feel more anxious and depressed. The stresses that have built up over the day tend to haunt you at night, leading to poor quality sleep, which creates hormonal disruptions and more stress the following day—a perfect recipe for the Modern Disease of the Modern Woman.

Creating an evening routine is essential for rebalancing and re-energising after a day. It allows you to release stress and reconnect with your soul.

A good evening routine lowers our stress levels and helps us into parasympathetic mode, which the body desperately needs to rest, repair, and heal. An evening routine can sound like a luxury self-care routine, but balancing your circadian rhythm with the internal master clock is essential for your health.

Neutralize Light

The suprachiasmatic nucleus (SCN) in your brain is very sensitive to light, and it controls your sleep and waking patterns. It constantly evaluates how much light your retina is exposed to. The SCN also controls your neural and hormonal signals and core body temperature; you can see why this is important when balancing hormones!

I advise my patients to wear polarising sunglasses, which are glasses that have red lenses. The red lens filters blue light input from fluorescent lighting, screens, phones, and television. Red lenses not only protect you from your computer screen and phone but also from the sun.

Dimming lights and avoiding screen time an hour before bed helps signal to the SCN that bedtime is approaching, which eases us into a beautiful slumber.

Neutralize Sound

If you have a dysregulated nervous system, are sensitive to noise and sound, and are struggling with stress, then your inferior colliculus (ICN) needs some love. The ICN in your brain is the gatekeeper to sound and how your nervous system reacts to it—using earplugs in a noisy environment or before bed can decrease your sensory overload. They can also help prevent and manage headaches. You can still hear everything when you wear earplugs, but it's dampened and less taxing on your nervous system, especially if you are struggling with sensory overload. Some women find that they are more sensitive to sound just before their period, and this can also be a problem during perimenopause.

The She-Sleep Routine

Create an electronic, Wi-Fi-free sleeping environment.

Remove all clocks, phones, and Bluetooth devices, and ensure the TV is off, not just on standby. Better still, get it out of the bedroom! Remember, you are an electrical being; your body and brain constantly send messages to each other via your spinal cord and nervous system. Your sensory nerves sense and feel everything, even what you can't see. Your heart, brain, and nervous system are electric; they have an electromagnetic field. Exposing your body and cells to constant electromagnetic radiation from phones, computers, and TVs affects your sleep and heart rate variability (HRV)—the timing between each heartbeat—and dysregulates your nervous system.

Walk

Take a brisk evening walk for 15-30 minutes. Some days, you might only manage 5 minutes—that's fine, but make sure to get outside and move. This isn't just great for your sleep; walking after a meal also helps lower blood glucose levels, burns fat, and reduces your risk of type 2 diabetes.

Breathe

Science shows us Diaphragmatic Breathing is one of the quickest and most effective ways to consciously influence our nervous system. This is the icing on the cake, the one thing you must take away from this book. It's the magical component that transforms many negative aspects of our health from negative to positive. It actively aids in fat burning, combating depression and burnout, and keeps us in a state of calm and present-moment consciousness.

Switch from short, shallow breathing to long, deep inhales and exhales, add sound to the out-breath and come home into your body. I promise this will reach and heal you in places you never knew needed attention. Nothing—and I mean nothing—regulates your nervous system and stress hormones like diaphragmatic breathing. It's essential for PMS, hormonal issues, and menopausal symptoms. Every woman should practise this; it's as crucial as brushing your teeth.

Also, take ten deep breaths from your diaphragm as you wind down in the evening. You can do this during your walk, after, or both. Breathing deeply calms the nervous system and instantly lowers stress levels. Connect with your heart centre and fill it with gratitude. It doesn't have to be for big things—often, the small things bring us the most pleasure and joy. Focus on positive thoughts and fill your heart with emotions like joy, love, and gratitude. Our thoughts and emotions directly affect our hearts, so choose them wisely and avoid negative automatic thinking that keeps us stuck in stressful patterns. Neuroplasticity allows us to change how we perceive and experience our lives. The brain's neural networks can change, grow, and reorganise, giving us the power to rewire our brains to function in ways that better support our lives and health.

Taking care of our hearts before sleep is crucial. Tachycardia, or an elevated heart rate, is often caused by shallow breathing and stress—in other words, the Modern Disease of the Modern Woman.

Tip:

If you are resistant to this type of breathing or have difficulty breathing deeply, I suggest working with a chiropractor or bodyworker to help remove the physical blockages. I find that many women are unconsciously afraid to breathe deeply and fully inhabit their bodies be-

cause they are scared of their feelings. Thus, they develop avoidance patterns, and the brain conjures up a myriad of reasons why you can't—but, trust me, you can! Please be honest with yourself and engage with this process because the emotions need to be felt and processed for you to feel fully healthy and alive in your body, mind, and soul.

Make time and schedule regular breathing breaks into your day. Link it to daily routines such as making dinner, walking, doing the laundry, or setting a specific time to connect deeper. I love to do this when I wake up, go to bed, and throughout the day.

Diaphragmatic breathing can be performed sitting, standing, or lying down. Place one hand on your diaphragm under your sternum and one on your lower abdomen. Inhale slowly and deeply for a count of four, then exhale slowly and deeply for a count of four. The slower and lower the breath, the better. Longer exhales stimulate the vagus nerve, activating the parasympathetic nervous system (rest and digest), taking us out of sympathetic dominance (stress). Growing evidence shows that the out-breath breaks the stress cycle, helping us relax while preventing disease and allowing optimal health.

I encourage women to make sounds on the out-breath. So many women are afraid of making noise and using their voices. I believe this is because, unconsciously, they are always in control and are afraid of losing control of their emotions, leaving them disembodied and holding back their voice and truth. Learning to hear and feel your own voice, feeling its vibration, taking up space and feeling the power of your emotions can be truly healing and transformational. It's so easy, yet women struggle to make the smallest of sounds. Practise taking up space in your body and life. Your life and health depend on it.

'You've got the words to change a nation
But you're biting your tongue
You've spent a lifetime stuck in silence
Afraid you'll say something wrong
If no one ever hears it, how are we gonna learn your song?'
—Emeli Sandé

Stretch it away!

When I'm stressed, I sometimes do light stretches, focusing on breathing and making gentle sounds. Hold each stretch for about a minute and let your breath ease the stress away. This calms your nervous system and prepares you for a restful night's sleep.

Journal

I like to write down everything on my mind—all the to-dos and thoughts swirling around. Get it out of your head and onto paper. When I'm done, I spend 5 minutes focusing on three things that went well that day. I also ask myself if there's anything I've learned. We often spend so much time focusing on what's not working that we forget to celebrate what is working.

These journal activities can take as little as 5 minutes. They release the anxiety that might be waiting to steal your sleep. This approach is grounded in neuroscience, guiding you from your limbic system to the neocortex of your brain. Your limbic system is centred on survival and fear-based emotions, which can overwhelm you and interrupt your precious deep sleep. It encompasses the internal conversations you engage in with people while lying in bed at night, all the remarks you wished you had made or regret making. It's the worst-case scenario we imagine and begin to believe, leading to nervous system dysregulation and stress. Journaling is an effective method for exercising the brain and soothing the nervous system. Gratitude and reflection are crucial for fostering greater happiness and abundance in your life and body.

Drink Water

Hydration is the secret weapon for keeping your cells healthy. Drinking around four glasses of water in the morning before food will help you hydrate and flush toxins through your body before you eat. Remember not to drink 15 minutes before and after eating; we need your beautiful gastric juices to work optimally. Try going to bed with a jug of water next to your bed so you can start drinking as soon as you wake up. I used to think water was boring because it had no taste, but the more you drink it, the easier it becomes. You can also add lemon, ginger, blueberries, cucumber slices, or essential oils to flavour your water—even herbs from the garden. Ensure the water is at room temperature, as this is better for your body to metabolise and use optimally. The more water we drink, the less water our body will hold onto. When we drink enough water, the body can let go of excess water in the cells, releasing harmful toxins. Water also helps keep you fuller between meals and helps plump out your skin. Women can overeat because they mistake the signs of dehydration for hunger pangs. Drink a glass of water and wait twenty minutes. If you're still hungry, then eat. Snacking on empty calories is how we become accidentally overweight and out of balance. Use water as your secret weapon; you will thank it as your bloated belly begins to disappear.

Add sea salt or Himalayan salt to your diet, and avoid processed table salt. Salt plays an important role in how our cells absorb water. Salt helps draw water into our cells, keeps them hydrated, and helps maintain optimal electrolyte balance.

She-tosis

Becoming metabolically flexible is the magic bullet we modern women need. I talked earlier about how counting calories is a fallacy and how all nutrients are not made equal. I want to go deeper now and discuss switching from sugar burning to fat burning and why this is important to our health.

Most women I met in my practise are stuck in sugar-burning mode, unable to burn fat. Again, this is not about dieting to be thin; I'm talking about being healthy on a cellular level, and this comes in all beautiful shapes and sizes. Stored toxic fat sends chemical signals around the body, causing more stress, cortisol spikes and hormonal disruption, leading to chronic inflammation, pain and stress, which I believe is the root cause of most diseases. I am talking about getting your body into ketosis or 'She-tosis,' a term I use in my clinic. Ketones are produced from fat cells when we switch from burning sugar to burning fat. They produce fewer waste products, including free radicals, and are an excellent source of fuel for the brain.

Because most of us are stressed, we eat food that picks us up and gives us a sugar spike. Even if it's low fat or low sugar, it is still sugar, and this leaves us a slave to sugar spikes—the highs and lows—and is very stressful on our bodies.

I'm not a fan of the run-of-the-mill keto diets out there. I think they are unhealthy and unrealistic and don't take into account our unique feminine biology or physiology. So, if you have tried a keto diet in the past and it hasn't worked for you, it's okay. It's not your fault.

Firstly, every healthy diet needs to consist of tons of vegetables, resistant starches, fibre, high-quality protein, and fat, plus other pre- and probiotic foods. Eating rashes of bacon, handfuls of fat, and cream is not what I am talking about, and I believe it will have devastating long-term health problems. Most of us can get caught up looking for short-term wins, but what we really want are long-term gains.

She-Fasting

Everyone is talking about fasting at the moment; it's the latest trend. However, fasting is far from new—it dates back to our most ancient ancestors. Our biology hasn't changed in the last 20,000 years; the only difference is that our ancestors were leaner and fitter, with no heart disease, diabetes, or high cancer rates. You were more likely to be eaten by a tiger than suffer from a chronic health condition. The difference today is that we've become like domesticated, cage-fed animals. If you think about it, do you ever see a chronically ill animal in the wild? Why is that? How do they move, eat, and think differently from those that are domesticated or kept in captivity? We are animals too, and our biology responds similarly depending on how we move, eat, and think—we are products of our environment. Feast and famine were how we survived; there wasn't a McDonald's or snack bar on every corner to eat from whenever we felt like it. We had to hunt for our food, and there were times when we didn't know where our next meal would come from.

This feast/famine lifestyle is what we now call fasting. The reason fasting has so many health benefits is that we are biologically designed to go without food for periods. We aren't meant to eat all the time, no matter what clever food marketing companies tell us. Ketones were how we stayed alert, alive, and helped us find our next meal.

Benefits of Fasting:

- Weight loss.
- Reduced blood sugar.
- Increased insulin sensitivity.
- Improved heart health.
- Better digestion.
- Lower risks of inflammation.
- Reduced cancer risk.
- Improved cholesterol levels.
- Improved brain function.
- Longevity and delay in ageing.
- Improved gut health.
- Reduced aches and pains.
- Aids detox process.

However, there is a distinct biological difference between how and when a woman should fast compared to a man. We have to take into consideration our hormones and cycles. Most women jump onto water fasts and fasting diets without considering their unique biochemistry and physiology, which can lead to increased stress in the body and hormonal imbalances. If fasting is done in a female-friendly way, you get all of the above benefits, plus:

- Hormonal balance
- Reduced anxiety, depression and burnout

The modern-day woman is stuck in sympathetic dominance, in a constant state of chronic stress. Our nervous systems are in constant fight-and-flight, and adding more stress through fasting can tip us over the edge if it's not done in a way that considers us as a whole, taking into consideration our unique feminine biochemistry. Cyclic fasting is the answer—using our unique cycle to determine how and when we fast.

She-Cycling

Week One—Menstruation

During the first phase of your cycle, your hormones allow for longer periods of fasting. This is an ideal time to try a 24-hour fast or go 16-17 hours without eating, known as time-restricted eating. After 16 hours, the body enters a state called autophagy, where it cleans up old, damaged cells, helping to prevent disease. For example, you might have your last meal at 6:30 pm on a Thursday and then not eat again until noon on Friday. If you're oestrogen-dominant, you might also consider a 3-day water fast. During this phase, your insulin levels are more balanced, making fasting easier on both you and your hormones. If you're new to fasting for this length of time, I recommend doing it with the guidance of a health coach who specialises in fasting.

During this time of your cyclic fasting, I recommend:

- Drinking green tea: It contains sirtuins that help combat free radicals, repair DNA damage, reduce chronic inflammation, and keep us young and healthy.
- Drink bone broth rich in glycine, which stimulates growth hormones that assist in muscle growth and repair.
- Dry body brushing and drinking lots of water to aid the detoxification process.
- Eat lots of spinach and dark leafy greens to increase iron consumption.
- Magnesium-rich foods can help with cramping on the first few days, or take a supplement.

Week Two—Before Ovulation

As oestrogen and testosterone levels rise, your hormones are changing, giving you more energy and making you feel great. This is the time to ease off longer fasts and switch to a more balanced approach. I recommend sticking to 16-hour fasts and avoiding 24-hour or three-day fasts, as these can impact ovulation. However, if you have PCOS, 24-hour fasts may be beneficial as they can lower insulin levels and increase luteinising hormone, helping you to release an egg and ovulate.

This phase is also important for building muscle. Women naturally lose muscle as we age, much faster than men, so it's crucial to focus on strength training. Protein synthesis is higher during this phase of your cycle, so you can concentrate on lifting heavier weights this week while increasing your protein intake and reducing carbohydrates.

Week Three—Luteal Phase

During this phase of our cycle, it's more difficult for women to do longer fasts. The metabolic changes happening in our biochemistry mean we need more calories for our developing endometrial lining. As progesterone begins to rise towards the end of the week, so does the urge to eat. Our bowel movements may slow down, we become more insulin resistant, and our serotonin levels drop, making us feel bloated, tired, irritable, and craving carbs—classic PMS symptoms.

PMS is often caused by high oestrogen levels combined with low progesterone. To help alleviate symptoms, focus on supporting your liver by detoxing, and increase your intake of fibre and magnesium to improve bowel movements. Longer water fasts can be beneficial during this time to assist with liver detoxification. Eat plenty of leafy green vegetables to support liver function, and drink lots of water to flush out excess toxins.

Women with PCOS often struggle even more with insulin resistance during this phase and may benefit from longer, more restrictive fasts. However, for most women, it's better to stick to a 12- to 14-hour eating window.

This is also the time to switch to slower, restorative exercises. Eat foods high in protein, and consider adding peppermint or chai tea while limiting caffeine. Dark chocolate, with at least 85% cocoa, can help curb food cravings. If you're having trouble sleeping, melatonin might be helpful this week.

Week Four—Before Your Menstruation

Insulin resistance peaks this week, leading to increased food cravings, mood swings, and sleep disturbances. This is the time to ease up on low-carbohydrate diets and reduce your fasting to a 12- to 14-hour window. Longer fasts during this phase can lower progesterone levels, and we want to keep these as high as possible at this stage of your cycle. Your endometrial lining is thickening and needs more protein and fat.

It's also important to support your gut microbiome, which requires extra care at this time, so include some prebiotic foods in your diet. Focus on eating good quality protein and foods high in fibre, as these will nourish the gut lining and help reduce cravings.

This week, remember to slow down, listen to your body, and get in tune with how it feels. Your body is your home, and it's important to feel comfortable living in it.

CHAPTER 20
SHE-PRACTISES—REAWAKENING YOUR 'SHE'

We often criticise ourselves harshly while ignoring and dismissing our feelings. Recognising our emotions is very healing. If we ignore our feelings and hide them away, they don't heal or change. It's like trying to hold back a huge wave. Eventually, the wave will crash over us, no matter what we do.

Reframing

Hiding our emotions and not expressing them drains our energy, making us tense and unwell. We must accept our feelings to heal properly. Looking at situations in a new light, or reframing, can help a lot. This means seeing things from a perspective of forgiveness, humility, and personal growth. We all make mistakes and have regrets, but that's part of being human. Learning to view ourselves and our actions with kindness and understanding helps us grow.

Make space and reflect:

- What could I have handled better today?
- How can I take what I learned today and start tomorrow anew?
- Reflect on why something happened the way it did. What is going on? How do you truly feel? What was the trigger?
- What words or images describe how you feel? Can you draw it or give it a colour? When we do this, we reframe the problem and see it as something inside of us that needs acknowledgement and love.

When we don't act as we wish we had, it's common to replay the situation in our minds, imagining how we could have handled it better. Reflect on why you couldn't act that way at the time, apologise to yourself, and forgive yourself. Self-reflection and visualisation can help you make a different choice if the same situation arises again.

It's easy to become overly defensive, especially when we're stuck in patterns that trigger old wounds, leading to negative cycles with others. Take a deep breath, try to really listen, and respond differently. Ask yourself if you're reacting defensively out of habit rather than expressing your true feelings.

Menstruation and PMS can heighten our defensiveness, making us feel attacked. During these times, be extra kind and patient with yourself. If possible, avoid tough conversations. If you need to, tell others it's not a good time for you, acknowledging their points but explaining you need to respond more calmly and not just emotionally. Then, step away if needed.

Ways to Come Back to Your Soul

- **Begin every day with intention.** Wake up, drink some water, light a candle, and sit in a comfortable position. Take five deep breaths in and five deep breaths out until you feel centred. Ask yourself in your journal, 'How can I make today feel more connected and sacred?' Repeat this practise before you go to bed, asking yourself, 'How was today magical and sacred? What can I bring more of into my life?'
- **Connect to your soul** and understand that you are more than just a mother, wife, daughter, or coworker. The roles we play and the masks we wear should not define us. We often attribute all our meaning to them and forget who we truly are, and this disconnection leads to discontentment. Breathe into this inner knowing—think it, feel it, know that you are all of it and more. I find going to a café to read, buying flowers, spending time in nature, and making nourishing food also help build this bridge back to me.
- **Get clear about what you want.** As women, we can feel guilty for wanting more, but our desires don't go away; they are there for a reason. Suppressing them takes energy and eventually affects your health. Desires are whispers from your soul, reminding you of who you are and who you were meant to be. Be clear about what you want from your relationships, friends, family, and career. Consider what changes you can make to bring you closer to where you want to be, knowing that this can change as you grow, and that's okay.

Practise Self-Love

Changing our patterns and making time for ourselves can feel overindulgent. We have many excuses and beliefs about why we can't or shouldn't. Here are the habits I try to incorporate into my life when I feel stressed, down, or need to reconnect with my femininity:

- Wear red lipstick. Yes, you read that correctly! I wear the brightest red I have on my lips, and I wear it boldly.
- Eat only when hungry, being wary of boredom and emotional eating.
- Consume food that nourishes your body.

- Say no more often and establish healthy boundaries.
- Dress in a way that expresses who you are, wearing clothes that make you feel sexy and alive.
- Look for the magic in the mundane, seek out symbols, write up your dreams, and make time for fun and laughter.
- Declutter and create space in your wardrobe and home.
- Make taking care of your body a sacred ritual.
- Connect to the sacred part of yourself.

Reawakening Your Inner 'She'

Do you remember her? Those big eyes, huge smile with gaps in her teeth. The way her stomach used to ache when you belly-laughed so hard you would almost pee your pants. The potions and mud cakes you made in the garden, the games you played, and the stories you concocted when no one was watching. The friends you had were both invisible and visible. There was trust in life, in yourself; there was lightness and joy. You loved without conditions or boundaries. You enjoyed discovering parts of your body, unafraid and proud of your own skin and everything your body was capable of.

This was you; this is you. She's still there inside, perhaps tucked away, maybe silent in a corner, or quietly entertaining herself. You've likely told her to be quiet, to leave, that you don't need her anymore. You're too occupied for fun; you haven't got the time, and people will mock you or take you less seriously if she were to emerge. She gazes at you with those large eyes brimming with love, acceptance, and the wisdom of time and accepts your words because her love for you is unconditional. She retreats into the shadows, forgotten like the many shattered, compromised dreams you once cherished. Your joy, spontaneity, passion, longing, and vitality are also concealed. Your creativity is halved, and your vulnerability, compassion, and joy, as well, for they are hers. You reject her, so you deny these aspects of life that nourish your soul, the elements you blindly seek. She is what you truly crave when you peer into the cupboard at night, wondering what you can eat to help fill this void and dull the sensation of loss.

You've forgotten her; you've forgotten you. You have forgotten that she is the most powerful part of you, the source of all your creations and life.

The fully embodied little girl you were before you learned it was unsafe to be is who you are. The part of your soul that was as real to you as your hands and feet, the energy in you that you let sink into the darkness, creating a void between your body and soul.

There was a time when you felt safe expressing your fire and soul, where you were your true self without expectations or conditioning. She's still in there, living in her secret garden, taking shade under the old oak tree.

Close your eyes and envision a locked gate before you. You approach to open the gate, which only you can unlock; it's slightly concealed by the overgrown ivy that has taken root over the years. You sense the way, you know it—you've always known it. She is in there waiting for you, like an untouched image of wholeness. As you enter, you observe her.

You imagine her lying on her stomach, head in her hands, reading and laughing. She turns around to gaze at the clouds and watches the shapes they form. She is dirty, and her hair is messy because she is having fun. There is a spark in her eye and a lightness in her body. She turns around, and as your eyes lock, the veil lifts. Your eyes connect, and you merge into her and she into you, becoming one. Emotion overwhelms you: laughter, tears, sadness, and grief for what you have lost and forgotten. She walks over to you, gives you the biggest smile, grabs hold of you, and pulls you into a deep embrace. You melt into one, whole again.

Many of us have ignored our inner child due to fear, rejection, trauma, and neglect. We've lost touch with our feminine side and our connection to our female body. Welcoming this part of us back and seeing the feminine as sacred can fill a gap in our healing. The parts of us that seemed too emotional, vulnerable, and weak were pushed away because we thought we needed to change to be loved and successful. We felt unsafe and lesser for being true to ourselves and might have blamed our feminine qualities for our problems and failures in life. Instead of facing challenges with our strength and light, we dimmed ourselves to fit in and be accepted, scared of standing out and embracing our power.

I encourage you to embrace and honour the feminine within yourself, the girl you once were, every day for the rest of your life. Reconnecting with and living true to her essence is key to shifting from just getting by to truly thriving. It's how we heal and lead a life that's abundant, aligned, and true to who we really are.

Practise:

1. Put in your ear pods or headphones.
2. Find a quiet space and search for the song 'She Used To Be Mine' by Sara Bareilles.
3. Immerse yourself in your body, listen to this song, feel what it evokes, and write a letter to your inner child.

CHAPTER 21
SHE-PRACTISES—EMBODIMENT

A rigid body = A rigid mind

To fully experience embodiment, you need to practise and take action, not just understand it intellectually. She-Practises are meant to activate your conscious awareness of your sensual embodiment and the awakening of your aliveness and feminine essence—a journey back to the centre of yourself. Embodiment involves unravelling, untaming, and stripping away beliefs, behaviours, and personas we adopt to survive. It means surrendering, feeling, and being in the body, trusting what we feel and intuit instead of striving to be a more improved version of ourselves based on a patriarchal blueprint.

Your feminine sacred wisdom lives in your body, not somewhere outside of yourself or in your head. Embodiment requires you to slow down, feel, and sense everything within you, the good and the bad. She—your higher Self—has always been there, waiting for you to wake up and come home. She is what will rebalance, rewild, and ultimately save you.

Our feminine sensual and sexual sides are often suppressed while we live in repetitive patterns, relying on addictive stress, and feeling burnt out, stiff, and in pain. Embodiment practises help you reach parts of yourself that your mind can't (or won't) access. This reduces stress, balances hormones, alleviates pain and prevents illness. We can't heal what we can't feel, and these practises help us embody and understand what is happening in our bodies. With these practises, your shakti, the fountain of youth, energy, and aliveness within will awaken.

Once you understand your neurological imprints and embodied patterns, you can rewire and re-establish aliveness and pleasure as your default setting, instead of stress and pain. Where you are now is a result of choices made from learned patterns based on a belief system, often running on autopilot for years. Embodiment helps break these habitual survival patterns, allowing you to thrive in your full potential.

She-Movement awakens your sexual energy and fuels the health of your entire body. This energy realigns you with the flow of nature and your inner feminine rhythms. An innate intelligence is activated, clearing out anything in your system that no longer serves you. This includes thoughts, behaviours, and patterns that keep you stuck, causing neurological and energetic disruption. She-Movement Therapy helps you access your sexual energy and cellular blueprint, removing what no longer serves you.

Everything you need to know about yourself is written within. Embodiment is the tool that helps you read your own autobiography. All the past numbness, stress, and tension are there, waiting for their story to be told and, if needed, rewritten.

Spiritual Bypassing

Spiritual bypassing happens when we identify with and understand spirituality as an idea or a belief rather than a lived embodied truth. To fully understand spirituality and consciousness, a lived experience is required. When a woman has become disconnected from her shakti and sexuality, it's much easier to bypass the body and stay in the head doing meditation and mindfulness. Spirituality then can become a crutch, a coping mechanism rather than something she embodies and then lives from a grounded, empowered essence.

We must delve deep within ourselves and feel everything, no matter how painful. This is how we heal. It's not just about the light, as many false gurus teach. There is always shadow, and there will always be shadow. You need to understand and learn to work with it, not against it. When we aren't conscious of the shadow, it controls us. Your greatest gifts and breakthroughs aren't in your head; they are in your body. This isn't about having more sex; it's about cultivating sexual energy and aliveness from within. When a woman awakens and harnesses her sexual energy, she re-empowers her nervous system and her emotional, physical, and spiritual body. She feels vibrant, alive, and deeply connected to the universe from an embodied heart, body, and mind.

The cost of being disconnected from your body is high. As we age, our spines lose their vitality and natural curves, so we start compensating for our imbalances and un-steadiness by standing more on one side than the other. We hike our hips, cross our legs, and hold the tension that we are trying so desperately to avoid. Emotionally, we become blocked and our shakti and life force get switched off. We become stressed, overworked, overwhelmed, and sick.

The pelvis, your inner 'cauldron,' is a container for everything that has happened to us emotionally. Everything gets locked away and stored in our tissues and cells until they just can't hold it all any longer. Signs and symptoms become the language the pelvis uses to get your distracted attention. She talks to us through pain, stiffness, period cramps, and a lack of libido—all because we are so weighed down and dense. But with She-Movement therapy, you can empty the pelvis of everything that's been weighing you down.

I am the sum of everyone—and every fear—I have ever known.

Your power does not live outside of you in the external world—it's inside of you. Healing and magic come when you discover that you still feel aligned and centred no matter what life throws at you. You don't need to lose yourself in overwhelm anymore! These practises will bring you back to the centre of yourself. Whether you're experiencing self-doubt, fear, beliefs, or shame, these practises enable you to feel the full spectrum of everything whilst still opening and flowing with life. Your body and spirit become unshakable no matter what is happening on the outside.

How many times have you tried to change something but have been taken down by your own negativity? This is because you are out of alignment, ungrounded, stuck in a cycle, and locked into a reality caged by your fears and 'what ifs'. I invite you to use these practises as a daily devotional practise, one that you will come to love. When we can open and remain fully in flow, feeling everything no matter what is going on around us or in our heads, we evolve our consciousness and connect to our magic. This is how we acquire a robust, fully functioning nervous system and manifest the life and body we deserve.

Having the tools and resilience to lean in deeper, maintaining the unshakable connection to self through embodiment and aliveness is how you get to dance through life, rather than struggling against it. You are the centre of the wheel! You are the creator of your own life and reality. These practises will awaken you to new possibilities and a deep presence in your life.

She-Movement

She-Movement lets you connect with your inner goddess, shakti, and sexual vitality. It uses breath, movement, and sound to awaken and rewire your unique feminine body, reigniting your sexuality and sensuality. These practises rebalance and recode your physical, mental, and emotional selves, reawakening your spiritual and sexual power.

> *'It is through the Goddess that you enter the world of spirit—*
> *she is your maze, and she is your guide.'*
> —Joseph Campell

She-Movement allows us to embody, feel, express, and release everything in our bodies. It gets our mind out of the way and helps us address the root cause of our feelings. Many diseases stem from issues and blocks in our tissues. Over time, these blocks build up, stagnate, and cause dis-ease. She-Movement helps release stored emotions and restores neural pathways, allowing the body to heal from the inside out. This therapy is personalised, letting you follow your own body's needs. I can guide you, but the journey is yours.

The body talks to us through symptoms. My answer is to get on the floor, move, shake, breathe, and sound it out. Your body wants and needs to be heard. This movement is like having a conversation with your body. When you find stiff, tense, painful areas, or feel blocked physically, get curious and move into and out of what you are feeling. Some movements may make you want to cry; let it out and release it. Don't bypass or avoid what needs to be felt.

There is a tendency to want to get somewhere, but I encourage you to be where you are in the moment instead of trying to reach a desired outcome. Learning to feel and embrace all our emotions is vital for your journey, allowing you to express and release what needs to be released so you can feel more vibrant and alive.

*The sacred third occurs when two dualities come together and meet in the middle—
something new is always birthed.*

Most of my patients know they are stressed, in pain, and have hormonal problems. They suffer from numbness, anxiety, and often feel overwhelmed, trying to avoid burnout. They have tried therapy and medication, but something still isn't shifting. They experience temporary mild relief but don't feel better, often feeling more numb and depressed, unsure of what's wrong.

She-Movement isn't about understanding why; it's about finding, feeling, and expressing emotions. This can't always be done with the thinking brain because emotions are feelings that need to move, and She-Movement moves them. In my experience, I can wake up feeling down, overwhelmed, and out of control. I come to the mat, light a candle, do five rounds of deep breathing, close my eyes, and let my body guide me home. I allow my body to express everything I have been repressing. This sacred movement bypasses my thinking brain and takes me straight to the problem, where I work with it and heal it.

Often, when I'm finished, I journal about how I feel or what came up for me. I may write a letter to myself from the Goddess or from my body, noting any words of wisdom I am ready to receive and ensuring I act on any guidance given.

She-Movement, alongside my sexuality practise, helps me clear away tension, frustration and stress. It releases any anger or blocked emotions I may have stored within the cells of my body. When I feel myself going into a pattern of behaviour or a thought process that I know is coming from stress or fear, I move it out so it doesn't fester. Disease can occur first in our energy body in the field that surrounds our physical body. Learning to move what needs to move helps prevent dis-ease and issues that show up in our tissues.

This practise has saved me many times. When I've felt low and alone, and my PMS made me feel like a madwoman, it helped me. It's changed how I show up in my relationships and how I feel about myself, my body, and my health. I no longer have the afternoon slump. My body feels energised, my brain is clear, and I feel alive. Doing this practise is like opening the curtains and windows in a stuffy, dark house and letting in light and air. I no longer feel heavy, stressed, and tired but energised, clear, and alive. I feel more present and grounded.

Illness and pain are stagnant, repressed energy that manifests in the physical body.

She-Movement Therapy: The Basics

Move What You Feel

This a powerful foundational practise, focusing on embodiment and releasing energetic and emotional blocks. It helps you become aware of your senses and how you feel. It brings you in touch with your sensuality and releases the powerful hormone oxytocin.

Choose music that reflects and mirrors how you feel, knowing this may change from day to day. If you're feeling mad, then play music with more of a beat. If you're feeling quiet, perhaps play some relaxing music. If you're feeling turned on and want to express your wild side, play sensual music with a beat. Ask your body how she wants to move. When the music begins, you will know intuitively if it is the right choice for you. Start by picking one song, set a timer and just move.

Begin by standing barefoot, grounding yourself into the earth. Feel your entire foot, including your toes, and begin to move your body. Imagine a beautiful egg full of light surrounding you that will hold you and your energy.

This is not a dance—it's not supposed to look a certain way, so the weirder and wilder the better! Simply feel and move how you feel. I like to start by rolling my neck and then my shoulders. Make sure that you actively move these areas as you exhale, unlocking any stored tension and bringing you further into your body.

Move your hips, exaggerating the movement; imagine you're touching the wall behind and in front of you as you circle them awake. Get the energy flowing, feel the way they love to sway and rotate. Use your hands to explore your inner thighs as they begin to open up. Notice any tightness, breathing into any numbness or stiffness, and allow a sense of surrender and openness to awaken the magic within your inner thighs.

Start to breathe more slowly and deeply into the lower belly and womb area, and begin making more noise on the out-breath. I like to breathe out and stick my tongue out like a lion or hiss like a snake. Remember, this is a rewilding, a re-awakening of your natural feminine animalistic instincts. You have been tame for too long! Touch your breasts and feel any sensations or pleasure that arises.

Continue to follow the sensations that arise in your body, trying not to overthink what you look like. Trust that your body intuitively wants and knows how to move. Jump up and down, side to side, fall to the floor, wail, stamp your feet, have a tantrum if that feels right (it often does), dance like no one is watching and let your feelings move your body back to wholeness. The key is to avoid structured movement, as this is not like normal exercising. We are breaking the rules when it comes to exercise as we have known it in the past. We are losing the tame masculine linear power movements and instead are freeing up how we move, think, and behave. We are going for non-linear, free-flowing movements. This can be messy in our conditioned mind, but it feels so good. Ignore any doubts or thoughts that you're doing it wrong and allow your body to guide you. As you do this, you may notice that you have started to hold your breath or aren't breathing deeply enough. I encourage you to return to the breath, breathe deeply and exhale out of your mouth, allowing for any stuck energy or sounds that need to move. Stick your tongue out, yawn, and release the jaw—this helps rid the body of built-up tension.

Ride your body like a wave. Each day, the current and tide will be different, so just get in the water, get in your body, and ride her.

When to do these practises:

- You find it hard to connect to your intuition and wisdom.
- You have stress and an overloaded nervous system.
- You feel numb or are unable to understand or express your emotions.
- You feel dysregulated.
- You are stuck in freeze in the body.
- You desire more sexual and sensuality in your life.
- You want more aliveness in your body and life.
- You want to learn the language of your body.
- You want to follow the path of feminine spirituality.

Benefits:

- Reintegrates trauma and grief patterns
- Breaks habitual moving and emotional patterns
- Relives pain and tension in the joints and muscles
- Eases perimenopause and menopausal symptoms
- Relieves depression, anxiety and frustration
- Connects the mind, body, and soul
- Releases tension
- Enhances sensual and sexual feelings and awareness
- Creates more fluidity of emotions

Happy Hips

The hips don't lie.

I have yet to meet a woman who is fully happy with her hips—how they look, feel, or perform. Yet, our hips are a crucial part of our feminine power, reflecting how we feel, what we believe, and how we show up in life. How they feel is far more important for your health than how they look. Interestingly, when we start to give some much-needed love to this area, we begin to appreciate the feminine, sensual beauty and pleasure they hold.

Many women focus on getting a good bum through heavy lifting, squats, deadlifts, lunges, and leg presses, which mainly work the joint forward and back. But there is so much more potential left unexplored. It's like visiting a beautiful mountain range and never going up to see the view, or going to the ocean and not feeling the water on your skin.

Your hips are synovial ball-and-socket joints designed for heavy weight-bearing and movement. They love to move, especially side to side, in circles, as well as flexion and extension. Both small and large ranges of movement are welcome—just move. Once these magic hip portals are unlocked, released, and embodied, you will begin to fall in love with the magic hidden in your hips. A women who is disconnected from her femininity will almost always have tight hips.

The following exercises address the lower body, specifically the hips. The psoas muscle plays an important role in our emotional healing journey, our stress behaviour and how this manifests as pain and rigidity. Tension and emotions stored in our hips reduce the blood flow and lymphatic drainage to our sexual organs and lower extremities. This tightness can cause pain and hormonal problems as well as disconnecting us from our intuition, sexual sensation, and feminine wisdom. By bringing movement and restoring balance in this area, we rebalance not just physically but mentally, emotionally, and spiritually.

Hip Circles and the Figure-8

Standing

Standing position should be done barefoot with your feet hip distance apart, bringing your hands to your hips. Begin with small circles, paying attention to any tight areas. Your hips may be especially tight if you sit behind a desk, so be patient. Soon, they will become more mobile and freer. After a few circles, feel into how the hips want to move—fast, slow, or a combination. Explore a Figure-8 movement, reaching into every part of your hips, remembering to switch directions. When you are finished, stand with your hands in the mudra of an upside-down triangle over your pelvic area, feeling the energy take root into the body.

Sitting

You can do this by circling on your sit bones when you sit at your desk at work. Add in the shoulders and neck, spending a few minutes connecting into the feminine within. Finish again with the upside triangle mudra.

On the Floor

Lay on the floor or yoga mat with your knees bent and feet on the floor. Rock your hips side to side to awaken the energy, then move the hips in each direction.

Butterfly Legs

Lay on your back with your knees bent. Place your feet together and start by slowly opening and closing the knees like a clam or butterfly. This helps to move tension and stress from the hip and pelvic area but can also bring up a lot of emotion. If you have a history of trauma or abuse, please go carefully with these practises—listen to your body and be kind to yourself.

Hip Thrust

Begin on your back with legs bent and feet hip-distance apart. Lift your pelvis to the ceiling into a bridge pose, then slowly lower back down. The lift is more of a thrust, and

I encourage you to make a noise on the exhalation as you rise. This helps release any stagnant energy hidden in the pelvic area.

Deep Pelvic Relaxation

This technique can be applied to all of the above exercises, and it can also be done at work, sitting at your desk, or any time you need to relax your body.

Start by bringing awareness to any part of your body that feels stiff. Is there tension, numbness or pain in your legs, hips, pelvis, or lower back? Feel your yoni and breathe deeply into your womb space.

Inhale and feel, staying with whatever arises in this moment without trying to change it. Go to the area where you feel the most tension, pain, or restriction. Tense and contract the area more, as if you have a squash ball in your hand and are squeezing it as hard as you can. This may bring up some emotion—breathe into it and stay present with the sensations that arise in your body.

As you exhale, relax and soften into the area physically and mentally. Be aware of how your body melts as you relax. You can do this to any area of the body that is tense. This technique is great for releasing stress and tension in the upper shoulder and neck area.

Bouncing

Start in a hip bridge pose. Begin bouncing your bottom up and down on the floor. It might feel like you're having sex, so go with it, feel whatever comes up, and make sounds. You can even stamp and scream if you encounter resistance or break down in tears—it's all okay. Just let the energy move. Remember, it's better for your health to get it out and flowing than to let it stay stuck and stagnant.

Bouncing can also be done standing with hips a little wider than foot distance apart. Your upper body is relaxed, let your arms hang and begin bouncing up and down. As you bounce, make sure your feet are rooted into the ground. Let your arms and head move with the way you feel, breathe, don't hold your breath and allow your body to surrender into the bounce, letting everything flow out of you that you want to release.

Child's Pose

Begin this movement with your eyes closed, in child's pose. Allow your neck, jaw, and whole face to relax. Close your eyes to the outer world and begin to come home to your inner world. Sometimes emotions will wash over, and you may need to sound or cry and lie in a foetal position, but when this passes, as it always does, return to your hands and knees and start by moving your body through the cat-cow pose. This is an easy way to embody your feelings, re-sensitize your body, and get the cerebral spinal fluid pumping. Imagine your spine pumping the spinal fluid from your brain throughout your nervous system, flushing out all the debris, stagnation and emotional neurotoxins that have built up throughout the day.

Next, allow your body to move in any way it wants, allowing your intuition and wisdom to awaken and guide the movement.

Although I find staying on my hands and knees for this practise the most beneficial, the closer I get to my animal nature, the more alive and untamed I feel. This is where I meet the real me and express the parts of myself that have no words. Thoughts and emotions come and go; I just observe and let the movement flow through me. I use an eye mask to keep my eyes closed and help me go deeper inside, blocking out any external distractions. I let myself be played like a musical instrument, discovering a new note and playing a different song each time.

*Visit **www.drmichelleboycedc.com/resources** for additional practises.*

Sexual Embodiment as a Sacred Practise

'And the day came when the risk to remain tight in a bud was
more painful than the risk it took to blossom.'
—Anaïs Nin

Let's talk about sexuality, sensuality, and all the pleasure waiting for you to awaken and explore. You are sitting on the treasure—you are the treasure. This connection is often the missing piece many women unconsciously seek. Sexual aliveness is your superpower, your energy, and the next level of She-Embodiment practises.

Sexual embodiment is about connecting with and awakening your pleasure and aliveness. I'm not just talking about sex, but feminine sacred sexuality—the kind we weren't taught in school or anywhere else. This hidden, ancient wisdom brings you back to life, balance, and health—the kind every woman should know.

This sexual energy, or shakti, as I often call it, is free-flowing energy that, once activated, can rewire your neurology and biochemistry. You will feel more alive and less stressed, and your nervous system will feel calm and balanced.

She-Movement may be enough for you right now, and that's okay. Be where you are and stay open to change in the future. Remember, the feminine is always cycling and never still. Think of it like peeling an onion—each layer is another surrender, another piece of armour removed that's been keeping you from yourself. It's a rewilding back to your instincts, feelings, and primal nature, untaming the conditioned and repressed person within. How deep you peel that onion is up to you. My advice? Let's go all the way!

Yoni Steaming

Preparation

Yoni steaming is an ancient healing and cleansing technique that has been upheld and passed on through ancient feminine healing traditions.

I learned this ancient practise when I trained as a scared sexuality teacher. It was taught to me through a beautiful ceremonial practise that I share with women who work in circles or one-on-one with me. It helps women release blocked emotions and tension held in the yoni and labia and is especially helpful after childbirth and to ease PMS and perimenopause symptoms.

Benefits

- Reduces menstrual cramps, bloating, and clots, easing PMS symptoms.
- Helps improve blood flow, reducing dark brown or black blood at the beginning and end of the menstrual cycle.
- Can help alleviate chronic yeast infections and vaginal odour.
- Regulates the menstrual cycle.
- Increases fertility.
- Helps with lower back pain.
- Relieves stress in the body and nervous system.
- Aids in healing the pelvic area after childbirth.
- Reduces symptoms of uterine fibroids, ovarian cysts, endometriosis, and PCOS.
- Helps heal haemorrhoids.
- Can alleviate menopausal symptoms such as dryness and pain during and after sex.
- Assists in clearing the womb of physical and emotional toxins.

When I first started Yoni steaming, I made my own setup using a small ceramic pot placed in my toilet. Now, I use a wooden box that I keep assembled because Yoni steaming has become a regular part of my life. This practise is especially helpful when I feel tense, emotionally blocked, or numb and just need to sit and reconnect with myself.

If you're new to Yoni steaming and want to try it, grab a small ceramic pot or saucepan (without a handle) that fits inside your toilet with the seat up. Fill the pot with hot water—not boiling, as we want to avoid discomfort. I like to add fresh or dried herbs from my garden, but you can use whatever you have at home. I recommend herb packs from a company called 'Steamy Chicks', available online if you decide to make this a regular practise.

Place your pot in the toilet and close the seat so you can sit on it (naked, without pants!). I find it helpful to use my dressing gown or a blanket wrapped around my waist to trap the steam.

Begin by breathing slowly—inhale for four counts and exhale for four counts. With each exhale, gently open your legs and Yoni a little more.

Feel the steam rising into your labia and Yoni, and breathe it up into your body. As you exhale, visualise negative thoughts, feelings, tightness, or stiffness leaving your body through your Yoni.

Each exhale is an opportunity to open and surrender deeper into your body. If emotions surface, allow them to rise—cry, laugh, make sounds, and release any anger or frustrations.

Stay with these feelings, aiming for about twenty minutes. Remember to keep breathing, allowing the steam to flow through you mentally, physically, and emotionally.

Sometimes, this practise triggers deep emotions, and I may sob from the depths of myself. I try not to analyse why I'm crying or what's wrong; instead, I let myself feel and release the emotions residing in my body. I direct the steam to areas of pain, numbness, or blockages, breathing deeply and letting go.

Other times, I feel relaxed and lighter—it's like opening a box of chocolates; you never know what you'll get. But if you trust and surrender, you'll always receive what you need.

*NOTE: Please avoid Yoni steaming if you are menstruating, pregnant, miscarrying, or experiencing a hot flush.

Yoni Massage

Exploring your sexuality connects you to ancient wisdom stored in your body and its sensations. Being sexually fulfilled and fluid enhances pleasure in all aspects of life.

The first step is to release any tension that is stuck in and around the yoni. I advise using a skin-friendly oil such as coconut oil and start exploring your labia, the inner and outer lips of the vagina, feeling for any tightness or numbness. The space between your vagina and anus can also be really tight, especially if you have childbirth scars in that area. As you begin to gently massage and explore your landscape, make sure you're relaxed, and breathe, remembering that the breath is just as important as the massage to help resensitise and bring blood flow back to this area.

I also advise using a handheld mirror to see what you look like down there. Become used to what is normal for you—this is your body and you need to know what it looks like…not just your gynaecologist! Feel and massage into the yoni, move your fingers left and right, feeling into any areas of numbness or tension. Sometimes if we sit cross-legged, one side of the vagina wall can be pulled and tight to one side, leading to hip and back pain. Some of you may find it easier to use a crystal or glass dildo to press into hard-to-reach places.

What about vibrators?

Breathing, relaxation and re-sensitization are vital to awakening your body to full orgasmic pleasure.

I don't advocate vibrators because it can lead to desensitising your yoni. Some women are only able to orgasm with a vibrator and not through sex with a partner. Self-pleasuring using a vibrator can become a quick a way to release tension and numb out, disconnecting you even more from your body. Pleasure and orgasms are not just about yang energy, with the climax being the only goal, usually performed quickly and efficiently so you can go about your day.

Vibrators don't allow for enough feminine Yin energy, which is more feeling, expanding, and sensual. In a nutshell, by only orgasming using vibrators, you are missing out on the amazing health benefits and intuitive rewiring of your sacred self. A vibrator bypasses the hormone-balancing effects of hormones, especially oestrogen and testosterone. If you are struggling with the Modern Disease of the Modern Woman, then I recommend using your hand, fingers, a jade egg, or a crystal dildo.

Your Orgasms

Orgasms are at the root of self-healing and self-love.

Being able to self-pleasure in different ways is empowerment, an important yet often overlooked part of what it means to be a fully awakened woman. I'm not going to beat around the bush here. You need to be having more orgasms. Orgasm is another important part of the health puzzle that's missing. Orgasms are not only extremely pleasurable but have life-changing effects on our physical, mental, and emotional wellness, as well as our biochemistry and physiology. It's usually the last thing on our list of priorities, and for some, it doesn't even make the list.

In magazines and the media, orgasm is often depicted as reaching a peak—a goal to be achieved, almost like a performance sport. But in reality, orgasm is a sacred, de-armouring experience that unfolds naturally. Women frequently lose themselves in meeting others' needs, putting their own desires to the bottom of the list. Between work, the school run, shuttling the kids around, household tasks, friends, and caring for loved ones, by the time bedtime arrives, we're completely knackered, longing only to collapse on the sofa, untouched and undisturbed, as our overstimulated nervous systems need a chance to unwind.

There's also the question of worthiness. You are worthy of pleasure, and if you've read this far, I hope you're beginning to see just how amazing and special both you and your body truly are.

Benefit of Orgasms

- Enhances pleasure!
- Increases circulation to the pelvis and internal female anatomy.
- Reduces chronic stress by detoxing cortisol from your system.
- Releases feel-good hormones and endorphins, lowering pain and depression.
- Rewires the nervous system from fight-or-flight to rest-and-digest mode.
- Rewires our biochemistry and physiology.
- Enhances the connection between pleasure and the brain.
- Reduces the body's perception of pain.
- Encourages healthy oestrogen metabolism, crucial in perimenopause.
- Reduces PMS symptoms, especially menstrual cramps, and helps regulate periods.
- Improves sleep quality.

- Increases intuition and feminine connection.
- Promotes heart health, providing a fantastic cardiovascular workout.
- Reduces headaches and other bodily pains.
- Boosts self-confidence.

Because many women are not experiencing enough orgasms, coupled with the challenges of perimenopause and menopause, there is a decreased sensitivity in our yonis and female anatomy. This results in fewer neural pathways for pleasure. Many of us are stuck on autopilot, rushing through life, with our foot constantly on the gas, trapped in negative thought and behavioural patterns, and often experiencing pain.

We frequently endure these negative patterns, whether physical or emotional. Some women have forgotten what it feels like to experience true pleasure, to embrace the fullness of their being. Instead, they are wired to feel pain, unable to access pleasure. This disconnect from our female anatomy and sexuality is a collective feminine crisis that no one seems to be discussing. I feel passionately about the need for women to reclaim their yonis, sexuality, and bodies because if we don't, others will.

This disconnection, coupled with society's fixation on disliking and disowning our bodies, is one of the major contributors to the increasing prevalence of female cancers. Women are not attuned to the signals from their bodies, often having no relationship with their yonis beyond an annual smear test or a brief sexual encounter. This lack of sexual intimacy and aliveness with ourselves can result in the development of cysts and the removal of organs within the medical system, often met with an attitude of, 'You don't need it, let's just cut it out.'

The truth is, you do need it—they are important, even though this isn't taught within the Western medical paradigm. Holistically, our body is always sending us messages, but we've disconnected from all communication. This disconnection, combined with the reduction and desensitisation of neural pathways, leads to numbness, pain, or a complete disinterest in sex. When we begin experiencing symptoms in our female organs, or when our hormones are out of balance and our menstrual cycles become erratic, it is often because energy is stuck, emotions are repressed, and blocks are preventing energy from flowing. Orgasm is one of the most effective ways to move and shift this energy, change your neurology, and rebalance your female biochemistry and physiology.

Once a month won't suffice. If you only used your legs once a month, they would feel weak, lack balance, and lose coordination. Your brain would have to create new pathways that would need to be strengthened by weekly or daily activity. You need to start thinking of your yoni in the same way. It's part of you—arguably the most intimate and intuitive part! Once activated, it will supercharge your life and health.

The more often you orgasm, the more neural pathways you create, which means you will feel more easily aroused, more frequently, and enjoy increasingly better orgasms. Your juices will flow again, and it will feel like someone has fixed that broken tap inside you that you'd forgotten to mend. You will experience the full spectrum of your emotions, becoming sexually and emotionally fluid, instead of feeling stuck, tired, dried up, and stagnant in various areas of life. In this case, practise really does make perfect!

If you don't use it, you lose it.

Remember, your vagina is a muscle and just like *every* muscle in the body, it needs to be strengthened or it will become weak and flabby. Due to the change in hormones that come as we age, our yoni and pelvic floor naturally become weaker. Coupled with childbirth and pregnancy, this area needs and deserves more attention and love than we give it. Pelvic floor problems affect most of us at some point in our lives, and many of us are unknowingly walking around with a slight prolapse.

Orgasmic Landscape

Your Vulva

Your Vulva is also known as the mound of Venus and is made up of all the external parts of your female genitalia:

- Mons pubis
- Labia majora
- Labia minora
- Clitoris
- Vestibular bulbs
- Vulva vestibule
- Bartholin's glands
- Skene's glands
- Urethra
- Vaginal opening (the gatekeeper)

Many women have shame when it comes to their vulva because they think it should look a certain way. Pornography and the media have given us a perfect image of how a patriarchal vulva should look. But guess what? It's not real! It's based on a belief system rather than on nature and how each woman is uniquely beautifully designed. Learning to love and appreciate your vulva is an important part of your sexual journey.

The pudendal nerve innovates a woman's external genitals and is responsible for pleasure and sensitivity. This can be activated through touch and massage, which helps prepare the vagina for penetration. When we allow for external stimulation, we activate the Bartholin's glands, which are mucous-secreting glands that lubricate the vagina and prepare her to be entered.

The whole of the vulva can be orgasmic—not just the clitoris. The inner and outer lips, the vagina opening, the perineum, and your anus are all places where you are able to feel pleasure and prepare the body to open.

So many women aren't ready to be penetrated and bypass the activation of their vulva because they feel numb or are disconnected. When we allow the body to talk to us, we will realise that there is a type of gatekeeper at the entrance to our vagina who has a clear *yes* or *no*. Feeling and embodying the *yes* or *no* of your vagina is often overlooked, but when we honour her voice, we build trust and are able to open and fully receive. When we don't listen, we tend to experience more numbness, tightness, and pain.

Your Clitoris

Your clitoris is the most superficial of your orgasmic portals and is the orgasm most women are familiar with. Clitoral orgasms normally come with a tensing of the body and are normally short and intense, followed by a short stress relief and sometimes emotional response. Your clitoris is made up of three parts:

1. The head
2. The shaft
3. The legs

What we are most familiar with is the head—the 'pearl,' as I like to call it—that gets stimulated by a finger or the tongue. Even though the head is important, it is only one part of the clitoral body and is literally just the tip of the iceberg. Underneath are the legs and shaft which make up most of the clitoral nerve network. What we were never taught in school is that the clitoral nerve network is just as large as the head of a penis and also has erectile function! Why would we have all these amazing pleasure nerve endings if we weren't built to experience pleasure?

Some women's clitoris is closer to the entrance of the vagina, which means it's easier for her to experience orgasms during sex. If this isn't available to you, it doesn't mean yours doesn't work—you just need more stimulation before you have sex.

For me, clitoral orgasms are the starter of a beautiful three-course meal, the spot orgasm as the main course and if I'm feeling really hungry, I go for dessert, a cervical orgasm. To be honest, I used to live on starters because I didn't know there was any main course or dessert but these days, I want dessert more often because this is what channels my physiology and biochemistry and reconnects me to my sacred self.

Home Play

Try experimenting with different pressures and ways you touch your clitoris. Use different strokes and speeds. Try using your non-dominant hand. Use feathers or water to feel any sensations that arise as you begin to move your body in your She-Movement practises.

Another tip is to try to relax your feet, legs, and pelvis as you slowly build up to orgasm. Allow your breath to move through your body slowly and fully, allowing your body to feel light. Every time you feel the urge to tense, breathe into the tension and allow your body to open into orgasm rather than be pushed into it.

Your Vagina

Your vagina is a powerful pleasure portal, brimming with magic and orgasmic potential, yet it is often one of the most misunderstood parts of a woman's anatomy. As our menstrual cycles and hormones fluctuate each month, and as we go through childbirth, perimenopause, and menopause, our feminine anatomy can change, impacting our pleasure and arousal. Each woman is uniquely different, which means our vaginas are, too. For instance, some women have their urethral sponge—containing erectile tissue—in different areas of the vagina, affecting sensitivity and pleasure. This is why you may experience dryness, pain, or numbness when you're not in the mood for sex. There's nothing wrong with you—it's just your physiology.

The nerve innervation in the vagina is different from that of the vulva, which is why we experience different types of orgasms. The pelvic nerve, which is internal, is responsible for cervical and full-body orgasms, along with the hypogastric and vagus nerves. Many women haven't yet experienced these types of orgasms because they aren't accustomed to using their nervous system in this way. Over time, creating new neural pathways can increase sensitivity and lead to more frequent and intense orgasms.

When your vagina is fully activated, it becomes a magnet for your desires, literally drawing what you want into your life. It's an essential tool for manifesting, yet many women aren't harnessing their sexual energy in this way. The vagina brings what you desire into your womb, where you have the power to birth your intentions into the world. Remember, your womb is not only for birthing physical babies, but for creating and birthing your true self and desires.

I want you to start turning up the volume of the voice that resides within your vagina. For years, we've silenced and repressed this inner wisdom and deep instinct through negative self-talk, numbing ourselves with birth control pills or an IUD, resenting our menstrual cycle, and generally speaking negatively to ourselves. We lack healthy boundaries, saying *yes* to sex when we really want to say *no*, and all of this is stored within us, waiting in the shadows, yearning for acknowledgement and healing.

Developing a loving relationship with your vagina, and everything you hold inside of her, is the key to your healing.

The Jade Egg

The jade egg has gained significant attention in recent years, and many women I speak to are curious about what it is and how it works. In my experience, the jade egg is a holistic practise that benefits women sexually, emotionally, and spiritually. It increases awareness of the sexual organs by building new neural pathways, heightening sensitivity, and awakening a deep consciousness and energy throughout the entire body. The jade egg can be used to heal blockages caused by past sexual traumas and address issues such as numbness, pain during sex, and trauma after childbirth. It helps alleviate PMS symptoms and, in my opinion, is an essential tool for women navigating perimenopause, menopause, and beyond, helping them use their sexual energy to support their overall health during this often challenging transition. The Yoni egg strengthens and revitalises the pelvic floor, and I've witnessed it help women with prolapse. However, it's best to work with a guide or jade egg practitioner who understands female anatomy.

You might wonder, 'Why use a jade egg instead of Kegel exercises for a weak pelvic floor?' This is a great question, as both can aid with urinary incontinence, pelvic floor issues, and prolapse. What I love about the jade egg is that it offers a unique healing system, working not only on the physical body but also on the mental, emotional, and spiritual levels. It's like comparing yoga to stretching—both are effective, but yoga feels different, and in my experience, it is different. The jade egg awakens aliveness within the body that you simply can't get from a basic stretch. Most women—and I would love to say every woman, though there's always an exception—experience better sex and orgasms after incorporating a jade egg into their practise. It's like a magic pill for sexuality without any of the unpleasant side effects.

A regular jade egg practise brings women into deeper alignment with their true selves. As they begin to peel back layers of conditioning and beliefs that no longer resonate, things and people that no longer serve them start to fall away. This is a powerful process, which is why I strongly recommend working with a jade egg teacher if you truly want to experience the full capacity of this sacred practise. A lot can surface during this process, and we need support and guidance to move through it. Otherwise, we might find ourselves thinking, 'It's not working,' or 'I don't feel anything,' or simply procrastinating and coming up with excuses for why it won't work for us. This resistance often comes from the reptilian brain, which is driven by fear and the desire for safety. Change and the unknown can be daunting for our reptilian brain, and this is when having the support of a good teacher can be invaluable.

Every woman carries some form of trauma in her vagina, whether from past partners, saying yes when we were truly too tired and wanted to say no, hating our periods and experiencing PMS, or internalising the patriarchal views we've been taught. There is so much there, even without the larger traumas, and it all sits within us, weighing us down. It needs to be cleared once and for all so that you can realign with the truth of who you are.

You can use any crystal egg, though I personally prefer jade for its strength and durability. However, if you develop a regular jade egg practise, you may find it both interesting and beneficial to work with the energy of eggs made from different healing crystals.

A Basic Jade Egg Practise

The jade egg is an excellent way to begin resensitising your vagina and reconnecting with this sacred part of your body. Before we explore a basic jade egg routine, I'd like to introduce you to the reflexology points within your vagina, if you're not already familiar. Just as the feet have meridians that mirror the organs in your body, so do your sexual organs. In the Taoist system, one of my sacred sexuality lineages, reflexology points within the vagina are activated during jade egg practise.

For example, the G-Spot area corresponds to your kidney reflexology points. When the kidneys are balanced, life flows smoothly, allowing us to trust and open ourselves to deeper connections. Moving further up in the middle of your vagina, you'll find the spleen and liver reflexology points, with the pancreas located a little further in. Deep within your vagina, at the cervix, is the reflexology point for your heart. Here's a fun fact: A man's penis mirrors the reflexology points of your vagina.

Imagine your vagina in three sections:

1. The opening of the vagina—Adrenal glands, thymus, pineal, and pituitary glands
2. The middle of the vagina—Kidney, liver, and spleen
3. The top of the vagina—Heart

Many of us think of the vagina as a single canal, but it's important to focus on working within its three distinct regions. This is crucial because some areas may feel painful or numb, and to strengthen, activate, and heal, we need to address the whole.

Before you begin, ensure you have an egg with two holes drilled at one end. Make sure it's clean—I like to use hot water and occasionally a bit of skin-friendly soap before and after use. You'll need some silk thread or non-toxic dental floss to thread through the holes in the egg. Make sure the thread is long enough so you can easily reach it when the egg is inside you.

Set the scene by putting on some relaxing music, lighting a candle, and perhaps wearing a long dress or skirt that gives you easy access to your yoni. Lie on your back with some large cushions on either side of your knees, bend your legs with your feet together, and allow them to open and rest on the cushions. Take your egg and place it at the opening of your vagina, with the widest part entering first. Breathe in, and as you exhale, gently allow the egg to slide inside. Sometimes, stimulating your breasts or engaging in self-pleasure can help your vagina open more easily. If you feel dry, especially for my peri- and menopausal ladies, use a skin-friendly lubricant to avoid any unnecessary discomfort or irritation. Over time, many women report needing less help with lubrication, and some none at all, as their sexuality awakens and their natural sexual fluids return.

Once you've inserted the egg into your yoni, use your fingers to guide it into the middle section. We're going to start in the middle. You can keep your fingers inside as you do the exercise, and after a while, you'll begin to notice how different areas of your vagina feel. There is a common assumption that the vagina is just one muscle, but as you work with the egg, you'll start to notice varying sensations and how the muscles grow stronger as you build new neural pathways.

When the egg is in place, begin to gently squeeze your vaginal walls around the egg. Don't worry if you don't feel much at first; over time, this will grow stronger. Using the jade egg is like resistance training for your vagina. Just as you can't strengthen any muscle without creating resistance, the vagina is no exception.

To begin, gently pull on the string you've tied through the bottom of your jade egg. Don't pull too hard—just enough to create resistance so that you need to squeeze the muscles around the egg to keep it in place. Inhale and squeeze for a count of three, then exhale and release for a count of three, but maintain a 10% hold on the egg as you release. When you squeeze, don't clench as if trying to crack a walnut—keep the movement gentle and controlled, using your breath as a guide. Repeat this movement 10 to 12 times.

Tip:

Ultimately, it's not just the jade egg that will heal you—it's the alchemy created when you combine it with sound, movement, and breath. Allow yourself to make sounds and move your body naturally, without forcing or over-controlling the experience. Feel the flow and let your breath and body guide you, as we are waking up your sexual energy alongside strengthening your yoni.

The reason for maintaining a 10% contraction between squeezes, without completely letting go, is to build up your sexual life force energy. Once you've finished, focus on circling that energy around your body—breathe in as you guide the energy up your spine, and breathe out as you send it down the front of your body, all while holding that 10% contraction. This technique, known as the microscopic orbit, helps circulate the Shakti energy that has awakened.

Next, move the egg towards the top of your vagina and repeat the same routine, finishing with three rounds of the microscopic orbit breathing.

Now, gently pull the egg towards the entrance of your vagina, but not so far that it falls out—just close enough to the opening while still being able to hold it inside. I often use the fingers of my other hand for support here.

After completing 10-12 rounds, push the egg back into the middle of your vagina. Take a moment to visualise your womb. Place your hands in a triangle shape, fingers pointing towards your pubic bone, and do three rounds of the microscopic orbit breathing. As you finish the third breath cycle, visualise a ball of white light filling your womb space, feel it under your hands and see it in your mind's eye. This is all the energy you've created, stored and waiting for you to use throughout the day.

Begin to notice how your energy shifts over time—do you feel more energised, more turned on, or more interested in sex? Pay attention as your yoni starts to wake up. This is the life force that will help you begin to create the life and body you desire.

Your G-Spot

The G-spot is made up of erectile urethral tissue and feels like a spongy, ribbed area on the anterior wall of your vagina, located about 5-8 cm inside. It's easier to find this pleasure spot when you are aroused, as it becomes erect when stimulated. In some women, the G-spot can fill with fluid that is released during a G-spot orgasm.

When you first begin to stimulate this area, it may feel uncomfortable, and you might feel the urge to urinate—this means you're in the right place! While these orgasms can take longer to achieve and may not feel as intense as clitoral orgasms, they offer health benefits that extend beyond just pleasure. In my experience, G-spot orgasms have played a significant role in my journey of self-love and awakening. The G-spot is a must for any woman who feels emotionally blocked, as it truly holds transformative healing power.

Home Play

To begin exploring, I recommend using a healing wand specifically designed to reach your G-spot. Surround yourself with pillows so you can fully relax and avoid any tension in your body. Use a skin-friendly oil, and prepare your body by massaging your breasts and vulva. Place the healing wand at the entrance of your vagina and tune in to whether your body gives you a *yes* or *no*—honour the answer it gives. If it's a *no* today, be patient. As your body regains trust, it will eventually become a *yes*.

If you receive a *yes*, use the healing wand to gently stimulate the area. The focus here isn't on climaxing, but rather on exploration, resensitisation, and getting to know yourself in ways you may not have before. Breathe into any areas of tightness or contraction, allowing your pelvis to relax and open. This process is one of surrender: stay open to how your body feels, explore what emotions are arising, and breathe into any sensations that come up. Let your body and its sensations guide you, rather than letting your mind dictate how you think it should feel. This is about moving out of your head and fully into your body.

Your Cervix

The idea that the cervix is numb is outdated.

Most doctors practising medicine today have limited knowledge when it comes to the cervix, beyond performing cervical smear tests. We've been taught that the cervix is simply something that opens during labour or a part of the body we need to monitor for cervical cancer. Well, if you're like me, you find smear tests uncomfortable! That's because there are nerves there, and if we can feel pain, we can certainly feel pleasure. The cervix is the gateway to the womb and is highly sensitive when touched.

Many women have never experienced a cervical orgasm, or they look puzzled when I mention it, as it's not something widely known, or they hold a belief that their body can't achieve it. Cervical orgasms have profoundly changed my life. I don't say this lightly—reconnecting to the cervical orgasm has opened me up and released emotional and energetic blocks I didn't even realise were there. Emotionally and spiritually, a lot of our suppressed feelings and hurts are stored in and around the cervix.

The deeper inside yourself you orgasm, the more profound the connection to yourself, energetically and emotionally. In my experience, cervical orgasms feel like waves of pleasure travelling through my entire body, cleansing and relaxing my nervous system. The effects can be felt for hours, even days after, as we release blocked emotions and create space for more energy to flow. These orgasms also flood the body with feel-good hormones and shift us out of the sympathetic 'fight or flight' mode that many of us live in daily.

Cervical orgasms require relaxation, openness, and a deep surrender to the wisdom within. With gentle and mindful sensitisation through stimulation using a cervical healing wand, your cervix can experience pleasure, and with time, love, and patience, cervical orgasms can be achieved. It takes time to rewire and build the neural pathways that have been often neglected in your cervix, but every woman has the potential to experience a cervical orgasm.

Full Body Orgasm

Yes, this does exist, and it's often accessible to women who are regularly in tune with their bodies and experiencing G-spot and cervical orgasms. It can occur spontaneously for some women, but if this is your goal, I would recommend following the path I have outlined for you.

When I trained as a tantra teacher, I experienced my first full-body orgasm. In the tantric practises that I teach, we use the technique of full-body energy activation. This practise awakens the orgasmic body by using bioenergetics, rewiring your nervous system to experience arousal, pleasure, and ecstatic energy, allowing you to feel the full orgasmic potential throughout your entire body. This technique is something I teach in a retreat setting, working with women who have already explored their sacred sexuality with me in previous sessions.

Perimenopause, Menopause and Sensual Aliveness

There is a narrative we've all been fed about women as they approach and enter this transitional phase of life, and I must say, much of it is myth and far from the complete truth. The reason it has become a reality for many women is that they've accepted this lie, often because they don't truly understand how their bodies work and the immense power of the female body. Until recently, there has been very little research or open discussion on this topic. A great deal of the advice has been hidden away, clouded by shame and humiliation, as women attempt to navigate the unknown changes that leave them feeling disconnected from themselves and their bodies. They feel frightened because they lack true knowledge and understanding of what is happening on a mental, physical, and emotional level.

The standard prognosis we are often shown as we approach 40 includes the following misconceptions:

- We are past our prime
- Our libido dies
- We gain weight

- We dry up, both inside and outside of our vagina
- We will need lubrication to have sex
- Metabolic disease will set in
- Higher risk of female reproductive cancers
- Our bodies will succumb to gravity
- We will feel old and stiff
- We will fall apart
- The best years are behind us
- We no longer matter
- And, of course, the stereotype of the 'lonely old cat woman' awaits...

This simply doesn't have to be the reality! Modern medicine offers us a wide range of options, from HRT and contraceptive pills to medication for depression and anxiety, as well as surgeries—including plastic surgery and even the removal of reproductive organs—to combat the effects of ageing. There's nothing inherently wrong with these options, and women should absolutely be free to choose, but I hope those choices come from a place of sovereignty, with full awareness of the facts, and not simply because they feel like they're falling apart.

As I've mentioned throughout this book, your body is innately intelligent and adaptive. If you're taking care of her, don't you think she has the capacity to regenerate? This is where mindset becomes crucial: what you believe, you become. You create your reality. Yes, getting older is natural, but that doesn't mean you have to feel old—that's just a perception.

Ageing isn't the enemy; it's a gift. We should feel excited and honoured to step into our wisdom years. In many cultures, including my own Celtic heritage, the older generation—especially women—are honoured for their wisdom and intuition. The womb, no longer releasing an egg each month, holds a deep wisdom and energy that enhances a woman's expansion, wisdom, and self-exploration. This isn't an ending; it's the start of a profound and sacred transition. In fact, for many women, it's a new beginning.

I believe women struggle with this transition because they see it as the end, rather than embracing it. Many women haven't been living in their full expression and aliveness, and by the time they reach their forties, they're burdened by unresolved blocks, shadows, and regrets that have piled up, creating roadblocks to the next stage of their lives.

When we hit forty, something magical and unsettling happens—we can no longer keep going as we used to. The masks we've worn begin to slip, and the weight we've been carrying becomes too much. Physically, mentally, and emotionally, we start to notice the cracks. Perhaps you realise you're in the wrong relationship or job, or wake up wondering who's staring back at you in the mirror. Frustration builds as the efficiency and drive you once had starts to fade. The body slows down, signalling that things need to be done differently.

For those who've constantly pushed themselves, ignoring their emotions, this can feel even more intense. Out of nowhere, you find yourself dealing with everything you thought you'd already worked through, feeling buried by your shadows and insecurities. One day, you're exhausted; the next, you're anxious or overwhelmed. Maybe you're taking the pill for PMS and now a mild antidepressant or anxiety meds to cope. Burnout feels near, but you're determined to keep going because this 'can't happen to someone like you.'

You start to feel aches and pains—stiffness in your back and neck, tension in your jaw and hands, and your PMS is worse than ever. You're emotional, crying over everything, and nobody seems to understand—not even you. Everything that once worked no longer does, and it won't, until you embrace the changes your body is asking for. This is the next stage of your evolution.

When I hit this transition (and I'm still navigating through it), I knew I had to let go of the superficial. I couldn't keep skimming the surface of life or staying on the edge out of fear. Back then, I was living with so much fear and shadow that I believed if I fully immersed myself, I'd sink. I held on to the belief that things like this didn't happen to people like me—I took care of myself, I was the one people came to for help. Being vulnerable wasn't in my nature; I was terrified of being seen as weak or not having it all together. This had to change. I had to be honest about my health, about where I was still bypassing and hiding the truth from myself.

I knew that my physical, mental, and emotional health was a reflection of where I'd been betraying myself—holding on to old patterns that I knew weren't serving me but was too scared to face. I desperately wanted to grow and evolve but didn't want to go through the deep work required. I was afraid. I knew it would be hard and inconvenient, like another dive into the underworld. For a few years, I was stuck dipping my toe in, but eventually, I reached a point where staying stuck was more painful than the fear of change.

Perimenopause brought me face to face with my deepest fears. I had to confront my insecurities about ageing—my looks, my body, my worth tied to youth and motherhood. At 43, I still wanted another child, even though I already had four, because I wasn't ready to move forward. But I had to accept and sit with these fears and insecurities. It took me six months, working with a Jungian coach, to finally confront these shadows. The journey taught me where I'd been stagnant in life and showed me the deeper flow and surrender required for the next stage of my journey.

All my work had led to this moment, but I had been trying to repress it out of fear— fear that the wave of change would overwhelm me. This is where my sacred practises and movement therapy were invaluable. My feminine soul needed breath, movement, and ritual during this powerful transition. I had to feel the full range of emotions, stay in the flow, and grow rather than retreat. My symptoms were showing me that I could no longer hold back what was inside of me; my intuition and ancient wisdom were pushing to be born, whether I liked it or not.

If you've ever given birth, you know you have to breathe into the contractions rather than resist them. That's what this transition has been like—birthing myself. Resistance only causes more pain. Through my practise, I learned to surrender, release blocks, and let go of resistance. It was tough, but I found the diamond within myself. And part of that diamond is what you're reading now—my work, my teachings. I've said yes to the life force inside me, and now I can offer more of my life's work while holding a deeper, awakened shakti for myself and others.

Looking back, I realise I was hiding behind being a mum because I was afraid of truly stepping out of the spiritual closet, claiming my place, and fully standing in my wholeness. My fears and excuses had kept me small. I was so afraid of rejection—wondering what others would say, if they'd like me, if they'd value my work—that it paralysed me, keeping me stuck in a safe but limiting space. Remember, growth, success, and everything your heart truly needs and desires lie on the other side of discomfort.

Here are some questions to ask yourself during this transition—be honest with yourself, as the truth will set you free:

- What is this stage asking me to change?
- Who is it asking me to be?
- Where have I been wasting my energy?
- What will fulfil me and make me feel alive?
- What feelings have I been blocking for years?
- What things, people or perfections do I need to let go of?
- What can't I let go of but know I should?
- Where am I stuck in my life?
- What's my story, and what do I want my new story to be?
- What is it that I don't want to do?
- What is my edge? What is the thing I think about but am afraid of doing or talking about?
- What lessons do I keep repeating?

Your dragon represents everything you are repressing. What does it look like to slay your dragon? Understand that the more weight you've carried and the longer you've held onto your blocks, the deeper you will need to go—this is a universal law. It may require more time, energy, and effort, but if you do the work, you will always resurface.

- What is your dragon?
- What is the challenge?
- Where is your dragon?

Now, take small steps each day and week to become the person you know in your heart, mind, and body you are meant to be. The train is leaving the station—get on it. Don't miss the opportunity, don't stay stuck in a dream; become the reality your soul yearns for.

Physical Manifestations

I believe extreme menopause symptoms are your body's way of shouting that something is wrong—that you're out of alignment and off track with where you're meant to be in life. The stagnant energy you've been running on just to get by needs to be released. Menopause is a transformation, a metamorphosis of the self. It's like the caterpillar entering the chrysalis before emerging as a butterfly; the in-between phase is messy and uncomfortable, but the butterfly always emerges, more beautiful and radiant than before. No longer struggling to crawl on the ground, she gets to fly and experience a whole new world.

When we've been disconnected from our bodies for years—wired, stressed, constantly overgiving, teetering on the edge of burnout while battling anxiety, depression, and hormonal imbalances—it's no surprise that by the time we hit forty, everything starts to fall apart. Our reproductive hormones are depleted, their energy consumed by survival mode. Is it any wonder that, for many women, this phase feels like the tipping point, the moment when everything unravels? It's the straw that breaks the camel's back. This is why so many women experience debilitating symptoms, such as:

- Hot flushes
- Heavy, clotting periods that flood
- Stiff, aching joints
- Back pain
- Headaches
- Restless legs
- Low libido
- Dry or numb vagina
- Pain during sex
- Pelvic floor dysfunction
- Rage, anger, and uncontrollable emotions
- Irritability and snapping at others
- Burnout
- Difficulty concentrating or zoning out
- Procrastination
- Small tasks feeling like huge efforts
- Depression
- Anxiety
- Racing heart, a constant feeling of dread
- Being easily startled and sensitive to noise
- Overthinking and inability to switch off
- Lack of energy
- Waking up exhausted, feeling dread
- Normal activities feeling overwhelming
- Loss of muscle and bone density
- Dry skin or acne
- Food intolerances
- Weight gain, especially around the middle
- Metabolic issues, such as high blood pressure and type 2 diabetes
- Heart problems
- Intestinal issues

- Sudden onset of autoimmune conditions like thyroid issues, MS, or arthritis
- Female reproductive cancers
- Resurfacing of past traumas
- Feeling like you're drowning or no longer at home in your body

I want to be absolutely clear: I'm not for a moment suggesting that these symptoms aren't real—they very much are, and some of them are a natural part of the perimenopausal and menopausal transition. However, they don't have to be as extreme as many women experience, nor do they have to be your inevitable fate. These symptoms have become so normalised that we've come to accept them as unavoidable, but for many, this phase of life can be much gentler. Menopause can be a powerful invitation to return to life, to realign with the person you're truly meant to become. Embrace the change—it's not an end but a new beginning.

Women who have a regular She-Practise experience a profound sense of awakening, alignment, and vitality. Stagnant sexual energy is cleared, and the Shakti life force is re-awakened, allowing energy to flow freely throughout the body. The more deeply a woman feels stuck, the heavier the issue, and the deeper she must go to release it. Depression, anxiety, and regrets often surface as psychological and psycho-spiritual manifestations of unprocessed and blocked emotions, but these are cleared and integrated through She-Practises. This process is one of unlearning and undoing, providing the ultimate reset. By releasing blocks and awakening Shakti, women experience a state of feeling fully alive, aligning deeply with their true selves.

Highly Sensitive Women and Menopause

Over the past thirty years, extensive research has highlighted that highly sensitive women may experience more intense peri-menopausal symptoms. These women may include:

- Empaths
- Carers
- Healers
- Intuitives
- Psychics
- Those with ADD/ADHD
- PTSD sufferers
- Individuals with unintegrated trauma
- And more...

I've always been highly sensitive, intuitive, and able to feel and read others' emotions and bodies, which is a gift I've honoured and used daily. However, there has been a downside to this. I would often feel anxious, overwhelmed, and drained, become hyper-vigilant, and live in fear and 'what ifs'. Before I started regular chiropractic treatments, my nervous system was very dysregulated. Fascinated by the nervous system, I explored neuroscience, the feminine brain, and my sacred work, which helped me learn to self-regulate. This alignment allowed me to thrive rather than just survive. My perimenopausal symptoms have become much more manageable since incorporating regular 'She' movement practises into my life.

If you know that you are a highly sensitive person, it's important to understand that regulating your nervous system is essential as you navigate your perimenopausal or menopausal journey. Knowledge is power! Having the ability to directly influence your nervous system and fully understand yourself and how your body works is truly empowering. Bringing your body out of survival mode will transform both your life and your health.

Your sexual life force energy is vital as we navigate this transition. I've previously mentioned that menopause can serve as a catalyst for spiritual awakening and heightened consciousness. When this energy isn't flowing and becomes stuck within the body, it can create menopausal havoc. Women who can truly move with and inhabit their sexual energy and shakti tend to experience menopause with more ease, finding greater pleasure and fewer symptoms, rather than crashing into the waves, gasping for air. When your sexual energy isn't flowing and being used to bring aliveness and alignment into your body, destruction and symptoms are inevitable, regardless of how many vitamins or pills you take.

Supporting women through this transition involves many factors—diet, nutrition, exercise, mindset, and shadow work are all essential. My hope for you is that you experience the most alive and embodied version of life through your body. Start by getting your nervous system checked by a chiropractor and begin practising 'She-Movement' therapy today!

CHAPTER 22
THE SACRED CONNECTION

As you close the final pages of *Your Body, Your Power*, you have journeyed through the depths of what it means to be a modern woman navigating the complexities of today's world. You've learned about the 'modern disease' of disconnection, the stress of constantly trying to prove yourself, and the toll it takes on your mind, body, and spirit. But through these teachings, you've begun to remember something essential—you are the authority on your own body.

Now, you understand that no one—whether a doctor, partner, or anyone else—can know your body as deeply as you do. This is your body, and it holds the wisdom of your power. You've reconnected with the sacredness of your feminine body, embracing the balance between your body, mind, and spirit. For perhaps the first time, you feel truly embodied, whole, and aligned, no longer fragmented by external expectations or stress.

You see yourself not just in parts but as an integrated whole. You realise that everything in your life—your thoughts, movements, emotions, and experiences—affects your well-being. You've tapped into a wellspring of energy that flows from within, awakening a deep connection to your womb and sexual vitality, a force you may never have known was there. This isn't just about sex; it's about creative life force energy, an ancient, primal connection to Mother Earth that flows through you.

In making peace with your body, you've unwound the tension that once kept you bound in stress and pain. Pleasure, once distant, is now within reach. You've learned to regulate your nervous system, supplement your health with intention, and honour your body's needs. This isn't about what your body looks like, but how it feels—how *you* feel in your body. You are more intuitive, grounded, and aligned with the cycles of the moon and the seasons of nature.

Your menstrual cycles have become a source of connection, not discomfort. PMS no longer rules your life because you've attuned to what your body needs. Your boundaries are clearer, your sovereignty stronger. You are no longer saying 'yes' when you mean 'no' because you have found the power of your own voice.

At the heart of this journey, you've rediscovered the sacred feminine within. Feminine spirituality is not something outside of you but a living, breathing part of who you are. God, or the Divine, is no longer distant but an energy flowing from the inside out, expressed through your body and your being.

You've come home to yourself. You laugh more, feel more, and understand that your emotions—while powerful—do not define you. You flow with the cycles of life rather than resist them, and you have cultivated practises that nurture your well-being. You have reclaimed your body, your power, and your life.

Just like Dorothy in *The Wizard of Oz*, you realise that everything you've been searching for was within you all along. The journey was about remembering who you truly are—a sovereign, powerful, and embodied woman.

This is your body, and it holds your power.

ACKNOWLEDGEMENTS

Firstly, I would like to acknowledge the true superstars of this book—my patients and clients at Chiropractic Optimal Health in the Netherlands, as well as those I support virtually across the world. You helped me birth this book; I have been the midwife helping to deliver this baby. Thank you for sharing your narratives and allowing me to serve the greater collective of women who are also striving to find healing from the Modern Disease of the Modern Woman.

My deepest gratitude goes to the incredible team at my clinic for supporting me in my mission to help all the women who walk through our doors. You are truly amazing!

I also want to extend heartfelt thanks to my parents, Tony and Pam, for your unwavering love and the invaluable life lessons you've imparted. Thank you for helping me to heal our own ancestral wounds.

To the wise women who came before me, especially Nana Olive and Nana Marge, you shaped my views and encouraged me to question my identity. Your unwavering belief in me has propelled me to heights I never thought possible.

Thank you to my friends and extended family for cheering me on over the past few years. I'm grateful for both the good and challenging moments, as each has contributed to my growth, helping me to show up as the best version of myself. It has been a humbling and transformative journey of healing. I have shed many layers while writing this book, experiencing countless rebirths along the way. Only true friendships could have withstood this journey and stood by me, so thank you for always allowing me to be myself and speak my truth.

Special thanks to Anastasia, whose love, encouragement, and positivity kept me afloat when I felt overwhelmed. Our weekly Tuesday chats are one of the highlights of my week.

To my teachers: Collette Corcoran—thank you for helping me make the unconscious conscious with your wisdom and guidance. To Ma Ananda Sarita and Ma Prem Tanmaya, whose teachings in Tantra have deeply influenced how I view women, our bodies, and the world.

A special acknowledgement and heartfelt gratitude to my publisher, friend, and writing angel, Astara Jane Ashley. I could not have achieved this without you. Thank you for your patience, support, and love as both myself and this book underwent our metamorphosis. Your invaluable insights and contributions have helped me in ways beyond measure. Thank you, dear sister, for believing in me when I wanted to give up and could not see the way forward. I look forward to creating the next book with you.

To my wonderful children—Olivia, Isabella, Sebastian, and Emilia Lily—you are my world. Thank you for your patience during the lengthy process of writing this book, which I know has felt like an additional sibling for the past few years. This book has accompanied us through weekends, evenings, and holidays. Thank you for giving me the time to do this and for enduring my distracted attention. You are my greatest achievement, and being your mother pushes me to expand my awareness, insight, and love in ways I never thought possible. I am so blessed to have you in my life and proud to call myself your mum.

Lastly, I wish to honour my true love and life partner, Vincent ten Klooster. You have been the most significant influence in my life every day for the past twenty years. You have supported and loved me both physically and metaphysically, always my biggest cheerleader. Thank you for seeing beyond my doubts, frustrations, and insecurities, and for believing in me when I didn't believe in myself. Your commitment to living authentically, speaking your truth, and standing by your convictions has inspired me and helped me soar. You are the wind beneath my wings, a true healer, a genius, a leader, and an amazing husband and father. I am immensely blessed to share my life with you and to journey through the sacred path of marriage by your side. From the depths of my heart, I love you, and I still believe you're the sexiest man in this world!

ABOUT THE AUTHOR

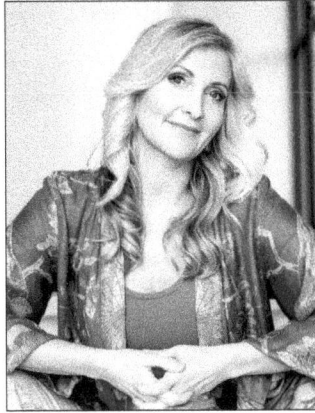

Dr Michelle Boyce, DC, is a practising chiropractor and functional medicine coach with over 20 years of experience. She is a healer, priestess, medical intuitive, and soul coach. Furthermore, she's a trained female health coach who specialises in hormones.

She believes that knowledge is power, and the power of the female body should be known and embodied by all women. Every woman has the right to know, understand, feel, and experience the power and aliveness in her body. Dr Michelle's mission is to help women feel at home in their bodies again and see the body as whole and holistic with its own innate healing intelligence.

By combining ancient wisdom with modern science, she educates women on female health, sacred sexuality, womb magic, tantra, and the ancient feminine mysteries of how to heal and transform your body. She covers a wide range of topics including food, herbs, movement, rituals, sacred practices, sexual awakening, and energy work.

Bringing together her wisdom and experience, she developed the 'Sheology' method in response to the epidemic she encountered among women she works with, which she calls 'The Modern Disease of the Modern Woman.' She helps women midwife their souls back to life by connecting mind, body, and spirit.

In order to support women—especially during perimenopause and menopause—to navigate life changes, heal their body, and reconnect to their power, she offers in-person and online courses, group and private coaching, and hands-on healing.

Dr Michelle was born in Wales and has lived in the Netherlands for 16 years, along with her husband Vince and their four children, Olivia, Isabella, Sebastian, and Emilia-Lily.

Learn more at **www.drmichelleboycedc.com**

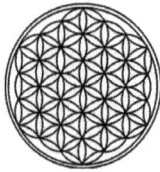

FLOWER *of* LIFE PRESS

Visit us at **www.floweroflifepress.com**

www.ingramcontent.com/pod-product-compliance
Lightning Source LLC
Chambersburg PA
CBHW080325270326
41927CB00014B/3104